HUMAN GENOME ANALYSIS PROGRAMME

Biomedical and Health Research

Volume 8

ISSN: 0929-6743

Human Genome Analysis Programme

Edited by

M. Hallen

European Commission , Directorate-General for Science,
Research and Development, Medical Research Unit, Brussels, Belgium

and

A. Klepsch

European Commission, Directorate-General for Science,
Research and Development, Biotechnology Unit, Brussels, Belgium

1995

IOS
Press

Ohmsha

Amsterdam, Oxford, Tokyo, Washington, DC

ISBN 90 5199 175 4 (IOS Press)
ISBN 4-274-90016-9 C3047 (Ohmsha)
Library of Congress Catalogue Card Number 94-077315
Publication no. EUR 16012

Publisher
IOS Press
Van Diemenstraat 94
1013 CN Amsterdam
Netherlands

Distributor in the UK and Ireland
IOS Press/Lavis Marketing
73 Lime Walk
Headington
Oxford OX3 7 AD
England

Distributor in the USA and Canada
IOS Press, Inc.
P.O. Box 10558
Burke, VA 22009-0558
U.S.A.

Distributor in Japan
Ohmsha, Ltd.
3-1 Kanda Nishiki - Cho
Chiyoda - Ku
Tokyo 101
Japan

LEGAL NOTICE
Neither the European Commission nor any person acting on behalf of the Commission is responsible for the use which might be made of the following information.

PRINTED IN THE NETHERLANDS

PREFACE

The opportunities for various genome projects have been discussed on the basis of advances in DNA sequencing technologies. In the mid '80s these discussions precipitated in concrete suggestions for proposing the need for a "Human Genome Project". In the United States the debate on "Big Science" in biology has received great public attention as in Europe, where its potential impact on mankind and specifically the expected medical benefits should become a major dimension of this endeavour. The fears and anxieties about the misuse of this new knowledge have existed since the very beginning, along with new hopes, especially for people suffering from diseases where no cure is yet available. The first initiatives concentrated on the establishment of a suitable research infrastructure in this area, i.e. making resources, which were developed by a small group of scientists, available to the European scientific community at large. These arguments eventually led to the European Commission being charged with developing a fundamental research programme on "Human Genome Analysis" (HGAP) under the Second Framework Programme to be implemented during the years 1990 to 1992.

The programme was adopted on 29 June 1990 with an initial budget of 15 million ECU (later increased by 0.6 million ECU) and prepared with the assistance of an "Ad Hoc Working Party on Human Genome Research", which established six study groups on (1) genetic (linkage) mapping, (2) physical mapping, (3) data handling and databases, (4) advanced genetic technologies, (5) training, and (6) ethical, social and legal aspects. The discussion on ethical, social and legal aspects of human genome analysis and its implications have played a significant role during the entire execution of this programme. An amount of 1 million ECU had been earmarked for these activities enabling the Commission to initiate and to participate in a broad debate involving scientists, doctors, theologians, philosophers, social scientists, legal experts as well as patients' organisations and others.

The main objective, however, was the establishment of a European infrastructure which allowed for a substantial contribution towards human genome research. This book contains the final reports of 26 research projects, including Resource Centres and "Single Chromosome Workshops" covering the following areas:
- Improvement of the infrastructure for human genome analysis:
  * **EURO**pean **GE**netic Mapping Project (EUROGEM)
  * Resource Centres (cosmid libraries, (complementary) cDNA libraries, yeast artificial chromosomes (YAC), Data Resource Centre, Danish Family Bank, and Single Chromosome Workshops)
- Transnational research projects:
  * Physical mapping/ordered clone libraries
  * Improvement of methods and basis for the study of the human genome

The considerable support and input provided to this programme by the members of the programme committee (CAN-HUG), the members of the working group on Ethical, Social and Legal Aspects of human genome analysis (WG-ESLA) and its implications and applications is gratefully acknowledged. In addition to those, the Commission services would like to thank the many experts who have assisted in the preparation and implementation of this programme, in particular Dr. Bronwen Loder.

Since the start of this initiative research on human genome analysis is now addressed in Area III within BIOMED 1, the current biomedical and health research programme. This "Area III" is the successor to the first "Human Genome Analysis Programme", which now emphasizes closer coordination in areas such as (1) the integration of physical and genetic linkage maps, (2) mapping cDNAs on YACs and cosmids in view of better understanding of diseases, their development and possible treatment, and (3) improvement of data handling and analysis. A total of 41 projects focusing on fundamental research are now being supported by this programme area.

Human Genome Research under BIOMED 2 in the forthcoming Fourth Framework Programme (1994-1998) will broaden the scope of activities with particular emphasis on the search for specific genes and the understanding of the functioning of genes, the research into improvement of treatment and better disease prevention in the future and finally research for the development and improvement of databases.

Brussels, November 1994   Manuel Hallen
                                                            Andreas Klepsch

European Commission
Directorate General XII
Science, Research and Development
Brussels, Belgium

Contents

Part 1

Improvement of the Infrastructure for Human Genome Analysis

Human Genome Analysis Programme
M. Hallen and A. Klepsch (Eds.)
IOS Press, 1995

THE EUROPEAN GENE MAPPING PROJECT
(EUROGEM)

N.K. Spurr and K. Nyberg
Clare Hall Laboratories, Potters Bar, United Kingdom

1. Introduction

The European Genome Mapping programme (EUROGEM) has completed its second year of contract. At the commencement of the project, the work of the Centralised Facility of a DNA Probe Bank for EUROGEM was outlined as follows:
- Acquisition of already existing probes
- Isolation of new markers detecting high levels of variation
- Computer records of all markers
- Distribution of markers to participating laboratories and analysis of feedback

The DNA probe bank facility undertook to distribute approximately 920 markers over the 24 month period. The markers were to be distributed in batches of 5-6 markers per laboratory at regular intervals. As the work involved in screening each marker varies considerably depending on how heterozygous the marker is, a tariff system was agreed on. In this system, a marker with a heterozygosity value up to 70% is equivalent to one. If the heterozygosity is above 70%, but below 80%, the marker is equivalent to two, and above 80%, equivalent to three. This tariff system has been used in this report to work out the number of "marker equivalents" each Network laboratory has received.

The contracts with the 22 Network laboratories were commenced on July 1st, 1991 and distribution started soon after this date.

The following report deals with the various aspects of the work of the Probe Resource Centre over the 24 month period from January 1991 to January 1993.

2. Distribution of Markers to the Network Laboratories.

The first batch of markers were sent out soon after the first EUROGEM meeting (August 19th, 1991). The batch consisted of 109 markers, of which 74 were DNA probes and 35 primer pairs for PCR based screening. At this time, the highly informative microsatellite markers were still rare, and most of the PCR based markers detected RFLP:s with two alleles. The DNA probes were sent dissolved in Tris-EDTA buffer; the concentration varied depending on the probe. All DNA probes were accompanied by a probe report form, which gives full details of the probe, including polymorphisms detected, information on the construction of the probe, the name and address of the originator and relevant literature references. The primers were synthesised in the Oligonucleotide Synthesis Unit at the Imperial Cancer Research Fund, Clare Hall. They were supplied to the Network laboratories fully deprotected and ethanol precipitated. The synthesis information form, as well as a copy of the reference, were supplied with the primers.

The second batch of markers were distributed in March - April 1992. This batch consisted of a total of 107 markers; 56 DNA probes and 61 PCR based markers. The increase of PCR based markers is notable; the proportion of highly informative microsatellite markers among these had also increased, making the informative value of the markers much higher.

The distribution of the third regular batch of markers was started in December 1992. The markers were sent to the Network laboratories as soon as we received them from the Oligonucleotide Synthesis Unit; at the time of writing this report, a few laboratories are still to receive their consignments. The batch was planned for distribution during the Autumn of 1992, but due to staff shortages and increasing demand within the Unit, they were unable to produce the primers in time. This batch consists of PCR markers only, and with a few exceptions the heterozygosity of the markers are above 70%.

In addition to the regular distribution a few laboratories have requested further markers. A total of 20 markers have been sent on request.

In 1992, Dr. Jean Weissenbach and colleagues at Généthon published information on 814 $(CA)_n$ microsatellite markers spanning the whole human genome (Weissenbach et al. (1992) Nature 359, 794-801). The Probe Resource Centre negotiated with Dr. Weissenbach for permission to use these in the EUROGEM project.

The first batch of markers purchased from Généthon was distributed in January 1993. A total of 207 primer pairs were sent to the Network laboratories. The markers are all highly informative and have previously been screened on 8 of the Centre d'Etude du Polymorphisme Humain (CEPH) families only. The typing of the remaining families with these markers will make a very valuable contribution to the construction of a high density linkage map which is the aim of this project.

The material sent out to the Network laboratories has been summarised in Table 1. The total weighted value of the markers sent out is 1008 probe equivalents, which slightly exceeds our commitment of 920.

3. Acquisition of Markers

3.1 DNA probes

The acquisition of existing DNA probes not tested on CEPH families was very important in the early part of the project, but it is becoming less so now, as most new markers published are PCR formatted. There are, however, a few exceptions, where requesting probes from the originators is still desirable:

- The inclusion of markers detecting polymorphisms in or close to genes in the screening is particularly valuable. A number of these markers are still only available as DNA probes, and new probes in this category are still published. We have tried to acquire as many as possible of these by writing to the originators.

- All markers designated as reference markers in 11th Human Genome Mapping Meeting have been requested from the originators. Just over one third replied and sent us the probe. We aim to include as many as possible of the reference markers which have not previously been typed extensively on the CEPH families in the EUROGEM project, and have already distributed 76 reference markers (of which 33 were DNA probes). There are still 31 reference markers waiting to be sent out; of these, 10 are DNA probes (Table 2).

- We have also received 36 minisatellite markers (see Table 3), for inclusion in the EUROGEM project, from Dr. J Armour at the University of Leicester. Most of these markers are highly informative, and they are fairly well distributed between the chromosomes (only chromosomes 2,4,9, and 11 lack markers in this collection). This has been a valuable resource of markers, and Dr. Armour has agreed to continue supplying us with new markers isolated in his laboratory. Their current screening programme has resulted in the detection of a number of polymorphic trinucleotide repeats which will be used in the EUROGEM project at a later stage.

Table 1

Markers distributed by the Probe Resource Centre

Laboratory	Batch 1		Batch 2		Batch 3 (**) (all PCR)	Requested		Généthon markers (all PCR)	Total weighted value
	Southern	PCR	Southern	PCR		Southern	PCR		
Bakker (Leiden)	3	2	2	3	2(+3)	-	-	9	≥ 47
Cann (CEPH)	2	3	1	4	5	-	-	9	≥ 46
Contu (Cagliari)	5	-	2	3	4	-	2	9	≥ 45
Estivill (Barcelona)	5	-	3	2	4	-	2	9	≥ 50
Ferguson-Smith (Camb.)	4	1	4	1	4	3	2	9	≥ 49
Gal (Lübeck)	1	3	5	-	4	-	-	9	43
Grzeschik (Marburg)	4	1	3	2	3	-	5	9	≥ 48
Harley (Cardiff)	3	2	4	2	(2)	-	-	10	≥ 45
Humphries (Dublin)	1	4	1	4	4	-	-	9	≥ 43
Kruse (Aarhus)	5	1	3	2	(4)	-	-	9	≥ 45
Lathrop (CEPH)	2	3	1	4	4	6	-	10	52
Lavinha (Lisbon)	5	-	4	1	(3)	-	-	9	≥ 48
McCarthy (Cork)	2	3	1	4	(3)	-	-	9	45
Moreno (Madrid)	5	-	2	3	(3)	-	-	10	≥ 48
Moschonas (Crete)	5	-	3	2	3	-	-	10	≥ 44
Povey (Galton)	3	2	2	3	6	-	-	10	50
Scheffer (Groningen)	2	3	1	5	(4)	-	-	10	≥ 45
Terrenato (Rome)	4	1	3	2	(3)	-	-	10	≥ 43
Vergnaud (Bouchet)	5	-	5	-	4	-	-	9	≥ 46
Weissenbach (Pasteur) *	2	3	-	-	-	-	-	-	≥ 6
Williamson (St Mary's)	3	2	3	2	(4)	-	-	10	≥ 52
Wright (Edinburgh)	3	2	3	2	(3)	-	-	9	≥ 40
Zakharyev (Moscow)	-	-	3	2	-	-	-	10	30

*   no further markers to be sent as requested by network lab.

**   ( ) = primers have been ordered and will be sent as we receive them

Table 2

The use of reference markers in EUROGEM

Chromosome	Sent		Still to be sent	
	PCR	DNA Probes	PCR	DNA Probes
1	2	1	-	-
2	1	1	-	-
3	2	5	-	-
4	3	-	-	-
5	1	-	1	1
6	2	1	-	-
7	4	2	-	-
8	1	1	-	-
9	2	-	1	-
10	2	3	-	-
11	3	3	2	1
12	2	1	-	-
13	1	-	-	1
14	3	1	1	-
15	2	-	1	-
16	3	1	5	-
17	2	2	1	-
18	-	-	-	-
19	1	-	1	1
20	-	-	-	-
21	2	-	1	1
22	-	2	1	2
X	4	9	6	3
Total	43	33	21	10

Table 3

Markers Supplied by Dr. J. Armour   (University of Leicester)

Locus	Probe Name	Heterozygosity	Location
D1S105	pMS601	74%	1
D3S1084	pMS628	49%	3q
D5S110	pMS621	92%	5p
D5S347	pMS635	74%	5
D6S86	pMS605	87%	6
D7S439	pMS602	60%	7p
D8S162	pMS502	90%	8
D10S90	pMS622	83%	10q26
D10S92	pMS614	77%	10p15
D12S40	pMS608	67%	12
D12S41	pMS618	83%	12
D12S42	pMS623	79%	12
D13S70	pMS604	64%	13
D13S103	pMS626	77%	13q
D14S44	pMS627	96%	14q
D15S86	pMS620	91%	15
D16S263	pMS624	36%	16
D16S264	pMS625	47%	16
D16S307	pMS637	56%	16p
D17S26	pMS638	83%	17q
D18S31	pMS440	83%	18q23
D18S32	pMS615	51%	18p11.3
D18S33	pMS616	51%	18q22-q23
D19S77	pMS610	80%	19
D19S176	pMS400	62%	19
D19S192	pMS207.2	65%	19p
D19S193	pMS301.2	70%	19q
D20S26	pMS617	79%	20
D20S73	pMS214.2	82%	20q
D21S155	pMS609	66%	21
D22S163	pMS607	90%	22
D22S164	pMS619	79%	22
DXS438	pMS613	35%	X
DXYS78	pMS600	91%	XY
DXYS82	pMS630	26%	Xp22.32; Yp11.3
DXYS89	pMS639	34%	Xp22.32; Yp11.3

3.2 PCR based markers

- We are continuing to screen literature and the GDB database for new highly informative PCR based markers. The number of new markers published are steadily increasing and the informative value is usually very high. The third batch of markers (see section 2), consisted entirely of markers collected from recent literature, and enough information for another batch is readily available.
- Reference markers: Most of the PCR based reference markers (see section 3.1), which had not already been typed extensively on CEPH families, were included in batch three. Some markers are waiting to be sent out later.
- Arrangements for screening Généthon markers: see section 2 of this report.

4. Identification of new markers at the Probe Resource Centre

4.1 Identification of di-, tri- and tetranucleotide repeats from sequence databases

Mono-, di-, tri and tetranucleotide repeat sequences have been identified from the EMBL and GenBank sequence databases. The sequences containing repeats were entered into a programme called Primers (available from Dr. C W Dieffenbach, c/o Henry M Jackson Foundation, Rockville, MD, USA). This programme is used to select PCR primer sets flanking the repeat sequences so that they fulfil certain selection criteria. The primers selected should be 18-22 nucleotides long, have a G-C rich 3' end, and a total GC content of between 45 and 55%. The amplified product should be shorter than 500 base pairs and longer than 100 base pairs. Homology of the primers selected is checked to prevent the formation of primer-self or primer-primer complexes. We have used this programme for most of the project, but we are not convinced of its usefulness, as "manual" selection often produces primers which work better.

The PCR primers selected were assessed and those judged most suitable were synthesised. Amplification of human DNA from random unrelated individuals and CEPH families was carried out, using a method developed partly within the scope of this project, in which ethidium bromide staining is used for visualisation of the PCR product (Watkins et al., 1991). The method is rapid and the results are easy to interpret as the stuttering caused by the incorporation of radiolabelled nucleotides is avoided.

We identified several new informative polymorphic markers with heterozygosity values frequently above 50%. The polymorphic sequences found were made up from di- and tetranucleotide repeats. We found no length variation of the poly A sequences studies. Those markers which had previously not been published were published in Nucleic Acids Research or Human Molecular Genetics (Warne et al., 1991; Watkins et al., 1991; Bodfish et al., 1992a; Bodfish et al., 1992b.) Two more dinucleotide repeat markers have been found and will soon be submitted to Human Molecular Genetics.

4.2 Screening libraries for tri- and tetra- nucleotide repeats

We have screened single chromosome Bluescribe libraries for positive clones using a synthetic (AAAT)15 oligonucleotide. The tri and tetranucleotide repeats are valuable alternatives to the very frequently occurring dinucleotide (usually (CA)n) repeats. Although the former are not as frequent and the screening may not lead to as many new markers, they have the advantage of being much easier to use. The screening has led to the identification of a number of positive clones which are at the moment being investigated. The results overall have been disappointing as the quality of the libraries appears to be rather poor, with a high proportion of religated vector as well as hamster contamination in some of the libraries. Studies on the (AAAT)n positive clones which we have identified so far will be completed, but otherwise the libraries will be abandoned in favour of a total human genomic library (Clontech). Work on this library has already started.

The great advantage of the monochromosomal libraries would have been the possibility to target chromosomes lacking in informative markers. However, screening a better quality library with a number of tri- and tetranucleotide repeat probes should result in a large number of markers which hopefully span the whole genome.

In parallel with this we are also investigating nonradioactive detection methods for library screening. The detection is based on chemiluminescence using a biotinylated probe with streptavidin linkage to alkaline phosphatase. The alkaline phosphatase dephosphorylates a dioxetane structure (Lumigen PDP) with the concomitant emission of light that can be detected on X-ray film. The method works well with pure DNA, and we hope to be able to modify it for use in colony and plaque screening. Results so far have been promising, but the bacterial debris still causes problems with non-specific binding.

4.3 Further isolation work

After initial success in finding new polymorphic markers from sequence databases, the production of new markers has been slower to start than anticipated. The screening for tri- and tetranucleotide repeats is however now well established, and we expect the screening programme to yield results in the very near future. The slowness has so far not hampered the project, as there has been a more than sufficient supply of published markers which we have been able to acquire for the Network laboratories.

5. Coordination of materials (in collaboration with CEPH)

The task of ensuring that the membranes sent out to each laboratory corresponds to the RFLP:s detected by the probes sent out has been the responsibility of the Probe Resource Centre. We also collected data on the probes which each laboratory wished to use as their own contribution to make sure they would receive the correct membranes for these.

As it was not possible to supply each laboratory with membranes for every probe, it was agreed that the Network laboratories would strip the filters after they had finished using them and have them ready to send to another laboratory on request. We compiled a list of which membranes each laboratory had received (Appendix 1) and distributed this to enable the Network laboratories to contact each other directly for the exchange of membranes.

We have also, as far as possible, endeavoured to collect information on which markers each Network laboratory is screening to avoid duplication of work.

6. Training

A workshop on PCR techniques was organised in collaboration with staff at CEPH and Généthon, and held at Généthon, on December 4th - 6th, 1991. The workshop was intended for those scientists who carry out the screening work and in particular for those who had little or no previous experience of PCR. The workshop practicals consisted of PCR analysis of microsatellites and VNTRs, using the non-radioactive staining technique described in section 4.1. In addition to the practicals, seminars and talks were given by staff from CEPH, Généthon and the Imperial Cancer Research Fund.

A separate CEC grant covered the expenses of the actual workshop, although the preparation was to a large extent carried out as part of the work of the Probe Resource Centre.

7. Data Collection for EUROGEM

It was recognised that each laboratory would require a fairly powerful computer in order to manage the typing data with a Sybase application (GENBASE) and to construct preliminary maps with LINKAGE, CRIMAP or similar software. SUN and DEC were the preferred suppliers and the final contract went to DEC to supply 24 Unix workstations, each with 424 MBytes of disk space and 12 MBytes of memory. A Pascal compiler licence was obtained for LINKAGE use and motif was added as an enhanced user interface.

The GENBASE software for data management was written by Jean-Marc Sebaoun from the CEPH in Paris. It is tightly bound to the EUROGEM requirements and also the necessary interaction with CEPH and the standard CEPH database. It has been written using the Sybase Relational Database Management System and provides and export facility to LINKAGE and Pedigree/Draw. It is undergoing continuous maintenance through feedback to CEPH.

Electronic mailing lists have been established at the Paris site, in order that material of general interest could be disseminated rapidly to all labs. They also enable discussion to take place between groups of people that would be much more difficult using telephone or fax.

Data entry has been carried out by individual laboratories and transferred by diskette, either to Paris or Clare Hall. To date we have received data from 6 laboratories, representing 100 systems typed on at least 8 of the CEPH families.

Bibliography

1. Watkins C, Warne D, Kelsell D, Beckmann J, Nyberg K, Spurr N. The use of PCR and ethidium bromide staining to detect length variation in short repeat units.
2. Warne D, Watkins C, Bodfish P, Nyberg K, Spurr NK. Tetranucleotide repeat polymorphism at the human beta-actin related pseudogene 2 (ACTBP2) detected using the polymerase chain reaction. *Nuc. Acids Res.* 1991;**19**:6980. *Technique* 1992;**3**:175-178.
3   Watkins C, Bodfish P, Warne D, Nyberg K, Spurr NK. Dinucleotide repeat polymorphism T in the human alpha-cardiac actin gene, intron IV (ATCC), detected using the polymerase chain reaction. *Nuc. Acids Res.* 1991;**19**:6980.
4. Bodfish P, Warne D, Watkins C, Nyberg K, Spurr NK. Dinucleotide repeat polymorphism in the human coagulation factor XI gene, intron B (F11), detected using the polymerase chain reaction. *Nuc. Acids Res.* 1991;**19**: 6979.
5. Bodfish P, Warne D, Nyberg K, Spurr N. Dinucleotide repeat polymorphism at the human erythroid alpha-spectrin (SPTA1) mRNA gene detected using PCR. *Hum. Mol. Genet.* 1992;**1**:287.

Contract number: GENO - 0001 - UK
Contractual period: 1 January 1991 to 31 December 1992

Coordinators
Nigel K. Spurr and Kerstin Nyberg
ICRF, Clare Hall Laboratories
Blanche Lane, South Mimms,
Potters Bar, Herts, EN6 3LD
United Kingdom
Tel: 44 71 269 3846
Fax: 44 71 269 3802

The work was carried out at the Probe Resource Centre, Imperial Cancer Research Fund.

Appendix 1

BamHI:	K-H. Grzeschik	
	F. Moreno	
BgII:	P. Humphries	
BgIII:	H. Cann	
	L. Terrenato	
DraI:	M. Ferguson-Smith	
	H. Scheffer	
EcoRI:	E. Bakker	F. Moreno
	X. Estivill	S. Povey
	A. Gal	H. Scheffer
	K-H. Grzeschik	G. Vergnaud
	H. Harley	J. Weissenbach
	T. Kruse	R. Williamson
HaeIII:	T. Kruse	
HincII:	J. Weissenbach	
	R. Williamson	
HindIII:	L. Contu	T. Kruse
	M. Ferguson-Smith	T. McCarthy
	K-H. Grzeschik	H. Scheffer
	H. Harley	A. Wright
HinfI:	E. Bakker	
	A. Gal	
	P. Humphries	
	S. Povey	
	G. Vergnaud	
	J. Weissenbach	

HphI:	H. Scheffer	
KnpI:	L. Terrenato	
PstI:	E. Bakker	M. Lathrop
	H. Cann	N. Moschonas
	H. Harley	L. Terrenato
	T. Kruse	A. Wright
PvuII:	H. Cann	S. Povey
	M. Ferguson-Smith	G. Vergnaud
	M. Lathrop	A. Wright
RsaI:	E. Bakker	
	H. Cann	
	M. Lathrop	
	J. Weissenbach	
SacI:	J. Lavinha	
	R. Williamson	
Sau3a:	L. Contu	T. McCarthy
(MboI)	X. Estivill	N. Moschonas
	A. Gal	H. Scheffer
	K-H. Grzeschik	G. Vergnaud
	H. Harley	R. Williamson
	T. Kruse	A. Wright
	J. Lavinha	
ScaI:	S. Povey	
StuI:	M. Ferguson-Smith	
XbaI:	X. Estivill	
Xmnl:	N. Moschonas	

Human Genome Analysis Programme
M. Hallen and A. Klepsch (Eds.)
IOS Press, 1995

MEMBRANE RESOURCE FOR EUROGEM

D. Cohen
Centre d'Etude du Polymorphisme Humain (CEPH), Paris, France

1. Objectives

The European Gene Mapping Project was conceived to establish, with European partners exclusively, a 5cM human gene map. Two resource centres were chosen and a network of laboratories was organized to carry out this work. A total of 22 laboratories was contracted to genotype each the panel of 40 CEPH reference families with 81 markers, in 24 months. The probe resource centre, located in the HGR laboratory (Human Genetics Resources Laboratory) at I.C.R.F. (Imperial Cancer Research Fundation, Clare Hall, U.K.) provided the different probes and markers. The CEPH., as Resource Centre for membranes and DNA, had to deliver to all EUROGEM participants the biological material necessary to screen their markers.

2. Project methodology

For PCR analysis, DNA from the 40 CEPH reference families was distributed in microtiterplates: 5 different families on each MTP, i.e. 8 different MTPs per laboratory. The plates were sent either frozen or with DNA in lyophilised form.

For classical hybridizations of Southern membranes, the DNA of the complete panel of the 40 reference CEPH family was digested, checked and then migrated under classical conditions. Most of the operations concerning DNA and reaction buffer distribution were automated. The electrophoretic migration and the electric transfer from the gel to the filter were automatically performed and linked using a prototype of a Multiblotter (Bertin-Labimap S.A.). Filters were prepared according to EUROGEM requirements with 22 different restriction enzymes: Msp1, Taq1, Hind 3, Eco RV, Eco R1, Pvu2, Pst1, Sac 1, etc.... All laboratories received membranes with MspI and Taq1 digests, and a further 3-4 membranes with digests of their choice according to the probes they had to use.

Particular caution was taken to insure the success of this project: the quality of all DNA conformed to the reference standards established at CEPH and the filters were optimized (reproducibility and reliability of sample size and migration conditions; clear and certain identification of the samples and membranes).

3. Work accomplished

During 1991-1992, the resource centre for DNA performed and distributed about 100 test-filters, 700 parental filters (22 enzymes, 80 parents) and more than 6000 membranes (average 110/week). The results appeared robust and efficient as data on 576 markers were submitted. These corrected data are now available in CRI-MAP format by anonymous ftp from mahler.clh.icnet.uk in /pub/eurogem/mapdata and from C.E.P.H. (Spurr et al., 1994).

References

- N.K. Spurr, S.P. Bryant, J. Attwood, K. Nyberg, S.A. Cox, A. Mills, R. Bains, D. Warne, L. Cullin, S. Povey, J.M. Sebaoun, J. Wiessenbach, H.M. Cann, M. Lathrop, J. Dausset, A. Marcadet-Troton and D. Cohen (1994). European Gene Mapping Project (EUROGEM): Genetic Maps based on the CEPH reference families. Eur J Hum Genet 2: 193-252.

Contract number: GENO-0002
Contractual period: 1 January 1991 to 31 December 1992

Coordinator
Professor D. Cohen
Fondation J. Dausset - C.E.P.H.
Human Polymorphism Study Centre
27 rue Juliette Dodu
F - 75010 Paris
France
Tel: 33 1 4249 9850
Fax: 33 1 4018 0155

Human Genome Analysis Programme
M. Hallen and A. Klepsch (Eds.)
IOS Press, 1995

EUROGEM NETWORK LABORATORIES

N.K. Spurr

Clare Hall Laboratories, Potters Bar, United Kingdom

The first two years of the European Genome Mapping Project (EUROGEM) have now been completed. The project formally started on July 1st, 1991, although initial difficulties in the distribution of DNA led to some delays at the start. Twenty-two laboratories signed subcontracts at the start of the project, and these have remained within the network for the duration. A further laboratory (Professor Mirzabekhov, Engelhardt Institute of Molecular Biology, Moscow) joined briefly in 1992, but due to a number of practical difficulties, for example the lack of a reliable postal service, the collaboration had to be abandoned.

The report deals with the work carried out by the 22 Network laboratories and the collaboration between these and the Probe Resource Centre during the period August 1992 - August 1993. Initially, the Network laboratories undertook to screen a total of 81 markers each over the two years, 27 during the first twelve months and 54 during the second half of the project. At the end of the first twelve months progress varied very much between the individual laboratories.

1. Markers supplied by the Probe Resource Centre

The Probe Resource Centre undertook at the beginning of the project to supply up to 50% of the markers used by the Network laboratories. The remainder was the responsibility of the laboratories themselves. In numbers, this meant approximately 920 markers supplied by the Probe Resource Centre over the 24 month period. This figure does not refer to the actual number of markers, but to the sum of the weighted values for each marker. The weighted value is based on the following tariff system which was agreed on at the beginning of the project:

Heterozygosity	Weighted Value
<70%	1
70% - 79%	2
≥80%	3

At the end of the first year, a total of ≥ 343 markers (weighted value) had been distributed. The final weighted value will probably be much higher, as in all cases where the heterozygosity of a marker was unknown the weighted value was taken to be =1 until further information was available.

The working methods and communication between the Probe Resource Centre and the Network laboratories established during the first year were continued for the second half of the project. During the first year two batches of markers were sent out, the second batch in March-April 1992. After that consignment a longer gap was seen to be necessary for the Network laboratories to be able to catch up. Five laboratories contacted us for more markers during this interval.

A third batch of markers was planned for distribution to all Network laboratories during the autumn 1992. This batch consisted exclusively of PCR based markers, which had been selected by continuous screening of literature and the GDB database. The informative value of these markers is usually very high; with a few exceptions the heterozygosity of these markers was >70% and their weighted values >1 accordingly. The primer sets for these markers were ordered from the Oligonucleotide Synthesis Unit at the Imperial Cancer Research Fund, and sent to the Network laboratories as soon as they became available. Unfortunately, due to staff shortages and the increasing demand for the services of this unit, at the time of writing a few laboratories have still not received their consignment.

Depending on the extent to which PCR based markers will be used within the project in the future, the capacity of our internal synthesis service may not be sufficient. Contact has been made with commercial companies and their quotations will be considered when the future work of the EUROGEM project has been decided on in more detail.

The slow distribution of the third batch of markers was compensated by a large consignment of high quality markers sent to all laboratories in January 1993. These markers are part of the set of 814 $(CA)_n$ microsatellite markers spanning the whole human genome which Dr. Jean Weissenbach and his co-workers at Généthon published in 1992 (Weissenbach et al. (1992) Nature 359, 794-801). Dr. Weissenbach agreed that the Probe Resource Centre would be allowed to purchase the primers for use within the EUROGEM project. The first consignment consisted of 207 primer pairs, which divided between the laboratories gave each laboratory 9-10 markers. In the distribution of these markers, the previously agreed assignment of chromosomes to laboratories could not always be adhered to, as the distribution of markers on the chromosomes was very uneven. However, all laboratories concerned agreed to screen markers on chromosomes outside their area of interest.

The information value of these markers was extremely high, with an average heterozygosity of 79%. The markers had previously been screened on only 8 of the CEPH families. The network laboratories were asked to give the screening of the remaining families with these markers priority before any other markers, and most laboratories have now concluded this task. The information gained from this work will make a very valuable contribution to the construction of a high density linkage map, which is the aim of the EUROGEM project.

2. Other materials supplied to the Network laboratories

In the first year of the project, membranes for Southern blotting were sent out from the DNA Resource Centre (CEPH, Paris) to each laboratory. The information on restriction digests required was supplied by the Probe Resource Centre and was based on the probes which were to be sent to the laboratories, and also on data on the probes which the laboratories wished to use as their own contribution. It was agreed that the Network laboratories would strip the filters after they had finished using them, and send them on to other laboratories on request. All Network laboratories received a list of which membranes each laboratory had been sent so they would be able to request the membranes directly.

We have received no reports on how this system has worked. It is possible that because of the greatly diminished use of DNA probes within the project, the membranes may not have been used to the extent which was originally anticipated.

3. European Gene Mapping Project (EUROGEM): Genetic Maps based on the CEPH reference families

Following the second EUROGEM meeting in Cork, Ireland 1-3 October, 1993, it was decided to prepare a set of genetic linkage maps for each human chromosome except chromosome Y for publication. This was completed in July 1994 and has been published recently in the European Journal of Human genetics. It is the culmination of the first round of the EUROGEM project.

The details of the data collection and map construcion are given below.

3.1 Genotyping and Data Collection

One of the requirements for those participating in this project was that all the genotype data produced during this project were to be made freely available. This was achieved by depositing all the data with CEPH for inclusion in their public database. To assist with this work a significant amount of time has been devoted to ensuring all laboratories had sufficient hardware and software. The laboratories were encouraged to establish a connection to the Internet network, and this was used to exchange information between laboratories and the co-ordinating centres. Only two laboratories at present are not connected to Internet and we aim to have a 100% connectivity during the second phase of the project which started in May 1994.

Each of the 22 network laboratories was supplied with a Unix workstation (DECStation 5000/25, Digital Corporation). This included a run-time version of the Sybase relational database management system (Sybase Inc), together with a Sybase application called GENBASE (Mark Lathrop and Jean-Marc Sebaoun, unpublished), and the version 6 CEPH database in Sybase format.

Each laboratory typed a number of markers across the CEPH panel, following the usual CEPH rules about typing informative families.. The data were collated mostly by the GENBASE software but some laboratories used the MS-DOS CEPH database programs, and uploaded electronically to a central ftp server (diamond.gene.ucl.ac.uk), accessible to all the network laboratories.

From here, the files were transmitted electronically to CEPH for inclusion in the main CEPH database. Those labs not networked at the time submitted their data on floppy disks.

The submitted data, in either Unix or PC dump format, were concatenated to a single file and then broken down into separate files by chromosome. Unix scripts (John Attwood, unpublished) were used to process these files into a format very similar to that used by the LINKAGE suite of programs, which were then analysed by the LINK2SUM program (John Attwood, unpublished) which performs the same checks and calculations as the original CEPH SUMDAT.EXE program. Allelic exclusions detected were reported back to the collaborating laboratories, the necessary corrections edited into the submitted data files and the LINKAGE format files regenerated. CRI-MAP input files were produced from these corrected files using the program LINK2CRI (John Attwood, unpublished) and placed on the ftp server for downloading by the laboratories making the maps.

In all, data on 576 markers were submitted. These corrected data are available in CRI-MAP format by anonymous ftp from mahler.clh.icnet.uk in /pub/eurogem/mapdata and from CEPH.

3.2 Map Construction

Following the data collection phase, a process of map construction was initiated. Each network laboratory was assigned one or more of the 2? autosomal chromosomes or chromosome X. The aim was to place the new EUROGEM markers on a well-supported framework map which could be composed of selected CEPH markers, Généthon CA repeats or Cooperative Human Linkage Center (CHLC) systems.

Laboratories made their own choice as to which framework to choose (CEPH or CHLC) and their reasons are detailed in the sections for each chromosome. The main task was to place as many as possible of the newly typed EUROGEM markers on the base map with 1000:1 support.

Each laboratory adopted a particular strategy for producing the map, described in the section for each chromosome. CRI-MAP version 2.4 was used by all but two of the laboratories. Map-building began in parallel with the elimination of allelic exclusions, with corrections being reported so that the data could be corrected and the CRI-MAP input files regenerated on a continuous basis. Most labs used the CRI-MAP 'build' routine to enlarge their maps. In the course of mapbuilding, intralocus recombinants were detected and reported back to the contributing laboratories who, in turn, fed corrections back to the central site. Considerable advantage was derived from most sites being connected to the Internet, as communication by electronic mail between labs was mostly very fast, and corrected datafiles could be downloaded within a few hours of requesting corrections. Additionally, help and advice from those more experienced in map-building could be obtained quickly and easily, and problems with using the software diagnosed and solved. As the maps stabilised, unusual clusters of recombinants could be detected using the 'chrompic' option of CRI-MAP, and further rounds of error-checking and correction were carried out. In cases where it was impossible to verify the data and strong doubts still remained as to their validity, they were removed from the data-files.

As well as regular checking throughout for local support of at least 1000:1 with CRI-MAP's 'flips2' option, the final maps were checked with 'flips4' to ensure that alternative orders had been sufficiently explored. For those markers which could not be placed with 1000:1 support, CRI-MAP 'all' runs were conducted for each to determine the range of positions that fell within the 3-unit support interval.

When complete, the CRI-MAP output files were uploaded by ftp and transformed into PostScript figures by a set of Unix scripts (John Attwood and Stephen P Bryant, unpublished). The framework maps were juxtaposed with 800-band ideograms (G. Spowart, unpublished) and a representative set of cytogenetic data chosen from GDB to map the relationship between the ideograms and the maps.

The support intervals for those markers which could not be placed uniquely were plotted separately. These figures were accompanied by a set of the individual chromosome reports. A representative map is shown in figure 1.

Legend to figure 1

Figure 1 shows the ideogram of human chromosome 2 along with the framework maps showing the order of markers supported at 1000:1. These orders and the recombination fractions between them are shown as male, female and sex averaged. The distances between markers is shown to scale. Loci haplotyped together are shown on the same line. Cytogenetic localisation of markers is shown for most chromosomes. This information was obtained from GDB and the localisations were derived using alternative techniques, mainly fluorescent in-situ hybridisation or somatic cell hybrid mapping. The markers typed during the EUROGEM project are indicated in bold type. Inset into each figure is a simplified representation of the framework map with markers equally spaced. To the right of these maps is indicated the positions of markers which could not be uniquely placed in the framework maps. The thickness of the bars indicates the statistical

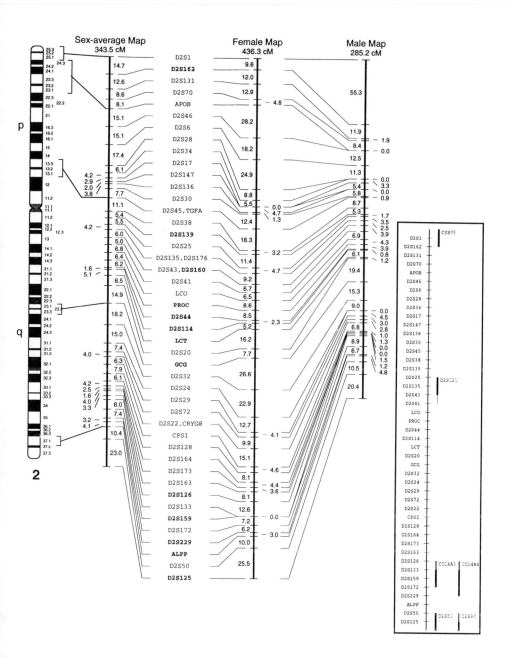

Figure 1.

support for each interval. The most likely interval, and others with a log-likelihood difference of less than 1 from it, is shown with a broad line. Intervals with a log-likelihood difference between 1 and 2 compared to the best have a narrower line. Intervals with a log-likelihood difference of between 2 and 3 compared to the best are indicated by a fine line. Dashed lines connect non-adjacent intervals.

Bibliography

Spurr et al, 1994. European Gene Mapping Project (EUROGEM): Genetic Maps based on the CEPH reference families. Eur. J. Hum. Genet. 2: 193-252.

Contract number: GENO 0007
Contractual period: 1 July 1991 to 30 June 1993

Coordinator
Dr. N.K. Spurr
ICRF, Clare Hall Laboratories
Blanche Lane, South Mimms
Potters Bar, Herts, EN6 3LD
United Kingdom
Tel: 44 71 269 3846
Fax: 44 71 269 3802

Participants
K.-H. Grzeschik, University of Marburg (D)
A. Gal, University of Kiel (D)
T. Kruse, University of Aarhus (DK)
F. Moreno, Hospital Ramon y Cajal, Madrid (E)
X. Estevill, Hospital de la Santa Creu I Sant Pau, Barcelona (E)
H. Cann, CEPH, Paris (F)
M. Lathrop, CEPH, Paris (F)
G. Vergnaud, Laboratoire de Génétique Moléculaire, Vert le Petit (F)
J. Weissenbach, Institut Pasteur, Paris (F)
N. Moschonas, IMBB, Heraklion (GR)
L. Contu, University of Cagliari (I)
L. Terrenato, University of Rome (I)
P. Humphries, University of Dublin (IRL)
T. McCarthy, University College, Cork (IRL)
E. Bakker, University of Leiden (NL)
C. Buys, University of Groningen (NL)
L. Archer, Universidade Nova de Lisboa (P)
H.J. Evans, MRC, Edinburgh (UK)
M. Ferguson-Smith, University of Cambridge (UK)
D. Hopkinson, University College, London (UK)
D. Shaw, University of Wales, Cardiff (UK)
R. Williamson, St. Mary's Hospital Medical School, London (UK)

Human Genome Analysis Programme
M. Hallen and A. Klepsch (Eds.)
IOS Press, 1995

THE ICRF COSMID REFERENCE LIBRARIES

D. Nizetic, G. Zehetner and H. Lehrach
Imperial Cancer Research Fund, London, United Kingdom

The integrated mapping of the target genomes by integration of data obtained through hybridisation using unique and complex probes has been a long-term strategy of the Genome Analysis Laboratory at ICRF (in further text: GAL).

A number of different laboratories including GAL have developed techniques and undertaken projects aiming at ordering genomic libraries using YAC, P1 and cosmid clones [1-4]. The end result is typically a number of contiguous DNA stretches (contigs) represented by ordered cloned fragments which are permanently stored at -70° C, and are individually accessible. An increasing number of genomic and cDNA probes is being genetically mapped to human chromosome maps and their relations to human polymorphisms and disease loci is being established by a large number of laboratories. To relate the clones in the contigs to the genetic, transcriptional, functional, sequence and other data accumulated in the world scientific community on human chromosomes as DNA molecules, reference collections of clones have to be hybridised to DNA probes (genes) which bear such information. The most efficient way to relate all these probes to ordered cosmids is by distributing high density replicas of retrievable chromosome specific libraries to all laboratories interested in obtaining cosmids around the probes of their interest. Autoradiograms as the result of screening are then sent back to the central laboratory together with the detailed information about the probe used. The positive clones and the data about the probe become an entry in the central database. In this way the clones to be ordered are already being related to the molecular genetic markers in parallel by many different labs which in return benefit from a rapid and technically easy "mail retrieval" of clones of their interest from the reference library [6,7].

The progress of work

Up to 2 years ago the status of the work at GAL was that the cosmid libraries had been constructed from flow sorted human chromosomes X and 21 each of which contained over 30 genomic equivalents, these had been picked into microtitre plates and duplicated. Libraries had been characterised both by analysing random clones and screening with genetically mapped probes. High density membranes had been prepared from microtitre plates such that two membranes or one membrane bear 4-5 genome equivalents of chromosomes X and 21, respectively. Such membranes have been distributed to more than 40 different laboratories (each chromosome) and over 100 single copy probes have been hybridised - the membranes for each chromosomes detecting in >90% of cases 1 - 10 positive cosmids per probe. The total number of positive clones detected up to a year ago on both libraries exceeded 4000.

For the last 2 years the EC has funded the construction of additional cosmid libraries for the human chromosomes 11 and 17 and the distribution of clones and membranes for four chromosomes (11, 17, 21, X). These goals have been achieved, and the facility extended even further.

The current status of the GAL reference library deliverables is that cosmid libraries for chromosomes 11 and 17, as well as additional chromosomes 6,13, 18 and 22 have been running for different time periods as reference libraries and 514 high density membrane sets have been sent to different laboratories in 10 European countries as well as a number of laboratories on other continents (see Appendix 1). A total of 1266 probes have detected over 10000 positive clones that have been sent to users as requested in 1508 individual requests. For about 80% of these deliverables the beneficiaries have been the European laboratories (see Appendix 1). Several contigs in the genetically important regions have been identified [5].

References

[1] Nizetic, D. *et al.* Construction, arraying and high-density screening of large insert libraries from human chromosomes X and 21: Their potential use as reference libraries. *Proc.Natl.Acad.Sci. USA* **88**: 3233-3237(1991).
[2] Nizetic, D. et al. An integrated YAC-overlap and 'cosmid-pocket' map of the human chromosome 21 Human Molecular Genetics **3**: 759-770 (1994).
[3] Hoheisel J.D. et al. High-resolution cosmid and P1 maps spanning the 14-Mbp genome of the fission Schizosaccharomyces pombe *Cell* **73**: 1-20 (1993) .
[4] Chumakov, I. *et al.* Continuum of overlapping clones spanning the entire human chromosome 21q. *Nature* **359**, 380-387 (1992).
[5] Dietrich A. et al. Molecular cloning and analysis of the fragile X region in man. *Nucl. Acids Res.* **19**: 2567-2572 (1991).
[6] Zehetner, G. and Lehrach H. The Reference Library System - sharing biological material and experimental data. *Nature* **367**, 489-491 (1994).
[7] Lehrach H. et al. in *Genome Analysis* Vol.1 (Cold Spring Harbor, New York) *Genetic and Physical Mapping*, 39-81 (1990).

Contract number: GENO 0003
Contractual period: 1 January 1991 to 31 December 1992

Coordinator
Dr. H. Lehrach
Inperial Cancer Research Fund
Genome Analysis Laboratory
44 Lincoln's Inn Fields
London WC2A 3PX
United Kingdom
Tel: 44 71 269 3308
Fax: 44 71 269 3068

Participants
Dr. D. Nizetic
University of London
Centre for Applied Molecular Biology
School of Pharmacy
29/39 Brunswick Square
London WC1N 1AX
United Kingdom
Tel: 44 71 753 5933
Fax: 44 71 278 1939

Dr. G. Zehetner
Imperial Cancer Research Fund
Genome Analysis Laboratory
44 Lincoln's Inn Fields
London WC2A 3PX
United Kingdom
Tel: 44 71 269 3571
Fax: 44 71 269 3645

Appendix 1

Report on the status of the ICRF reference library deliverables for human chromosome cosmid libraries.

Chromosome	Country	Probes	Contacts	Requests	Clones
11	Belgium	1	1	1	3
	Germany	2	2	2	65
	Netherlands	2	2	2	4
	UK	72	20	76	472
	Israel	1	1	1	17
	USA	5	3	5	62
13	Belgium	2	2	2	2
	Germany	4	3	4	20
	Switzerland	1	1	1	16
	UK	26	6	26	167
	P.R. China	1	1	1	10
	USA	1	1	1	2
17	France	2	1	2	54
	Germany	22	6	22	215
	Italy	1	1	1	8
	UK	106	31	109	881
	USA	18	3	18	241
21	Belgium	4	2	5	6
	France	76	4	76	692
	Germany	2	2	2	2
	Italy	2	2	2	5
	Netherlands	6	2	7	93
	UK	91	9	94	6043
	USA	37	10	39	180
	Israel	1	1	1	3
22	Belgium	2	2	2	2
	France	15	2	16	68
	Germany	4	2	4	23
	UK	28	9	29	206
	USA	2	1	2	50
X	France	60	14	64	822
	Germany	137	14	141	774
	Italy	42	3	42	134
	Sweden	7	4	7	213
	Netherlands	23	10	23	99
	UK	176	56	182	1301
	USA	129	43	130	758
	Australia	6	2	6	30
	Canada	12	2	12	27
	P.R. China	12	1	15	128
Total (Europe)		916	212	1051	12390
Total (all)		1141	281	1175	13898

Human Genome Analysis Programme
M. Hallen and A. Klepsch (Eds.)
IOS Press, 1995

THE HGMP RESOURCE CENTRE cDNA PROGRAMME

K. Gibson
HGMP Resource Centre, Cambridge, United Kingdom

A cDNA Resource has been created from which users can gain rapid access to any cDNA of interest. The Resource is now largely established and changes since the last report (November, 1992) have been largely numerical in nature. This report concerns primarily the changes at the Resource Centre which are salient to the EC cDNA programme.

1. Clone Resource

Clones have proved to be of interest either because their sequence indicates them to be related to sequences of interest to the user or because they have been probed by the user and thus identified to originate from the users region of interest. The level of interest has been greater in the clones for probing rather than the sequences, reflecting the rate and manner that they are available to users. The 5760 clones from conventional phage libraries, including liver, brain (cortex), bone marrow, placenta and rhabdomyosarcoma, have been made available primarily as sequences since it has proven to be technically difficult to probe grid phage.

The technology for normalising cDNA libraries developed at the centre has proven to meet its aims. Essentially, sequence analysis has demonstrated that cDNAs can be divided up into separate populations with minimal overlap between each population. This makes it possible to pick and grid large numbers of cDNAs with a high representation of many different human genes. Furthermore, it has been demonstrated that the technology substantially biases (32 fold) against abundant cDNAs, reinforcing the view that a replete collection of genes is within reach with minimal redundancy. Using this technology 21,000 normalised cDNA clones were added to the collection from average 15 week menstrual age brain (15,400 clones), liver (1,500 clones), kidney (96 clones) and adrenal (5,100 clones) tissues. This has been supplemented by clones from fetal liver and a mixture of six tissues. Mixtures are important to avoid the wasteful overlap of cDNAs originating from more than one tissue. The normalised clones are in a modified version of the plasmid vector, bluescript KS$^+$, which has proven to be ideal for gridding. The 21,000 normalised clones therefore, were augmented by 20,000 clones from a conventional library. This library was prepared originally by the group of Hans Lehrach (ICRF) from the pancreatic duct cell tumour cell line, PATU 8902. However, difficulty has been experienced in sequencing clones from this library.

Characterisation of cDNAs by partial sequencing has been confined to those occurring as positives on the high density grids. This ensures their integration with physical mapping because the probes used have already been physically mapped, for example YACs.

2. cDNA Database

The relational database, for the purpose of acting as an electronic reference library for cDNAs, prepared in Sybase™ and mounted at the Resource Centre has now been utilised as an archive for sequences and libraries from other members of the consortium. This necessitated the development of appropriate of file transfer procedures, usable over the electronic networks.

In order to aid users through familiarity, the database has the same 'feel' as the Genome Database (GDB). Currently data concerning 23 libraries and over 4,000 sequenced clones is stored.

Network access to the database continues to be available throughout the world by internationally accepted means: registration as a user to obtain a suitable password and account.

Sequences from the database have been forwarded to the public databases (E.M.B.L.) for further use access. This does not include relational data which it is only appropriate to store locally but may in future become available through I.G.D.

3. Partial sequencing

A further 1200 sequences have been produced by the Resource Centre as part of the gene identification programme by producing expressed sequence tags. Comparison of these sequences to the public databases confirms that ca. 60% of the sequences are entirely new. The normalised clones have proven to be a highly efficient and effective Resource for pursuing this strategy with latterly over 70% of the sequenced clones giving rise to reads greater than 350 bases and over 98% accuracy. This has allowed us to set these figures as extremely stringent quality control parameters before submission to E.M.B.L. It is also encouraging for the representation of the gridded arrays.

The programme icatools has proven to be of great utility for characterising the frequency classes of the sequences obtained and will therefore allow only unique sequences to be submitted to E.M.B.L.

Contamination with non human sequences has not been detected.

4. High density cDNA grids

Grids of normalised cDNA clones have continued to be distributed. On average, 2 sets of 22,000 clones are distributed per month. cDNA clones are requested at a rate of over 35 per month from the grids. The grids are precious and therefore we encourage their reuse as far as possible.

The low level of repeat sequences reported originally has been confirmed. There is a tendency for users probes to identify these sequences. In future a database will identify such clones and eliminate them from screenings.

5. Normalised cDNA libraries

In the human there are ca. 50 tissues and 200 cell types. Different cDNAs are obtained from a tissue at widely differing levels. In addition, there is a high degree of overlap between cDNAs obtained from different tissues. These factors combine to make it highly unlikely that a majority of human cDNA can be identified by procedures based upon random picking. More importantly, it makes the highly desirable objective of providing in the short term, the majority of human cDNAs on grids, an unlikely eventuality. In order that these problems can be overcome, we have developed a "normalisation" procedure during which a large population of cDNAs are divided into sets which have a low degree of overlap. Furthermore, the method is applicable to cDNAs prepared from complex mixtures of tissues, thus avoiding much of the redundancy introduced by overlaps between tissues. Suitable use of the subsets gives a high yield of unique cDNAs, which demonstrate a low degree of overlap between different subsets, as determined by the proportion of antisense sequence similarities (normalised cDNAs were cloned directionally) between exclusively different subsets (2.5%), as opposed to the same subsets from different tissues (9.8%).

The normalised cDNAs continue to be distributed. Clones are now sequenced once they have been demonstrated to hybidise to a physically mapped proble. Up to 99% of the clones from a subset, have inserts in a unique orientation. Ca. 70% of human cDNAs are available. A greater emphasis has been placed on screening the subsets by direct hybridisation, whereby positives are PCR amplified after hybridisation to the clone of interest.

CpG island libraries have been obtained from Professor Adrian Bird to complement the "normalised" cDNAs. The CpG island libraries should be perfectly normalised since they are prepared from genomic DNA but only represent about 60% of human genes since the remainder of genes lack such islands. They are being made available similarly to the normalised cDNAs.

6. Full Length cDNA Libraries

Neither CpG islands nor normalised cDNAs represent full length transcripts. These have therefore been complemented by obtaining 50 high quality, full length libraries from Dr. Dai Simmons at the I.M.M. Oxford and these are being distributed. The current rate is 41 libraries per month.

7. Future direction

The services will continue to be provided along the lines described with technical innovations being passed on to the user as the innovations are developed.

CIRCULAR RNA MOLECULES CONTAINING HUMAN SEQUENCES

D. Marazziti, E. Golini, A. Gallo, R. Matteoni and G.P. Tocchini-Valentini
Istituto di Biologia Cellulare, CNR, Roma, Italy

We have developed a method for isolating rare sequences from the pool of human sequences expressed in brain or, indeed, any other tissue.

The method takes advantage of the fact that, although the intervening sequence in natural pre-tRNAs is small (8-60 nucleotides), the presence of abnormally large introns does not prevent the halves from folding correctly and producing the L-shaped conformation characteristic of the mature domain [1,2]. We inserted a collection of human frontal brain (HFB) cDNA molecules at the HpaI site of the intron of yeast pre-tRNA $^{Leu}3$ gene; a large number of the T7 transcripts derived from the stretched genes were correctly cleaved by the XL splicing endonuclease, an enzyme that recognizes features of the mature domain [3,4]. The pre-tRNAs can, therefore, tolerate inserts over 1000 bases long and still fold correctly. Correct folding of the mature domain means that the RNA molecules will have 5' and 3' termini that are very near to one another as a result of the presence of complementary sequences which lead to the formation of an acceptor stem helix. We are able to utilize the T4 ligase to connect the termini of the transcripts and to obtain circular RNA molecules [5]; their circularity was verified by linearization with XL RNaseP, an enzyme that regenerates the original termini.

The circles can be readily separated from linear molecules; digestion with RNase H can be used to linearize molecules containing sequences complementary to specific oligodeoxynucleotides.

The library that resulted was plated and clones were randomly selected for analysis by cDNA sequencing.

References

[1] H. Swerdlow and C. Guthrie. J. Biol. Chem. 259: 5197, 1984.
[2] M.C. Lee and G. Knapp. J. Biol. Chem. 260: 3108, 1985.
[3] A. Otsuka, A. de Paolis, G.P. Tocchini-Valentini. Mol. Cell. Biol. 1: 269, 1981.
[4] E. Mattoccia, M.I. Baldi, D. Gandini-Attardi, S. Ciafré and G.P. Tocchini-Valentini. Cell 55: 731, 1988.
[5] T. Pan, R.R. Gutell, O.C. Uhlenbeck. Science 254: 1361, 1991.

THE PARTIAL SEQUENCE ANALYIS OF HUMAN cDNAS

Progress Report by Dr. Arnold and Dr. Domdey
Genzentrum München, Germany

A: cDNA-ANALYSIS

B. Obermaier, S. Stachowitz, B. Blum, and H. Domdey

1. Summary

More than 1,000 cDNA clones from a commercially available cDNA library [oligo(dT) and random primed] from the left ventricle of human heart and from a self-made cDNA library [oligo(dT) primed] from atrium were analysed by partial DNA sequence analysis. Similarity searches against the nucleic acid and protein databases resulted in the identification of more than 500 new and hitherto unknown partial mRNA sequences transcribed in the human heart. 11% of the sequenced clones showed similarities between 50 and 95% to known human mRNAs or DNAs or to mRNAs of other species. Although the majority of these inserts represented only repeated elements of the human genome, a reasonable number (around 1/3 of them) have to be considered as new members of already known gene families and are therefore of special interest. 16% of the analysed inserts were identical (more than 95% similarity) with already known human genes. Most of the known human mRNAs were represented only once; on the other hand, some tissue specific sequences were highly abundant, like the cDNA inserts coding for the human ß-myosin heavy chain. The remaining 28% of the analyzed inserts coded either for mitochondrial or ribosomal mRNAs.

All new and hitherto unknown cDNA sequences as well as those which showed only similarities to other mRNAs or DNAs - but were not identical - have been transferred to the EMBL database, after having them compared with each other using the program QUICK-SEARCH in order to avoid two-or severalfold submission of the same sequence.

All cDNA clones are available as DNA samples from our laboratory.

2. Results

For the heart ventricle cDNA library, a commercially available cDNA library (Stratagene) was chosen. The mRNA had been isolated from the left ventricle of a 22 year old male. cDNA synthesis had been primed with oligo(dT) and random primers. Due to the use of random primers, this library supposedly contains a high number of coding sequences next to the sequencing primer sites. Coding sequences are extremely convenient for computational analysis, i.e. for the comparison and identification of genes, especially when the more specific peptide comparison programs are used.

The library in which the cDNA had been inserted in the *Eco*RI side of the Lambda ZAPII vector, was converted as a whole to pBluescript plasmids. Tansfection into *E.coli* XL-1 Blue and plating on X-Gal containing medium revealed, however, a high background of just vector DNA (about 50% of the colonies). Furthermore, since restriction analysis from isolated plasmid DNAs showed that most of the inserts were only 100-500 nucleotides in length, a size selection was carried out by electrophoresis of a large pool of undigested plasmid DNA on an agarosegel and selective retransformation with DNA containing inserts larger than 500 base pairs. During this step, the vector DNA without insert was eliminated, too. This also reduced the background of blue, only vector-DNA carrying colonies to less than 10%.

The template-DNA for all sequencing reactions was prepared by the alkaline lysis procedure, followed by purification of the plasmid DNA via Quiagen column chromatography. Part of the double-stranded cDNA clones were sequenced manually with ^{35}S-labeled dATP, T7 DNA polymerase (Pharmacia) and the T3- or T7-primers. The other part of the cDNA-clones was sequenced with Taq DNA polymerase and the cycle sequencing protocol with the help of an automated DNA sequencing system from Applied Biosystems. This system allows to use either fluorescently labeled standard primers or unlabeled primers in combination with dye-labeled dideoxynucleotides. The average length of readable sequences was around 290 nucleotides (between 153 and 344) for the classical radioactive method, and around 338 nucleotides (between 162 and 520) for the "automated" sequencing procedure.

Since the first sequencing round showed that 39% of the inserts were derived from DNA coding either for mitochondrial or ribosomal RNA, a colony hybridization with probes isolated from clones containing mitochondrial and ribosomal cDNA-inserts was made. A total of 3000 colonies were picked into microtiterplates, incubated in LB/amp medium and then transferred to nylon-membranes and hybridized with ^{32}P-dCTP labeled probes covering the entire mitochondrial genome and the ribosomal 18S and 28S RNA genes. Clones, which gave no detectable positive signals on the autoradiogram were used as sequencing templates. This preselection through hybridisation increased the number of new and unknown sequences from 40% to 52%, while mitochondrial and ribosomal cDNA clones were reduced from 31% down to 14% (Table 1).

Table 1
Total number and characteristics of partially sequenced cDNAs derived from human heart ventricle mRNA

	A	B	C
total no. of analyzed cDNA-inserts:	278 (100%)	546 (100%)	824 (100%)
cDNAs identical with			
- human mitochondrial RNAs:	66 (24%)	63 (12%)	129 (16%)
- human ribosomal RNAs:	46 (17%)	55 (10%)	101 (12%)
- known human mRNAs:	45 (16%)	93 (17%)	138 (17%)
cDNAs with similarities to			
- human mRNAs and DNAs:	7 (3%)	26 (5%)	33 (4%)
- mRNAs of other spezies:	4 (2%)	24 (4%)	28 (3%)
cDNAs witout any obvious similarities :	110 (40%)	285 (52%)	395 (48%)

A, sequences before colony hybridization with mitochondrial and ribosomal probes;
B, sequences after colony hybridization with mitochondrial and ribosomal probes;
C, total sequences.

Initially, the obtained cDNA sequences were examined for similarities in the nucleic acid databases (EMBL and GENBANK) with the FASTA program, which does a Pearson and Lipman search for similarity between a query sequence and any group of sequences. Sequences which had a high score of similarity to any other species were translated to the more sensitive amino acid level and compared to the protein databases MIPS and SWISSPROT.

Significant similarities with more than 95% identity to nucleic acid database entries of known human DNAs, mRNAs or proteins are listed in Table 2. These matches of at least 95 % were considered to indicate that the partial cDNA sequence corresponds directly to the known human gene, mRNA or protein. Most of the 60 known human mRNAs are represented only once, however, the human ß-MHC mRNA for ß-myosin heavy chains, e.g., represents around 20 % of all obtained, already known human heart cDNA-sequences. To avoid continuous sequencing of these cDNAs in the future, it will be necessary to add the corresponding probes to the mitochondrial and ribosomal hybridisation probes.

Table 2
Similarities (identities 95%) of the human heart ventricle cDNA inserts to known human DNAs, mRNAs or proteins

Database entry	Frequency
1) Human beta-myosin heavy chain	23
2) Human desmin gene	15
3) H. sapiens mRNA titin	6
4) Human cardiac alpha-myosin heavy chain	3
5) Human beta globin region on chomosome 11	3
6) Human mRNA for ventricular myosin light chains	3
7) Human alpha-B-crystallin	3
8) Human adenosine deaminase	2
9) Human DNA for insulin-like growth factor	2
10) Human expressed sequence tag similar to Pig Aconitase	2
11) Human von Willebrand factor mRNA	2
12) Human Na+,K+ /ATPase isoform alpha-III gene	2
13) Human nonerythroid alpha-spectrin	2
14) Human desmoplakin I mRNA	2
15) Human TCB gene encoding cytosolic thyroid hormone-binding protein	2
16) Human mRNA for muscle phosphofructokinase	2
17) Human skeletal alpha-actin	2
18) Human heparan sulfate proteoglycan mRNA	2
19) Human pM5 protein mRNA (collagenase)	2
20) H. sapiens glutathione peroxidase	1
21) Human mitochondrial transcription factor 1 mRNA	1
22) H. sapiens, alpha-2 (VI) collagen	1
23) Human beta-adrenergic receptor kinase 1	1
24) Human laminin B1 chain mRNA	1
25) Human fibroblast mRNA for aldolase A	1
26) Human mRNA for lactate dehydrogenase B	1
27) Human mRNA for slow skeletal troponin C	1
28) H. sapiens ASM gene for acid sphingomyelinase	1
29) Human calcium-ATPase	1
30) Human mRNA for plasma gelsolin	1
31) Human moesin mRNA	1
32) Human mRNA for actin-binding protein	1
33) Human microtubule-associated protein	1
34) Human x-linked phosphoglycerate kinase gene	1
35) Human mRNA for T-cell surface glycoprotein E2	1
36) Human mRNA for 90-kDa heat-shock protein	1
37) Human mRNA for alpha actinin	1
38) Human neuroleukin mRNA	1
39) Human cAMP-dependent protein kinase type I-alpha subunit	1
40) Human novel protein AHNAK mRNA	1

41) Human gene for plasminogen activator inhibitor 1   1
42) Human skeletal muscle alpha-tropomyosin gene   1
43) Nucleotide and deduced amino acid sequences of the cDNA for the
       large subunit of human mCANP   1
44) Human angiogenin gene   1
45) Human alkaline phosphatase   1
46) Human prothrombin gene   1
47) Human myc-oncogene exon 1 and exon 2   1
48) Human proalpha 1 (I) chain of type I procollagen mRNA   1
49) Human p53 gene for transformation related protein p53   1
50) Human cytovillin 2 mRNA   1
51) Human mRNA for F1/ATPase beta subunit   1
52) Human mRNA for cardiac troponin I   1
53) Human skeletal muscle alpha-tropomyosin   1
54) Human CCAAT-box-binding factor   1
55) Human mRNA for cysteine proteinase inhibitor   1
56) Human collagen type 1 pro-alpha-2 mRNA   1
57) Human alpha-tubulin mRNA   1
58) Human insulin-responsive glucose transporter mRNA   1
59) Human hexabrachion mRNA   1
60) Human mRNA PCTAIRE-1 for serine/threonine protein kinase   1
61) Human gene for the light and heavy chains of myeloperoxidase   1
62) Human hexokinase 1 mRNA   1
63) Human transposon L1.2   1
64) Human alpha-fodrin gene   1
65) Human putatively transcribed partial mRNA   1
66) Human lysozyme mRNA   1
67) Human 20-kDa myosin light chain   1
68) Human endogenous retrovirus type c oncovirus   1
69) Human breast carcinoma non-myc 3.8pScR1 sequence with LINE-1 insertion   1
70) Human DNA for Alu element C3N3   1
71) Human L1Heg repetitive element from the intergenic region of the epsilon
       and G-gamma globin genes   1
72) Human transposon-like element p2 solo LTR with inserted Alu element   1
73) Human long interspersed (LI) repetitive DNA from clone pHSRV-H-107   1
74) Human expressed sequence tag (EST 01627) similar to ribosomal protein L1a   1
75) Human expressed sequence tag (EST00287) similar to *Neurospora*
       processing/enhancing protein precursor   1
76) Human expressed sequence tag (EST 01367)   1
77) Human expressed sequence tag (EST00169)   1

The similarities of probably higher interest are those with smaller percentages of identity, since they might indicate new members of already existing protein families or proteins sharing specific domains with others (Table 3). This might also be true for the proteins listed in Table 4 which show similarities to known DNAs, mRNAs or proteins which have already been identified in other species.

From this library, also a set of 395 cDNAs was obtained with none of them displaying any significant similarities or homologies with any nucleic acid or protein in the available databases.

The heart atrium cDNA library was synthesized by standard procedures in our laboratory. The mRNA had been isolated from tissue of different patients. cDNA synthesis was primed with oligo(dT) and cloned in one orientation in an *EcoRI/XhoI* cleaved Lambda ZAPII vector. The library again was converted as a whole to pBluescript plasmids from which the cDNA-inserts were analyzed as described above. The corresponding data are presented in Tables 5 -8.

All new and unknown cDNA sequences as well as those which showed similarities to other species have been transferred to the EMBL database, after having them compared to each other with the program QUICKSEARCH in order to avoid two- or severalfold submission of the same sequence.

Additionally we have started full-length cDNA-sequencing of some selected clones. Since the the cDNAs which show similarities to already known DNAs or mRNAs of man or other species, we have concentrated our efforts on this specific groups. Furthermore, we hve started to analyze the expression of selected genes by Northern blot analysis using RNA from human heart and other control tissues.

Table 3
Similarities (identities between 50 and 95%) of the human heart ventricle cDNA inserts to known human DNAs or mRNAs

	Clone	Database entry	Id / nt	Id (Sim) / aa
1)	HSDHEHB10	Human cytochrome P450 gene exons 1 und 2	73% / 287	26% (44%) / 98
2)	HSDHII021	Human plasminogen activator inhibitor-1	54% / 260	23% (48%) / 78
3)	HSDHII094	Human mRNA for nebulin	58% / 254	38% (61%) / 87
4)	HSDH14A08	Human mRNA for alpha-actinin	73% / 307	73% (83%) / 78
5)	HSDH14C04	Human mRNA for carboxylesterase	60% / 265	56% (71%) / 85
6)	HSDHEAD02	Human poly(A)-binding protein mRNA	71% / 330	81% (90%) / 109
7)	HSDH15G04	Human Hpf4 mRNA (DNA binding Protein)	84% / 129	81% (84%) / 43
8)	HSDH14D01	Human expressed sequence tag (EST01579)	68% / 158	
9)	HSDH23E11	Human chromosome 4 sequence-tagged site St S4-54	64% / 262	
10)	HSDH15C01	Human chromosome 4 sequence tagged site sts4-238	73% / 335	
11)	HSDH14A10	Human cathepsin G gene	71% / 217	
12)	HSDHEAB12	Human tumor necrosis factor receptor, 3´flank	75% / 114	
13)	HSDH22G01	Human C5a anphylatoxin rceptor mRNA	68% / 192	
14)	HSDH22H12	Human carboxylpeptidase M 3' end	80% / 129	
15)	HSDHEI093	Human c-fms proto-oncogene for csf-1 receptor	54% / 217	
16)	HSDH25C01	Human platelet glycoprotein II b gene	71% / 262	
17)	HSDHEHA11	Human glandular kallikrein gene	75% / 138	
18)	HSDHEFB11	Human h-lys gene for lysozyme (upstream region)	69% / 292	
19)	HSDHCF008	Human endogenous retrovirus-like sequence	72% / 116	
20)	HSDHECB06	Human hypoxanthine phosphoribosyl transferase	74% / 258	
21)	HSDHEGD11	Human beta globin region on chromosome 11	73% / 138	
22)	HSDHEI073	Human adenosine deaminase gene	83% / 153	
23)	HSDHEKL09	Human thymidylate syntase gene	86% / 125	
24)	HSDH22G07	Human lysozyme mRNA	62% / 146	
25)	HSDH15B04	Human plasminogen activator inhibitor-1	75% / 092	
26)	HSDH15D02	Human gene for c1-inhibitor	78% / 152	
27)	HSDH14D03	Human beta globin region on chromosome 11	89% / 138	
28)	HSDH14D08	Homo sapiens erythrocyte membrane protein	82% / 164	
29)	HSDH28A04	Human beta globin region on chromosome 11	82% / 321	
30)	HSDHE0034	Human DNA region with homology to D. melanogaster heat shock protein	71% / 205	
31)	HSDH25C04	Human recognition surface antigen (CD4) 5' end	78% / 301	
32)	HSDHEBD03	Human kpni repeat mrna	76% / 326	
33)	HSDH22B11	Human alpha satellite and satellite 3 junction DNA Sequence	62% / 263	

11)	Identity starts after polyadenylation signal
12)	No significant identity on protein level
13)-14)	Untranslated regions
15)-17)	Identities within introns
18)-26)	Alu repeats
27)-31)	Identities within repeat regions
33)	Alpha satellite repetitive element

Table 4

Similarities of the human heart ventricle cDNA inserts to known mRNAs from other species

	Clone	Similarity to	Id / nt	Id (Si) / aa
1)	HSDHEKL71	Rabbit mRNA for titin	62% / 122	51% (59%) / 41
2)	HSDHEKL74	Rabbit mRNA for titin	91% / 120	90% (92%) / 40
3)	HSDHII045	Rabbit mRNA for titin	59% / 270	64% (76%) / 89
4)	HSDHII044	Mouse mRNA for talin	90% / 332	84% (88%) / 85
5)	HSDHEEC09	C. elegans unc-22 gene for twichin.	57% / 175	40% (56%) / 60
6)	HSDHEEF07	R. norvegicus mRNA for H36-alpha7 integrin alpha chain	81% / 331	31% (52%) / 114
7)	HSDHE0051	RNDP150 Rat DP-150 mRNA for 150K dynein-associated polypeptide	82% / 262	85% (90%) / 88
8)	HSDHEEC07	Drosophila melanogaster brahma protein mRNA	62% / 299	64% (80%) / 72
9)	HSDHEFD08	Chicken tensin mRNA	72% / 221	26% (46%) / 137
10)	HSDHEI062	Rat NGF-inducible putative secreted protein	77% / 193	44% (61%) / 62
11)	HSDHEI077	Mouse myeloid differentiation primary response mRNA encoding MYD116 protein	67% / 233	20% (42%) /101
12)	HSDH23F11	M. musculus mRNA for I47 clone	78% / 245	56% (69%) / 81
13)	HSDHE0190	Rat mRNA for smooth muscle myosin RLC-B	81% / 187	
14)	HSDHEAC09	Rabbit sarcolumenin protein mRNA	82% / 301	
15)	HSDHEDD03	Rabbit sarcolumenin protein mRNA	65% / 326	
16)	HSDHEEB07	Chicken urokinase-type plasminogen activator	67% / 167	
17)	HSDHII005	Pig heart aconitase mRNA	70% / 258	
18)	HSDH22B07	S. cerevisiae (CDC14) gene	91% / 172	
19)	HSDHEDD08	Mouse MHC (H-2) S region complement		
20)	HSDHII024	SV40/Mouse hybrid pv4 late region DNA	74% / 121	
21)	HSDH25B05	B. bovis WC1.1 mRNA	64% / 274	
22)	HSDH14A04	Mouse L1Md-A2 repetitive element with two open reading frames	73% / 259	
23)	HSDH14F09	rev Mouse alpha-B crystallin mRNA component C4 gene	89% / 119 60% / 134	
24)	HSDHEFE12	Rabbit DNA for L10c4 repeat	60% / 204	
25)	HSDHEGF07	Mouse DNA with homology to EBV IR3repeat, segment 2, clone Mu2	63% / 216	
26)	HSDHEI091	Nucleotide acid sequences of the cDNA inserts of the chicken rsk-cb clone AV36 (A) and the mouse rsk-mo-1 clone Mufa	78% / 189	
27)	HSDH23E04	Pig heart aconitase	94% / 336	
28)	HSDHEKL24	Rice complete choroplast genome	55% / 255	

13)-18)	Identities in untranslated regions
19)-21)	No significant identities on protein level
22)-28)	Identity within repeat region

Table 5

Total number and characteristics of partially sequenced cDNAs derived from heart atrium mRNA (oligo(dT)-primed without preselection per hybridization)

total no. of analyzed cDNA-inserts:	345	(100%)
cDNAs identical with		
- known human mRNAs:	49	(14%)
- mitochondrial RNAs:	94	(27%)
cDNAs with similarities to		
- human mRNAs and DNAs:	43	(13%)
- mRNAs of other species:	30	(9%)
cDNAs without obvious similarities:	129	(37%)

Table 6

Similarities (identities >95%) of the human heart atrium cDNA inserts to known human DNAs, mRNAs or proteins

Database entry	Frequency
1) Human Wilm's tumor-related protein (QM) mRNA	3
2) Human sceletal muscle alpha-tropomyosin (htm-alpha) mRNA	3
3) Human fibrillarin mRNA	2
4) Human peptidylglycine alpha-amidating monooxygenase mRNA	2
5) Human expressed sequence tag (EST01784) similar to 60K filarial antigen	2
6) Human mRNA for beta-actin (Nucleotide sequence of the rabbit alpha-smooth-mucles and beta-non-muscle +actin mRNA)	2
7) Human ribosomal protein L3 mRNA 3' end	2
8) Human mRNA for nuclear P68 protein "Nuclear protein 1 with sequence homology to translation initiation RT factor eIF-4A";	1
9) H. sapiens partial cDNA sequence; clone 819	1
10) Human expressed sequence tag (EST01826) similar to ribosomal protein S10	1
11) Human protein tyrosine phosphatase (PTPase-alpha) mRNA	1
12) Human gene for atrial natriuretic factor	1
13) Human mRNA for fibronectin receptor beta subunit; glycoprotein	1
14) Human set gene	1
15) Human Ews=Ets and Fli-1 homolog	1
16) H. sapiens glutathione peroxidase gene	1
17) H. sapiens son-a mRNA repetitive sequence	1
18) H. sapiens mRNA for nuclear factor IV	1
19) H. sapiens partial cDNA sequence clone 01d01	1
20) H. sapiens beta-myosin heavy chain gene	1
21) H. sapiens gene for interleukin-2 (5' flanking region) repetitive sequence	1
22) Human deoxycytidine kinase mRNA	1
23) Human muscle creatine kinase gene	1
24) Human ferritin L chain mRNA	1
25) Human hsc70 gene for 71 kd heat shock	1
26) Human class I alcohol dehydrogenase	1
27) Human mRNA for mitochondrial ATP synthase (Fq-ATPase) alpha subunit	1
28) Human mRNA for calcium dependent protease	1
29) H. sapiens putatively transcribed partial sequence, UK-HGMP sequence ID AAABLIE; single read	1
30) Human cytochrome bc-1 complex core protein II mRNA	1
31) Human acidic ribosomal phosphoprotein P0 mRNA	1
32) Human HepG2 3'-directed *MboI* cDNA	1
33) Human mRNA for myosin regulatory light chain	1
34) Human mRNA for cytoplasmic beta-actin	1
35) Human tumor antigen (L6) mRNA	1
36) H. sapiens dek mRNA	1
37) H. sapiens partial cDNA sequence	1
38) Human mRNA for coupling protein G(s) alpha	1
39) Human chondroitin/dermatan sulfate proteogycan	1

Table 7

Similarities (identities between 50 and 95%) of the human heart atrium cDNA inserts to known human DNAs or mRNAs

	Clone	Database entry	Id / nt	Id (Sim) / aa
1)	HSDH0C59	H. sapiens NAP (nucleosome assembly protein) mRNA	70% / 260	46% (68%) / 56
2)	HSDH0B36	Human slow skleletal muscle troponin	71% / 256	72% (84%) / 88
3)	HSDHEW18	Human initiation factor eIF-4 gamma	72% / 261	55% (68%) / 87
4)	HSDHE005	Human zinc finger protein 41 (ZNF41) gene	68% / 325	49% (71%) /128
5)	HSDH0A56	Human retinoblastoma suspectibility gene exons 1-27	59% / 257	
6)	HSDH0C02	Human dystrophin gene	59% / 232	
7)	HSDH0C76	HUMRTPGEF Homo sapiens cDNA	78% / 265	
8)	HSDH0C37	Human interleukin 11gene	81% / 301	
9)	HSDH0053	Human CD1 R2 gene for MHC-related antigen	79% / 193	
10)	HSDHAB11	Human beta-tubulin pseudogene	82% / 269	
11)	HSDH0B16	Human mRNA for adipogenesis inhibitory factor	81% / 221	
12)	HSDH0B60	Human amplified VK gene	74% / 162	
13)	HSDH0F04	H. sapiens gene for mitochondrial ATP synthase c subunit	79% / 235	
14)	HSDHD49A	Human gene for tyrosine d aminotransferase	79% / 286	
15)	HSDHD38A	H. sapiens DNA for cGMP phosphodiesterase	82% / 175	
16)	HSDHD80A	H. sapiens son-p-f1 DNA sequence	73% / 260	
17)	HSDHAB27	Human debresoquine 4-hydoxylase	80% / 218	
18)	HSDHAB16	Human placental protein 14 (PP14) gene	78% / 270	
19)	HSDHD41A	Human insulin receptor (allele 1) gene	80% / 239	
20)	HSDHE004	H. sapiens gene for antithrombin III	77% / 133	
21)	HSDHAB19	Human L1 repetitive sequence with a region homologous to a mouse ORF	75% / 260	
22)	HSDH0A26	Human medium reiteration frequency repetitive sequence	78% / 152	
23)	HSDHE032	Human L1Heg repetitive element	86% / 214	
24)	HSDH0B08	Human beta-myosin heavy chain gene	76% / 172	
25)	HSDHD57A	Human CYP2D7AP pseudogene for cytochrome P4	79% / 172	
26)	HSDHE007	Human carcinoma cell derived Alu RNA transcript	90% / 139	
27)	HSDHD70A	Human thymidine kinase gene	84% / 283	
28)	HSDH0C33	Human dispersed Alu repeats	74% / 432	
29)	HSDHD33A	Human HepG2 3'-directed MboI cDNA, clone s1	81% / 102	
30)	HSDHD34A	Human HepG2 3'-directed MboI cDNA	85% / 357	

5)-16)	Identities in untranslated regions
17)-20)	Identities within introns
21)-29)	Identity within repeat region
30)	No significant identity on protein level

Table 8

Similarities (identities between 50 and 95%) of the human heart atrium cDNA inserts to known mRNAs from other species

	Clone	Similarity to	Id / nt	Id (Si) / aa
1)	HSDHB062	Chicken cofilin mRNA	92% / 164	100% (100%) / 29
2)	HSDH0A72	Mouse phospholipase A-2-activating protein	87% /229	75% (81%) / 99
3)	HSDE0C05	Ovine 6-pgdh mRNA for 6-phosphogluconate dehydrognase	74% / 343	25% (46%) / 59
4)	HSDH0A55	Mouse GA binding protein	82% / 368	77% (84%) / 107
5)	HSDHD76A	Rat clathrin heavy chain mRNA	88% / 343	91% (91%) / 67
6)	HSDHD43A	Mouse single stranded DNA binding protein	77% / 249	34% (44%) / 69
7)	HSDHD48A	Rat mRNA for ribosomal protein L38	83% / 285	88% (91%) / 68
8)	HSDABA23	Chicken cofilin mRNA	82% / 309	
9)	HSDHEW19	Rat rhoB gene mRNA	71% / 302	
10)	HSDH0A45	Bovine cAMP-regulated phosphoprotein mRNA	72% / 271	
11)	HSDH0E01	Murine Glvr-1 mRNA	77% / 396	
12)	HSDABA08	G. gallus PR264 mRNA	55% / 291	
13)	HSDHA058	R. rattus mRNA for brain neuronal myosin heavy chain	53% / 264	

8)-11) Identities in untranslated regions
12)-13) No significant identities on protein level

B: cDNA SEQUENCE-ANALYSIS

F. Schwager and G. Arnold

1. ESTs of Human fibroblast cell line WI38

In this project, a commercially available cDNA library representing the expressed genes of the cell line WI38 was chosen. The cell line WI38 derives from embryonic lung tissue. The library is oligo dT primed and cloned unidirectionally into the vector lZAPII. Aliquots of the library were converted to pBluescript plasmids in the *E. coli* host XL1 blue. Template preparation was done by alkaline lysis and Quiagen column chromatography. The library was subjected to sequence analysis without any preselection. The sequencing strategy was similar to the one outlined before, however, only classical sequencing techniques were used, and the obtained autoradiogramms were scanned and further analyzed with the BioImage DNA sequence film reader and identification system. Sequence data analysis was carried out as before. Table 9 shows the total number of sequenced templates until July 1993, and their distribution. The WI38 library contains a reasonably low background of vector and ribosomal sequences. A fairly high fraction (57%) of the sequences analyzed did not show similarities (> 95%) to sequences of the EMBL database. The fibroblast cell line is not regarded to be highly specialized as compared to, e.g., lymphocytes or neuronal cells. Therefore, the number of new genes detected in the library is surprisingly high. The redundancy of mRNA derived sequences (i.e., non-mitochondrial, non-vector, non-ribosomal sequences) in the library is only 7,9 %. The new and unknown cDNA sequences as well as those which show homologies to other species are currently transferred to the EMBL database.

Besides the sequences shown in Table 9, another 300 human fibroblast cDNAs have sequenced but have not passed database analysis so far.

Table 9
Total number and characteristics of partially sequenced cDNAs derived from human fibroblast cell line WI38 (31.7.93)

Total number of cDNA inserts	316	100,0 %
homologies to		
-Vector sequences	9	2,7 %
-Human mitochondrial sequences	26	8,2 %
-Human ribosomal RNA	1	0,3 %
-Known human mRNAs	57	18,1 %
-mRNAs of other spezies	43	13,6 %
no obvious similarities	180	57,1 %
Redundancies	(25)	(7,9 %)

2. ESTs of Human stomach mucosa

Gastric mucosa is a tissue which is very poorly characterized at the molecular level so far. The tissue consists of several histologically well defined cell types and is the locus for synthesis of various proteins for the digestion pathway, for transport proteins like the vitamin B12 transporter "gastric intrinsic factor", and for HCl secretion.

Gastric mucosa was prepared from a small healthy part of the fundus region of a human patient, whose stomach had to be surgically removed almost completely, as a consequence of stomach cancer disease. After RNA preparation and poly A$^+$ RNA isolation via two rounds of chromatography on oligo-dT columns, a unidirectional cDNA library was constructed using the cDNA synthesis system of Stratagene and the cloning vector λZAPII (EcoRI and Xho cleavage sites).

From 3,3 μg total ds cDNA obtained, an aliquot of 150 ng was ligated into λ vector and packaged *in vitro*. 5.04x10^5 clones were obtained, corresponding to 1.1x10^7 primary λ clones available *in toto*.

To proof the characteristics of the library, 87 clones were converted to plasmids and sequenced as described for the WI38 cell line. It turned out that 24 clones (28 %) represent pepsinogen mRNA, and another 38 clones (44 %) represent an insertion not identified so far. This finding is consistent with the observation of at least two distinct bands in a denaturing gel electrophoresis of the gastric mucosa mRNA. Therefore, the redundancies observed seem to be a *bona fide* reflection of the mRNA distribution in the tissue, rather than a cloning artefact.

For further sequence analysis of the library, a pre-selection of the clones for the two major mRNA species will be performed on the colony level prior to preparation of the sequencing templates.

THE GENEXPRESS cDNA PROGRAMME

C. Auffray
CNRS, Villejuif and GENETHON, Evry, France

The Genexpress Programme team has developed an integrated approach for the molecular analysis of the human genome and its expression, mainly in neuromuscular tissues.

1. Hybridization signatures

cDNA clones have been spotted on high density filters and hybridized with a variety of probes: total cDNA from various tissues, ribosomal, mitochondrial, Alu and L1 repeats, microsatellites, actin, tubulin and other unique sequences. 8592 clones of a human T-lymphocyte cDNA library and 12152 clones from a human skeletal muscle cDNA library have been analyzed as bacterial colonies using film autoradiography and visual scoring. A selection of 1366 cDNA clones from skeletal muscles and 960 clones from a normalized infant brain cDNA library have been analyzed as PCR amplified inserts and purified plasmid DNA, respectively. The results have been captured using phosphor screens and quantified using a specifically designed software. Clones have been classified in four categories according to the strength of hybridization with total cDNA probes.

2. Sequence signatures

a) Analysis of cDNA insert end sequences from the T-lymphocyte cDNA library led to the detection by us and other groups of a large fraction of sequences derived from yeast and unknown bacterial contaminants. This information was circulated widely since the spring of 1992 and led to the identification of *Leuconostoc* species at the origin of the contamination in this and other libraries. Subsequently PCR-based quality controls have been implemented to check for the presence of undesirable sequences of endogenous (ribosomal, mitochondrial) and exogenous (viral, bacterial, yeast) origins at all stages of cDNA library construction and analysis. An adapted validation and analysis process has been developed to circumvent the recurrence of similar problems.

b) 6248 valid sequences, including 1595 multiple versions, have been derived from the end of skeletal muscle cDNA inserts. Primary redundancy analysis defined 2904 unique sequences which were analyzed against the protein and nucleic acid databases using the BLAST and FASTA families of programmes. 26% (751) correspond to known human genes, 25% (733) are related to known entries in various species, whereas 49% (1420) show no significant similarity and are considered new, unknown sequences. A total of 1482 sequences have been deposited at the EMBL Data Library in 1993.

c) 15727 sequences have been derived from the ends of infant brain cDNA clones. This library which is size-selected, oriented and normalized has been constructed by Dr. Bento Soares at Columbia University and arrayed in 96-well plates by Dr. Greg Lennon at the Lawrence Livermore DOE Genome Center. Redundancy analysis indicates that 11800 sequences are unique, of which 12% (1405) are already known in man, 19% (2264) are related to known entries and the remaining 69% (8131) unknown.

d) An in-depth secondary analysis process is being performed to detect chimerism and overlapping sequences derived from transcript families before submission to the electronic databases.

3. Chromosomal assignment

Primer pairs have been designed to allow PCR amplification of the corresponding human genes from monochromosomic human-rodent somatic cell hybrids. A total of 1830 eSTS markers (615 derived from skeletal muscle and 1215 derived from infant brain cDNA end sequences) have been developed and allow the detection of unique chromosomal locations. In addition 199 eSTS markers detect 2 chromosomes, and 51 detect 3-7 chromosomes but may be in part artifactual due to the impurity of the somatic cell hybrids.

4. Distribution of reagents and technical assistance

130 cDNA clones, 31 sets of filters (including those containing the 40,000 PCR product of the normalized infant brain cDNA inserts) and 1105 eSTS primer pairs have been distributed, and technical assistance provided to 26 European laboratories: France 16 (Généthon, CEPH, Institut Pasteur, CNRS, INSERM, Hospitals) UK 5, Belgium 1, Germany 1, Netherlands 1, Austria 1, and 18 non-European laboratories: USA 13, Australia 2, Canada 1, Israel 1, New Zealand 1.

The Genexpress Programme team has implemented efficient, low-cost, protocols to obtain finished sequences from cDNA inserts using a combination of primer walking and nested deletion methods, to build a fine resolution gene map by integration into the cytogenetic, genetic and physical maps of the human genome using PCR-based and hybridization methods, and is seeking to collect expression profiles by RT-PCR and *in situ* hybridization.

The data collected in this integrated approach should facilitate the identification of the genes which govern physiological traits and their impairment in genetic diseases, starting with limited information on the chromosomal location, site of expression or structure, and complement the positional cloning paradigm.

Contract number: GENO - 0004/0028
Contractual period: 1 January 1991 - 31 December 1992

Coordinator
Dr. K. Gibson
HGMP Resource Centre
Hinxton Hall
Hinxton CB10 1RQ
United Kingdom
Tel: 44 223 494 500
Fax: 44 223 494 512

Participants
Professor G. Tocchini-Valentini
Istituto di Biologia Cellulare
Viale Carlo Marx 143
I - 00137 Roma
Italy
Tel: 39 6 827 3287
Fax: 39 6 827 4642

Professor G. Auffray
College de France
GENETHON-GENEXPRESS
1, rue de l'Internationale
F - 91000 Evry
France
Tel: 33 1 69 47 2965
Fax: 33 1 60 77 8698

Professor Dr. H. Domdey
Laboratorium für Molekulare Biologie
Am Klopferspitz 18a
D-8033 Martinsried/München
Germany
Tel: 49 89 740 17403
Fax: 49 89 740 17448

Human Genome Analysis Programme
M. Hallen and A. Klepsch (Eds.)
IOS Press, 1995

RESOURCE CENTRE FOR YAC LIBRARIES

D. Cohen
Centre d'Etude du Polymorphisme Humain (CEPH), Paris, France

1. Objectives

The objectives of this project, Resource Centre for YAC libraries, were: to establish YAC library screening centres and to screen the available YAC libraries upon request of applicants from EC countries. The characterized YAC clones were sent to the EC applicants for their own further study.

During the contract period CEPH had to perform at least 250 screenings.

2. Project methodology

The CEPH YAC library was constructed from a lymphoblastoid cell line as described (Albertsen et al., 1990). This library contains 50,000 clones (average size: 430 kb)

CEPH stored the YAC library in an ordered manner in 96 well microtiter plates (MTP). For security, we made three copies of the YACs and stored them at -80°C. This storage is very efficient and, we found that only 1.2 % do not grow.

The procedure that we have developed to characterize positive YACs, is based on PCR screening of three dimensional YAC DNA pools.

The 50,000 YAC clones were grown, individually, in AHC selective medium in MTPs, in order to generate 4 sets of YAC DNA pools for screening by PCR. YACs cultures from 8 individual MTPs were pooled to give primary pools. YACs from individual MTPs were mixed to give secondary MTP pools. YACs from the rows and the columns of the same 8 MTPs were pooled to give tertiary pools. Then, the DNA was extracted, tested by PCR and aliquoted. This simple procedure determines the position of the positive YACs in the library.

Upon request, CEPH sent the DNA from the primary pools to EC applicants, to be tested with their PCR primer sets.

When positive primary pools were found by the EC applicants, CEPH performed the secondary and tertiary pool screenings. The positive YACs were grown and characterized before sending to the relevant laboratories for further analysis.

3. Work accomplished

Since 1990, more than 300 collaborations have been established between CEPH and laboratories requesting screenings and/or YACs. In most of the cases we sent them primary pools; in some cases YACs already characterized.

The CEPH YAC library has been primordial to characterize disesase genes like fragile X (Heitz et al., 1991, Hirst et al.,1991, Verkeck et al., 1991), familial adenomatous polyposis coli (Joslyn et al., 1991, Groden et al., 1991), Kallmann syndrome (Legouis et al., 1991), Charcot-Marie-Tooth disease (Valentijn et al., 1992, Timmerman et al., 1992, Matsunami et al., 1992, Pentao et al., 1992), Menkes disease

(Mercer et al., 1993); Huntington disease, isolate and characterize of the N-myc amplicon in neuroblastoma (Schneider et al., 1992); characterize the alipoprotein and plaminogen genes and region (Malgaretti et al., 1992); construct of a YAC contig across the Huntington disease region (Bates et al., 1992), X pseudoautosomal region (Slim et al., 1992) and Charcot Marie Tooth and Smith Magenis diseases region (Chevillard et al., 1993); define the region involved in adrenoleukodystrophy (Feil et al., 1991), Friedreich ataxia (Fujita et al, 1992) and Prader-Willi/Angelman syndrome (Kuwano et al., 1992), study the organisation of the myosin heavy chain isoforms (SoussiYanicostas et al., 1993); characterize KRAB-zinc finger proteins genes (Bellefroid at al., 1993) (Table 1).

Table 1: CEPH YAC library used for:

gene isolation:

> fragile X
> familial adenomatous polyposis coli
> Charcot-Marie-Tooth
> Menkes
> Kalmann
> N-myc amplicon in neuroblastoma
> alipoprotein and plaminogen genes
> Huntington

YAC contig across:

> Huntington disease region
> X pseudoautosomal region
> Charcot Marie Tooth and Smith Magenis disease region
> MHC region
> long arm of the chromosome 21
> hereditary renal carcinoma t(3;8) translocation breakpoint

define the region involved in:

> adrenoleukodystrophy
> Friedreich ataxia
> Prader-Willi/Angelman syndrome
> MEN 2A

study the organization of the myosin heavy chain isoforms

characterize KRAB-zinc finger protein genes...

In addition, the CEPH YAC library has been used in a large number of physical mapping projects concerning genes in all the following inherited diseases or, diseases with an inherited predisposition: (table 2).

CEPH also isolated for the first time the entire Major Histocompatibility Complex in terms of overlapping clones and prepared the first physical map of the HLA class I region in YACs. (Abderrahim et al., 1993).

CEPH developed a new approach to isolate chromosome specific YAC subsets (Chumakov et al., 1992). It is based on the hybridization with Alu polymerase chain reaction (PCR) products. Screening of YACs with Alu PCR products amplified from hybrid cell lines containing only human chromosome 21 allowed identification of chromosome 21 specific YACs. The majority of clones were confirmed to be on chromosome 21 by the presence of specific STSs and by in situ hybridization. These results indicate that when a Megabase insert human genome YAC library is available, it can be rapidly and accurately subdivided into chromosome specific sublibraries and, will permit quick assemby of large contigs.

CEPH also reported a whole genome approach for mapping the human genome (Bellanne-Chantelot et al., 1992). 22,000 YACs have been fingerprinted to obtain individual patterns of restriction fragments detected by a LINE-1 (L1) probe. More than 1,000 contigs were assembled. We demonstrated that, by using large insert YACs, a whole genome approach becomes feasible and, will quickly permit covering more than 90 % of the human genome.

Table 2: CEPH YAC library currently in use for the search of:

breast and ovarian cancers	Norrie
Limb-girdle muscular dystrophy	DiGeorge
spinocerebellar ataxia	von Hippel-Lindau
nephronophtisis	multiple endocrine neoplasias
retinis pigmentosa	tuberous sclerosis
spinal muscular atrophy	multiple sclerosis susceptibility
Treacher Collins	Ewing
nephroblastoma	tumor suppressive genes
ataxia spinal cerebellar	translocation breakpoints
Wilms	Alzheimer
hypophosphatemia	Miller-Dieker
ataxia telangiectasia	ret protooncogene
paraganglioma	arterio-hepatic dysplasia
trisomie 21	Ivemark
Batten	X linked hypophosphatemic rickets
polycystic kidney	Coffin-Lowry
Marfan	retinoblastoma
hemochromatosis	Werner
BOR	campomelic dysplasia
Alagille	medullary cystic
diabetes	Best's macular dystrophy
Wilson	

The YAC Screening Consortium

Participants	Facility details	Libraries[1]	
CEPH Centre d'Etude du Polymorphisme Humain 27, rue Juliette Dodu F - 75010 Paris	PCR screening: 3D pools and superpools. Primary pools on request. Final screen sec/test pools in house.	CEPH YAC CEPH Mega YAC	P, D P, D
HGMP Human Genome Mapping Project Resource Centre Watford Road UK - Harrow HA1 3UJ	PCR screening: All pools of 3D system provided. No in-house screening (Temporarily suspended through overwhelming request). Filter screening: High-density filters provided at cost price.	ICI St. Louis ICRF (4x/4y) St. Mary ICRF	P, D, F P, D P, D P, D P, D
ICRF Imperial Cancer Research Fund 44, Lincoln's Inn Fields UK - London WC2A 3PX	Filters only: no in-house screening. All libraries provided on 22x22 cm filters (ca 80.000 clones). Clones provided from feedback data on filterhyb.	CEPH YAC CEPH Mega YAC ICRF (4x4) St. Mary ICRF Whitehead	D, F D, F D, F D, F D, F D, F
Istituto Genetica e Biochemica ed Evolutionistica Via Abbiategrasso 207 I - 27100 Pavia	PCR sceening only: (super)pools upon request Final screen in-house. Optional: FISH-mapping, YAC subcloning	CEPH Mega YAC ICI	P, D P, D
University of Leiden Faculty of Medicine Department of Human Genetics Wassenaarseweg 72 NL - 2333 AL Leiden	PCR screening: In-house screening in 2 stage super/subpools. Filter screening: High density screening (Beckmann, 6x6 per 96 well position, 3500/filter) In-house screening and filter sets on request. Optional: FISH-mapping, YAC subcloning.	CEPH Mega YAC ICI St. Louis St. Mary ICRF	D, F D, F D, P D D, F

Table 3

[1] P = PCR screening; D = direct clone request; F = Gridded filter screening.

CEPH also was the first to isolate a whole human chromsome in terms of overlapping YACs (Chumakov et al., 1992). In total 198 STS (104 anonymous , 50 polymorphic, 21 Not I-linking clones and, 21 derived from known genes) were used to screen the library. 810 clones were isolated and characterized. They cover all the long arm of human chromosome 21. This result demonstrates the good representativity of the library and indicates that this strategy can be performed for all the other chromosomes.

In addition, the CEPH YAC library was distributed to ICRF (London).

Since 1991, CEPH has been a 'Resource Center for YAC libraries', funded by the EC. The contract period for this project was expected to be 24 months and, we proposed to perform at least *250* screenings.

Actually, the database contains information about *1,490* screenings (more than five times the expected number). More than 5,740 YACs have been characterized and sent to various laboratories, more than half European, for analysis. This is an underestimate, since we also sent candidate YACs and, the return of information is slow and, confirmation sometimes requires several months. The sizes of more than 3,000 YACs are presently known and, the location of 363 have been determined by Fluorescent In Situ Hybridization (FISH).

CEPH YAC Library references (Avril 1993)

- Abderrahim H., Sambucy J-L., Iris F., Ougen P., Billault A., Chumakov I., Dausset J., Cohen D. and Le Paslier D. (1993). Cloning the human Major Histocompatibility Complex in YACs. Genomics, submitted.
- Albertsen H.M., Abderrahim H., Cann H., Dausset J., Le Paslier D., and Cohen D. (1990). Construction and characterization of a yeast artificial chromosome library containing seven haploid genome equivalents. Proc.Natl.Acad.Sci. USA 87: 4256-4260.
- Bates G.P., Valdes J., Hummerich H., Baxendale S., Le Paslier D.L., Monaco A.P. Tagle D., MacDonald M.E., Altherr M., Ross M., Brownstein B.H., Bentley D., Wasmuth J.J., Gusella J., Cohen D., Collins F. and Lehrach H. (1992). Characterization of a Yeast Artificial Chromosome contig spanning the Hungtington's disease gene candidate region. Nature Genetics 1:180-187.
- Bellané-Chantelot C., Barillot E., Lacroix B., Le Paslier D. and Cohen D. (1991). A test case for physical mapping of human genome by repetitive sequence fingerprints: construction of a physical map of a 420 kb YAC subcloned into cosmids. Nucleic Acids Research 19: 505-510.
- Bellané-Chantelot C., Lacroix B., Ougen P., Billault A., Beaufils S., Bertrand S., Georges I., Gilbert F., Gros I., Lucotte G., Susini L., Codani J-J., Gesnouin P., Pook S., Vaysseix G., Lu J., Ried T., Ward D., Chumakov I., Le Paslier D., Barillot E. and Cohen D. (1992). Mapping the whole human genome by fingerprinting Yeast Artificial Chromosomes. Cell 70: 1059-1068.
- Bellefroid E., Marine J., Ried T., Lecocq P., Riviere M., Amemiya C., Poncelet D., Coulie P., de Jong P., Szpirer C., Ward D. and Martial J. (1993). Clustered organization of homologous KRAB-zinc finger genes highly expressed in human T lymphoid cells. Embo J. 12: 1363-1374.
- Buonavista N., Balzano C., Pontarotti P., Le Paslier D. and Golstein P. (1992). Molecular linkage of the human CTLA-4 and CD28 lg-superfamily genes in yeast artificial chromosomes. Genomics 13: 856-861.
- Chevillard C., Le Paslier D., Boyer S., Ougen P., Billault A., Passage E., Mazan S., Bachellerie J-P., Cohen D. and Fontes M. (1993). Construction of a YAC contig spanning the region duplicated in the Charcot-Marie Tooth disease and the distal end of Smith-Magenis critical region: involvements in the molecular mechanism of these diseases. Human Molecular Genetics, submitted.
- Chumakov I.M., Le Gall I., Billault A., Ougen P., Soularue P., Guillou S., Rigault P., Bui H., De Tand M-F., Barillot E., Abderrahim H., Cherif D., Berger R., Le Paslier D. and Cohen D. (1992). Isolation of chromosome 21-specific yeast artificial chromosomes from a total human genome library. Nature Genetics 1: 222-225.
- Chumakov I., Rigault P., Guillou S., Ougen P., Billault A., Guasconi G., Gervy P., Le Gall I., Soularue P., Grinas L., Bougueleret L., Bellané-Chantelot C., Lacroix B., Barillot E., Gesnouin P., Pook S., Vaysseix G., Frelat G., Schmitz A., Sambucy J-L., Bosch A., Estivill X., Weissenbach J., Vignal A., Riethman H., Cox D., Patterson D., Gardiner K., Hattori M., Sakaki Y., Ichikawa H., Ohki M., Le Paslier D., Heilig R., Antonarakis S. and Cohen D. (1992). A continuum of overlapping clones spanning the entire chromosome 21q. Nature 359: 380-387.

- Crété N., Gosset P., Théophile D., Duterque-Coquillaud M., Blouin J.L, Vayssettes C., Sinet P. and Créau-Goldberg N. (1993). Mapping the Down Syndrome chromosome region: establishment of a YAC contig spanning 1.2 Megabases. Eur.J.Hum.Genet. 1: 51-63.
- Dausset J., Ougen P. Abderrahim H., Billault A., Sambucy J-L., Cohen D. and Le Paslier D. (1992). The CEPH YAC libary. Behring Inst. Mitt. 91: 13-20.
- Dittrich B., Knoblauch H., Buiting K. and Horsthemke B. (1993). Characterization of a DNA sequence family in the Prader-Willi/Angelman syndrome chromosome region in 15q11-q13. Genomics 16: 269-271.
- Feil R., Aubourg P., Mosser J., Douar A-M., Le Paslier D., Philippe C. and Mandel J-L, (1991). Adrenoleukodystrophy: a complex chromosomal rearrangement in the Xq28 red/green color pigment gene region indicates two possible gene localizations. American Journal of Human Genetics 49: 1361-1371.
- Fujita R., Sirugo G., Duclos F., Abderrahim H., Le Paslier D., Cohen D., Brownstein B., Schlesinger D., Mandel J-L. and Koenig M. (1992). A 530 kb YAC contig tightly linked to Friedreich ataxia locus contains five CpG clusters and a new highly polymorphic microsatellite. Human Genetics 89: 531-538.
- Gemmill R., Mendez M., Dougherty C., Paulien S., Liao M., Mitchell D., Jankowski S., Trent J., Berger C., Sandberg A. and Meltzer P. (1992). Isolation of a yeast artificial chromosome clone that spans the (12;16) translocation breakpoint characteristic of myxoid liposarcoma. Cancer Genet. Cytogenet. 62: 166-170.
- Glesne D., Collart F., Varkony T., Drabkin H. and Huberman E. (1993). Chromosomal localization and structure of the human type II IMP dehydrogenase gene (IMPDH2). Genomics 16, 274-277.
- Goldberg Y., Rommens J., Andrew S., Hutchinson G., Lin B., Theilmann J., Graham R., Glaves M., Starr E., McDonald H., Nasir J., Schappert K., Kalchman M., Clarke L. and Hayden M. (1993). Identification of an Alu retrotransposition event in close proximity to a strong candidate gene for Huntington's disease. Nature 362: 370-373.
- Groden J., Thliveris A., Samowitz W., Carlson M., Gelbert L, Albertsen H., Joslyn G., Stevens J., Spirio L., Robertson M., Sargeant L, Krapcho K., Warrington J., McPherson J., Wasmuth J., Le Paslier D., Abderrahim H., Cohen D., Leppert M. and White R. (1991). Identification and characterization of the familial adenomatous polyposis coli gene. Cell 66: 589-600.
- Heitz D., Rousseau F., Devys D., Abderrahim H., Le Paslier D., Cohen D., Vincent A., DellaValle G., Schlessinger D., Toniolo D., Oberle I. and Mandel J-L. (1991). Isolation of normal sequences that span the Fragile X site and identification of a CpG island involved in Fragile X expression. Science 251: 1236-1239.
- Hirst M., Roche A., Funt T., Mackinnon R., Bassett J., Nakahori Y., Watson J., Bell M., Patterson M., Anand R., Poustka A., Lehrach H., Schlesinger D., D'Urso M., Buckle V. and Davies K. (1991). A YAC contig across the Fragile X site defines the region of fragility. Nucleic Acids Res. 19: 3282-3288.
- Joslyn G., Carlson M., Thliveris A., Albertsen H., Gelbert L., Samowitz W., Groden J., Stevens J., Spirio L. Robertson M., Sargeant L. Krapcho K., Wolf E., Burt R., Hughes J.P., Warrington J., McPherson J., Wasmuth J., Le Paslier D., Abderrahim H., Cohen D., Leppert M. and White R. (1991). Identification of deletion mutations and three new genes at the familial polyposis locus. Cell 66: 601-613.
- Kuwano A., Mutirangura A., Dittrich B., Buiting K., Horsthemhe B., Saitoh S., Nikawa N., Lebdetter S., Grenberg F., Chinault A. and Lebdetter D. (1992). Molecular dissection of the Prader Willi/Angelman syndrome region (15q11-13) by YAC cloning and FISH analysis. Human Molecular Genetics 1: 417-425.
- Lairmore T., Dou S., Howe J., Chi D., Carlson K., Veile R., Mishra S., Wells S. and Donis-Keller H. (1993). A 1.5 megabase yeast artificial chromosome contig from human chromosome 10q11.2 connecting three genetic loci (RET, D10S94 and D10S102) closely linked to the MEN2A locus. Proc.Natl.Acad.Sci. USA 90:492-496.
- Legouis R., Hardelin J-P., Levilliers J., Claverie J-M., Compain S., Wunderle V., Millaseau P., Le Paslier D., Cohen D., Catarina D. Bougueleret L, Delemarre-Van de Waal H., Lutfalla G., Weissenbach J., and Petit C., (1991). The candidate gene for the X-linked Kallmann syndrome encodes a protein related to adhesion molecules. Cell 67: 423-435.
- Malgaretti N., Acquati F., Magnaghi P., Bruno L, Pontoglio M., Rocchi M., Saccone S., Della Valle G., D'Urso M., Le Paslier D., Ottolenghi S. and Taramelli R. (1992). Characterisation by yeast artificial chromosome cloning of the linked apolipoprotein(a) and plasminogen genes and identification of the apolipoprotein(a) 5' flanking region. Proc.Natl.Acad.Sci. USA 89, 11584-11588.
- Matsunami N., Smith B., Ballard L., Lensch M., Robertson M., Albertsen H., Hanemann C., Müller H., Bird T., White R. and Chance P. (1992). Peripheral myelin protein 22 gene maps in the duplication in chromosome 17p11.2 associated with Charcot-Marie-Tooth 1 A. Nature Genetics 1: 176-179.
- Mercer J., Livingston J., Hall B., Paynter J., Begy C., Chandrasekharappa S., Lochart P., Grimes A., Bhave M., Siemieniak D., and Glover T. (1993). Isolation of a partial candidate gene for Menkes disease

by positional cloning. Nature Genetics 3: 20-25.
- Mole S., Mulligan L., Healey C., Ponder B. and Tunnacliffe A. (1993). Localisation of the gene for multiple endocrine neoplasia type 2 A to a 480 kb region in chromosome band 10q11.2. Human Molecular genetics 2: 247-252.
- Pentao L, Wise C., Chinault A., Patel P. and Lupski J. (1992). Charcot-Marie-Tooth 1 A duplication appears to arise from recombination at repeat sequences flanking the 1.5 Mb monomer unit. Nature Genetics 2: 292-300.
- Schneider S., Zehnbauer B., Taillon-Miller P., Le Paslier D., Vogelstein B. and Brodeur G. (1992). YAC cloning of the MYCN amplicon in human neuroblastoma. Mol. Cell Biol. 12: 5563-5570.
- Serova O., Pautier P., Chappuis S., Wang Q. Vuillaume M., Sylla B., Le Paslier D., Feunteun J. and Lenoir G. (1993). Physical mapping of the BCRA1 region on chromosome 17q21: linkage between D17S579 and D17S509. Hum. Genetics, submitted.
- Slim R., Le Paslier D., Compain S., Levilliers J., Ougen P., Billault A., Donohue S.J., Klein D.C., Heitz D., Bernheim A., Cohen D., Weissenbach, J. and Petit C. (1993). Construction of a yeast artificial chromosome contig spanning the pseudoautosomal region and isolation of 25 new sequence-tagged sites. Genomics, in press.
- Soussi-Yanicosta N., Whalen R. and Petit C. (1993). Five skeletal myosin heavy chain genes are organized as a multigene complex in the human genome. Human Molecular Genetics, in press.
- The Huntington's Disease Collaborative Research Group. (1993). A Novel gene containing a trinucleotide repeat that is expanded and unstable on Huntington's disease chromosomes. Cell 72: 971-983.
- Timmerman V., Nelis E., Van Hul W., Nieuwenhuijsen B., Chen K., Wang S., Ben Othman K., Cullen B., Leach R., Hanemann C., De Jonghe P., Raeymaekers P., Van Ommen G., Martin J., Müller H., Vance J., Fischbeck K. and Van Broeckhoven C. (1992). The peripheral myelin gene PMP-22 is contained within the Charcot-Marie-Tooth disease type 1 A duplication. Nature Genetics 1: 171-175.
- Tunnacliffe A., Liu L, Moore J., Leversha M., Jackson M., Papi L, Ferguson-Smith M., Thiesen J. and Ponder B. (1993). Duplicated KOX zinc finger gene clusters flank the centromere of human chromosome 10; evidence for a pericentric inversion during primate evolution. Nucleic Acids Res. 21: 1409-1417.
- Valentijn L., Bolhuis P., Zorn I., Hoogendijk J., Van den Bosch N., Hensels G., Stanton V., Housman D., Fischbeck K., Ross D., Nicholson G., Meersbock E., Dauwerse H., Van Ommen G., and Baas F. (1992). The peripheral myelin gene PMP-22/Gas-3 is duplicated in Charcot-Marie-Tooth disease type 1 A. Nature Genetics 1: 166-170.
- Verkerk A., Pierreti M., Fu Y., Sutcliffe J., Huhl D., Pizzuti A., Reiner O. et al. (1991). Identification of a gene (FRM-1) containing a CGG repeat coincident with a breakpoint cluster region exhibiting length variation in Fragile X syndrome. Cell 65: 905-914.

Contract number: GENO-CT91-0020 (SSMA)
Contractual period: 1 January 1991 - 31 December 1992

Coordinator
Professor D. Cohen
C.E.P.H.
Centre d'Etude du Polymorphisme Humain
Human Polymorphism Study Center
27, rue Juliette Dodu
F-75010 Paris
France
Tel: 33 1 42 49 98 50
Fax: 33 1 40 18 01 55

Participants
Dr. D. Toniolo
CNR
Istituto di Genetica Biochemica
ed Evoluzionistica
via Abbiategrasso 207
I - 27100 Pavia
Italy
Tel: 39 382 527 967
Fax: 39 382 422 286

Professor G.-J. van Ommen
Department of Human Genetics
Sylvius Laboratories
NL - 2300 RA Leiden
The Netherlands
Tel: 31 71 27 6293/ 27 6000
Fax: 31 71 27 6075

Dr. T. Vickers
HGMP Resource Centre
Watford Road
UK - Harrow HA1 3UJ
United Kingdom
Tel: 44 81 869 3809
Fax: 44 81 869 3807

Dr. H. Lehrach
ICRF
Genome Analysis Laboratory
44 Lincoln's Inn Fields
UK - London WC2a 3PX
United Kingdom
Tel: 44 71 269 3308
Fax: 44 71 405 4303

Human Genome Analysis Programme
M. Hallen and A. Klepsch (Eds.)
IOS Press, 1995

THE EUROPEAN DATA RESOURCE FOR HUMAN GENOME RESEARCH (EDR)

S. Suhai
European Data Resource for Human Genome Research, Heidelberg, Germany

1. Introduction

1.1 Goals and services of EDR

The general goal of the Data Resource is to provide informatics support for the European human genome research community, especially for the laboratories participating in the ongoing Human Genome Analysis programe (HGA) of the Commission of the European Communities (CEC). It is implemented as a Resource Centre for the data handling (data acquisition, management, analysis, and distribution) aspects of human genome research, focusing mainly on European on-line database and analysis services, user training, and specific developments. Several large scale research programs are running world-wide, including most member countries of the European Communities, aimed at the capture and interpretation of the genetic information contained in the human genome. They may vary in experiment techniques and research strategies but they all produce enormous volumes of data. It is the task of specific databases to store machine-readable representations of these data in a persistent form, efficiently accessible for queries, analyses, and updates. Furthermore, appropriate software analysis programs will have to be developed to make sense of the stored data, to visualise, assess, compare, or otherwise process it. Therefore, computer-aided methods of the interdisciplinary research field *genome informatics* will play a central role in genome mapping and sequencing projects.

Realising this close connection between experimental genome research and computational methods, the CEC appointed the Deutsches Krebsforschungszentrum (DKFZ) in Heidelberg to serve as the Data Resource for the European Human Genome Analysis Programe. The Commission identified data and analysis services, training of users, promotion of network communication, and new developments in database integration and interfacing as the main goals of this Resource Centre. In this way, it has to complement other, experiment oriented, resource centres implemented within the same programe (DNA-Probe Bank for the European Human Genome Mapping Project, Membrane Resource for the European Gene Mapping, European Consortium on Ordered Clone Libraries, and the European Consortium on cDNA Libraries).

According to the contract between the Commission and DKFZ, the Resource Centre had to meet the following major objectives:

1. Providing on-line access to the most important databases in the field of genome mapping, sequencing and analysis. Beyond appropriate network services and general information retrieval tools (eg, WAIS, Gopher, News, etc.), the Resource Center had to install up-to-date software for the scientific evaluation of genomic data (genomic sequence analysis, genetic mapping, etc.) and make available specific servers in Heidelberg for the efficient processing of the data by a large user community through network.

2. Extensive user support including telephone hot-lines, electronic-mail, a regular newsletter, database and software documentations, training workshops, technical courses and scientific meetings.
3. Organisation and hosting of specific developers' workshops on new aspects of genome computing. Providing scholarships at post-doctoral and senior scientist levels, respectively, to promote collaborative European research projects whose developments will be installed at the Resource Center and made available for all users.
4. Implementation of a collaborative European research and development project, the Integrated Genomic Database (IGD), with participation of CNRS, DKFZ, HGMP-RC, ICRF and MRC, aims at integrating genome related data from multiple resource databases. It provides for a common and extensible data model and a query language interface, distributes the data over computer networks, and provides for high level (graphical, where possible) tools for end users to view and manipulate data, to compose queries, to communicate with the network, and to call services both locally and remotely to the users computer. These tools should enable the scientists to store retrieved data locally, annotate them and merge them with their own private experimental data.

1.2 Embedment of EDR into the biocomputing environment at DKFZ

As the institution hosting the Resource Center, DKFZ assists the activities of EDR through its scientific research capacity and experience in the field of biocomputing. About one half of the research groups at DKFZ work in the field of molecular biology and genetics. They provide a valuable experimental background and close (in-house) co-operation for the development and testing of new computer aided tools in genome research. The Department of Molecular Biophysics (MBP) has been developing and implementing biocomputing methods and software for the past ten years. The co-workers of MBP provide experience in nucleotide and protein sequence analysis, in the design and implementation of genome related new databases, in the computer aided modelling of the structure and function of gene products, and in the application of new informatics tools (e.g. artificial neural networks, genetic algorithms, and object oriented database structures) to genome research. They have developed a UNIX based version of the GCG programe package of the University of Wisconsin and complemented it with several additional methods developed partly at MBP or acquired through academic co-operations. They regularly maintain this software environment on two CONVEX computers (one of which is devoted to extra mural users) and complement it with the latest versions of all important genetic databases.

The computer hardware of the Data Resource is integrated into the in-house (Ethernet based) computer network of DKFZ and it will mostly be maintained by the experts of the Computer Center (Zentrale Datenverarbeitung, ZDV). The Local Area Network (LAN) of DKFZ integrates several classes of computers. The co-workers of the ZDV also provide help in UNIX related problems and with relational and object oriented databases. The administrators of the ZDV take care of the user accounts of the Data Resource. This management expertise is an important pre-condition for the success of the Data Resource. DKFZ also has up-to-date connections to national and international computer networks that automatically support users of the Data Resource. DKFZ provides in-house facilities for education and training. Its lecture halls are at the disposal of the Data Resource for the sake of its conferences and training workshops. A specific computer course room with a large number of networked PCs provides adequate facilities for biocomputing courses. In-house printing and graphical services (for the production of manuals and training materials), and one of the largest biomedical libraries in Europe complement the above infrastructure. The Department for General Administration of DKFZ provides the necessary administrative support for the smooth management of the project.

The Department of Molecular Biophysics (MBP) at DKFZ conducts active research in the field of theoretical biophysics and genome informatics. The focal points of its research activities are the development of computer-aided molecular modelling methods for the simulation of biomolecular structural problems, the development and application of new informatics tools (artificial neural networks, genetic algorithms, object oriented database structures, etc.) for the prediction and analysis of the three-dimensional structure and of the function of gene products, and the design and implementation of comprehensive genomic databases. Beyond their own research, the co-workers of the MBP participate in several co-operative research projects conducted together with several experimental departments of DKFZ to be able to test the newly developed methods and to contribute to the solution of actual problems in cancer research. The three major scientific focal points of biocomputing are: molecular biological sequence analysis, biomolecular structure analysis, and genome analysis.

MBP implemented and maintains a comprehensive environment for DNA and protein sequence analysis, HUSAR (Heidelberg Unix Sequence Analysis Resources). Its coworkers have been supporting a large scientific user community in the past years (250-300 regular users at DKFZ and 120-150 users distributed at several faculties of the University of Heidelberg). During the years 1989-1992, the co-workers of MBP established, in co-operation with the Central Data Processing department of DKFZ (ZDV), the German national node of the European Molecular Biology Network, EMBNet. This node provides biocomputing support (hardware, software, and networking) for scientists of over 80 universities and research institutions scattered over the whole country. The Data Processing Center (ZDV) of DKFZ runs one of the largest biocomputing facilities in Germany. It has four mainframe scientific computers (CONVEX Models 3440, 220, and 210, and IBM 9000, respectively) and it maintains an in-house Ethernet network to which about 50 workstations and 600 PCs are connected. During the past years, the ZDV has built up connections to all important national and international computer networks and it is steadily improving these connections in co-operation with national and European authorities. The networking group of the ZDV provides an invaluable technical support for the related activities of the Data Resource and its experts regularly contribute to the training and education of the users.

DKFZ accommodates about 250 PhD students and provides an excellent infrastructure for education and training. A major in-house lecture hall (for 300 persons) and five smaller ones (for 40-50 persons) are equipped with all the necessary technical tools to support demanding workshops and training courses (including interactive computer sessions). A large number of major workshops and conferences take place each year at DKFZ, so there are enough experienced personnel to organise and manage such events. Furthermore, since a substantial part of the resources of DKFZ originates from extra mural funding, its administration has the necessary experience to smoothly manage such a support.

2. Report on the activities of EDR

In the first period of its existence, the main activities of the *Data Resource* concentrated on
- building up the appropriate hardware platform,
- establishing inter network communication,
- implementing the standard software environment,
- developing and implementing specialised (database and analysis) software for genome related problems,
- user support, training and development workshops.

The progress report below summarises our major accomplishments in the above fields during the period of June 1, 1991 to July 31, 1993. The report will be organised to reflect the structure of the Technical Annex to our contract with the Commission. Section 2.1 will provide an overview of the hardware set-up of EDR, Section 2.2 the networking and communication aspects, Section 2.3 the implementation of standard software tools, Section 2.4 the development of specific software for genome data integration, and Section 2.5 the activities related to the training and support of the user community.

2.1 Hardware configuration of EDR

A SUN 4/470 Sparcserver with appropriate configuration (64 MB memory, 4 GB disk storage, tape, printer, etc.) was installed in summer 1991 and connected to the Ethernet network. It plays the role of the central SYBASE and GDB (Genome Data Base) server for all European scientists interested in the services of the Data Resource. The type and configuration of this server has been determined by the requirements of the GDB administration in Baltimore. The column OMIM/GDB users in Figure 1 shows that currently about 510 users regularly have access to this computer. On average, 250 connections per month are established with an average session time of 18-20 minutes.

A CONVEX 210 minisupercomputer with 64 MB memory, 4 GB disk storage and appropriate network connections is the second major computer of EDR. Fifty per cent of the capacity of this machine is assigned to (and funded by) the genome computing project mainly serving the database OMIM (On-line Mendelian Inheritance in Man), several sequence and structure databases (EMBL, GenBank, Swissprot, PDB etc.) implemented in the database management system IRX (Information Retrieval Experiment), and the sequence analysis package HUSAR (Heidelberg Unix Sequence Analysis Resources). In an exploratory phase preparing the implementation of EDR, OMIM has been installed on this machine in 1990. The capacity of this machine is nearly exhausted with more than 950 registered users and up to 1.7 million CPU seconds per month. On the other hand, the number of the users (Figure 2) as well as their computer time are still steadily increasing. This will make it necessary to think about the extension of the capacity of this machine in the near future. A Sparcstation I with 32 MB memory and 1.2 GB disk capacity has been purchased as a development tool for graphical front-end software and for SYBASE programing. Two SUN IPC Sparcstations with 16 MB memory and 200 MB disk and four PCs with network connection have been installed for general program development. The major part of the hardware installations was performed during the first four months of the contract period, while the software implementations extended over the whole two years as planned in the time schedule.

Month	No. of users (total)	HUSAR users	OMIM/ GDB users	No. of active users	CPU (Sec)
90/09	81	76	39	6	4275
90/10	104	99	50	25	29620
90/11	148	141	67	53	114418
90/12	167	160	76	57	128289
91/01	172	165	77	56	72457
91/02	210	202	91	70	265427
91/03	228	219	95	84	272601
91/04	252	241	98	84	421932
91/05	282	271	107	97	771675
91/06	306	295	113	127	553841
91/07	318	307	119	126	829217
91/08	331	320	127	116	502678
91/09	348	336	136	121	580554
91/10	363	351	149	134	740385
91/11	411	398	180	167	815739
91/12	436	423	200	152	848034
1991 (gesamt)	436	423	200	258	6951142
92/01	459	444	216	157	655270
92/02	513	495	248	178	990672
92/03	531	512	262	202	1328701
92/04	557	537	274	198	1128986
92/05	593	572	296	219	1242816
92/06	634	590	306	229	1069609
92/07	652	612	319	244	1147766
92/08	652	630	325	228	889350
92/09	682	657	345	245	967165
92/10	718	692	367	255	1317377
92/11	739	713	384	271	1597232
92/12	769	742	409	270	1202679
1992 (gesamt)	769	742	409	452	13541300
93/01	805	776	431	292	1312640
93/02	820	790	437	306	1403198
93/03	856	826	451	322	1644942
93/04	874	843	463	321	1558590
93/05	874	843	463	319	1445437
93/06	921	890	489	330	1176628
93/07	962	931	509	339	1735986

Figure 1

Total amount of accounts: 632

Belgium	8
Denmark	5
Finland	3
France	15
Germany	509
Greece	5
Ireland	3
Israel	1
Italy	19
Luxembourg	1
Netherland	10
Norway	3
Poland	1
Portugal	8
Russia	1
Slovakia	1
Spain	6
Sweden	2
Switzerland	9
UK	22

Figure 2

Distribution of GDB/OMIM user account associated with (EDR) European Data Resource for Human Genome Research Project.

2.2 Networking and Communication

The DKFZ network has been integrated over the past two years into European network structures through the Mannheim and Düsseldorf nodes, respectively, into WIN (Wissenschaftsnetz), through Düsseldorf into EuropaNet, and through Bonn (GMD) into EBONE. EuropaNet is the continuation of the pilot project EMPB providing an X25 based network with IP services. It is managed by PTT Telecom of Holland and provides national connection capabilities from 64 kbit/sec to 2 Mbit/sec.

The following list presents a selection of the European cities where EDR has a number of co-operating scientists and with which communications have been effectively established:

Belgium	(Diepenbeek, Brussels, Gent, etc.)
Denmark	(Aarhus, Copenhagen, Risskov)
Finland	(Helsinki)
France	(Paris, Marseille, Rennes, Strasbourg, etc.)
Greece	(Athens, Crete)
Ireland	(Dublin, Cork)
Italy	(Roma, Bologna, Pavia, Pisa, etc.)
Luxembourg	(Luxembourg)
Netherlands	(Amsterdam, Leiden, Rotterdam, etc.)
Norway	(Oslo, Bergen)
Poland	(Warszawa)
Portugal	(Lisboa, etc.)
Slovakia	(Bratislava)
Spain	(Madrid, Barcelona, etc.)
Sweden	(Stockholm, Goeteborg, etc.)
Switzerland	(Basel, Bern, Zurich, etc.)
United Kingdom	(London, Glasgow, Cambridge, Edinburgh, etc.)

Information is being accumulated with respect to international institution connectivity attained from direct telephone/e-mail/computer session contacts. This information assists in helping new users to establish connectivity with our institution and solving problems with existing users. In spite of improvements in internet connectivity, we still maintain access through the German Datex-P (in France TRANSPAC). This allows users to use normal telephone/modem connections when using our services. Our co-workers within DKFZ have performed careful measurements to characterise the speed of the network connections. Statistical information has been accumulated specifically for Internet capabilities detailing the connectivity packet travel times between DKFZ and several European host gateways for the European Community. While the average network response time in milliseconds (msec) between DKFZ and nodes in Germany, in Middle Europe, in North Europe show an excellent-to-good connectivity (500-800 msec), further improvements had to be made within the group South Europe, which could be achieved in July 1993. Figure 3 gives a summary of approximate data packet travel times between DKFZ and major European cities. This information assists in the understanding of network trends and in finding weak links (bottlenecks) in the European network.

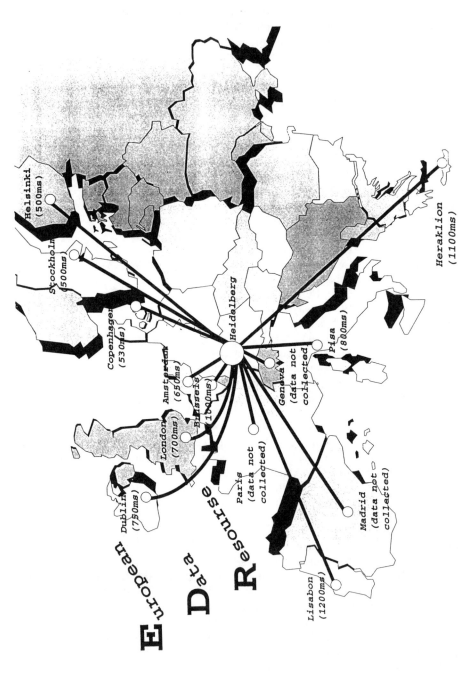

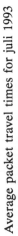

Figure 3

Average packet travel times for juli 1993

2.3 Implementation of standard software

Figure 4 gives an overview of the general structure of the standard software environment of EDR. For the handling of genome data, the relational database management system SYBASE has been implemented on the SUN 4/470 Sparcserver and on the Sparcstation I in June 1991. GDB Version 4.1 has been installed on the Sparcserver in August 1991, updated to Version 4.2 in May 1992 and further updated to Version 5.0 in June 1993. A batch interface to the user registration software of Baltimore has been developed at EDR in October 1992. Recently, we opened our server for access by the graphical GDB front-end running under SUNVIEW.

The CEPH program package for linkage analysis has been installed in April 1992 on the Sparcserver. Since the parallel use of these programs by several scientists leads to a very heavy load on the Sparcserver, in the next phase of the project we are planning to move it to the CONVEX 210 which may provide a more appropriate architecture for these applications. We have ported the IRX (Information Retrieval Experiment) environment from its SUN version (kindly provided by NCBI/NLM/NIH) to the CONVEX and implemented a program interface to it on a client/server basis. From early 1992, the following databases have been made available in their IRX version:
- EMBL Nucleotide Data Library
- SwissProt Protein Sequence Database
- GenBank
- PIR Protein Sequence Database
- ICRF Reference Library Database

The Resource Center provides on-line access to all important genome-related databases including genome mapping databases (like GDB, RLDB), phenotype databases (like OMIM), bibliography databases (based on Medline), macromolecular structural databases (Protein Data Base, Cambridge Crystallographic Database), nucleotide sequence databases (EMBL and GenBank), protein sequence databases (Swissprot and PIR), specialised sequence databases (REBASE, PROSITE, etc.), and further comprehensive genome databases of the human and other model organisms (IGD, ENTREZ, ACEDB, GBASE, FLYBASE, etc.). We specifically emphasise GDB as the official database of the genome mapping community world-wide. We install and support "experimental and raw data" databases (e.g., RLDB from ICRF, the GENET-HON Database) of major data producers (experimental resource centres) as they become publicly available. Figure 5 presents a list of the most important databases that are available on-line at EDR.

The Resource Center installed and developed tools for data acquisition, validation, and electronic submission. It will distribute sequence submission tools (e.g. Authorin) and develop and distribute electronic tools to submit genomic data directly to GDB. The development and distribution of an enhanced version of such tools for GDB editors is in preparation. The latter would enable the GDB editors to download a (sub)copy of GDB, do local editing, and propagate the changes to the central GDB installation. This could also be used effectively by Single Chromosome Workshops.

On-line access is provided to major analysis tools and packages covering the structural and sequence data, genetic and physical mapping data. This includes the HUSAR package (Heidelberg Unix Sequence Analysis Resources) for nucleotide and protein sequence analysis, the LINKAGE package for genetic mapping analysis, the ICRF package for the physical mapping, and LDB and SIGMA for heterogeneous genome map integration and management (the two later packages are currently being implemented). These tools will be complemented by general utility tools for file management, transfer, editing, graphics, etc. We will also support off-line versions

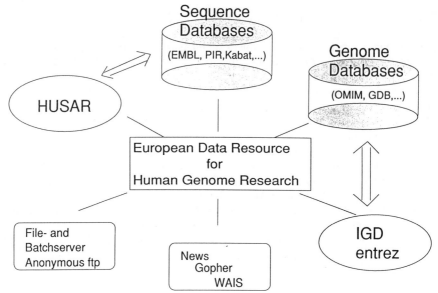

Figure 4

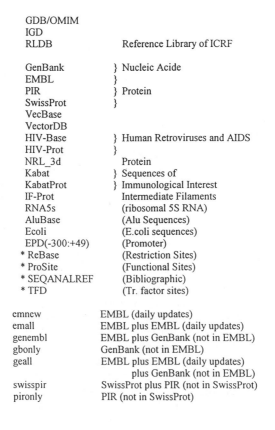

Figure 5

Databases available

(e-mail and batch) for selected services. We provide general information retrieval tools to enable users to access relevant information over wide area computer networks (e.g. WAIS, Gopher, Archie, News). Users also have access to electronic mail and file transfer services. We are co-operating with European partners and agencies to improve the overall network connectivity in Europe and to start building up a 2 Mbit connection for the Data Resource.

Database and analysis applications will be distributed between shared and dedicated server computers to avoid slowdowns and collisions caused by some of the applications (e.g. sequence database search or multipoint linkage analysis). This distribution will be transparent to the users. At the present time we distribute the workload between two computer servers (CONVEX and SUN). We are currently working on the installation of two additional specialised servers, one for the sequence database search and one for the genetic analysis. All major sequence and structure databases relevant for genome research (EMBL, GenBank, SwissProt, PIR, PDB etc.) are available for users on the CONVEX 210 and they will be regularly updated through the network (some of them daily). The HUSAR (Heidelberg Unix Sequence Analysis Resource) program package (including the GCG programs of the University of Wisconsin) provides a convenient and versatile environment with analytic tools for most problems relevant to genome research. During the project, new versions of several programs in HUSAR have been implemented (e.g., CLUSTAL, FASTA, MAP, FRAMES, etc.) and a number of completely new programs have been included (like PRIMER, GENETRANS, BOXALIGN, TREE, BLASTN, TBLASTN, etc.). A detailed definition of these programs is provided in the new version of the HUSAR manual. A new menu user interface has also been developed to facilitate the use of the system.

2.4 Development and implementation of specialised software

As a first step, the object oriented database ACEDB of the C. elegans genome project (developed by Richard Durbin, MRC and Jean Thierry-Mieg, CNRS) has been implemented on the Sparcstation. It served as a prototype database for the development of the user front-end to the Integrated Genomic Database (IGD). In May 1992, Version 4.2 of the Genome Database (GDB) was implemented in ACEDB and the database Entrez of NCBI was installed for internal use. The software development tools ER Draw and SDT (Lawrence Berkeley National Laboratory) were installed as object oriented programing and database development tools on the Sparcstation. Furthermore, in co-operation with the Institute for Parallel Computer Architecture's of the University of Stuttgart, the comprehensive software environment SNNS (Stuttgart Neural network Simulator) for neural network modelling of genomic information has been installed.

One of the major projects of EDR was to develop an open software system to handle human genome data. The system, called IGD, integrates information from many genomic databases and experimental resources into a comprehensive target-end database (IGD TED). Users will use front-end client systems (IGD FRED) to download data of interest to their computers and merge them with their own local data. FREDs will provide persistent storage of and instant access to retrieved data, friendly graphical user interface, tools to query, browse, analyse and edit local data, interface to external analysis, and tools to communicate with the outside world. The TED will be implemented using both relational and object oriented technologies in parallel; it will be accessible over the network (on-line and off-line) as a read-only resource for multiple clients. Tools are being developed for automated updating of the TED from its resource databases and data sets, which include major databases for nucleotide and protein sequences and structures, genome maps, experimental reagents, phenotypes, and bibliography, and sets of raw data produced at genome centres and laboratories.

Beside character-based access via Gopher, WAIS, FTP, and several query language interfaces to the TED, we are developing a specialised front-end client, IGD FRED, with its own database manager, based on the ACEDB program. The FRED will support graphical display methods for sequence feature maps, chromosomal genetic and physical maps, and for experimental objects like clone grids, etc. FRED data will be coupled with rules and knowledge via PROLOG interface. FRED will also provide interface to important analysis software packages, and tools to submit data to external databases in their own format. The IGD schema models objects and processes in considerable detail, so that scientists will be able to use the FRED as a laboratory notebook. At the same time, and in the same environment, they will link their experimental data to public reference data coming from the TED. This will enable the FRED to be used as a single editorial interface to multiple genomic databases.

The development of IGD is a collaborative project (with participation of CNRS, DKFZ, HGMP-RC, ICRF and MRC) aimed at integrating genome related data from multiple resource databases, providing a common and extensible data model and a query language interface, distributing the data over computer networks, and providing for high level (graphical, where possible) tools for end users to view and manipulate data, compose queries, communicate with the network and call services both local and remote to the user's computer. These tools will enable the user to store retrieved data locally, annotate them and merge them with private experimental data.

IGD takes the data from established, both public and experimental, databases (EMBL, GenBank, SwissProt, PIR, GDB, OMIM, RLDB, Probe). The data model comprises records of experimental entities (clones, probes, libraries), records of experimental processing (library construction, hybridisation, sequencing), records and results of the analyses (genetic and physical maps, feature maps of sequences), relationships between these entities, bibliography and cross-references to other databases.

IGD will only compile data from the resource databases. All eventual updates or data submissions will be redirected to them as well. IGD will perform no data verification other than syntax checking. It can thus be seen as a materialised and coherent view on all the resource databases (see Figure 6) for the general structure of IGD). The IGD system model is open and modular, i.e. the framework is capable of including data from new databases with different database management systems (hierarchical like GCG sequence data, relational like GDB, IRX text retrieval like OMIM, object oriented), and for supporting multiple data query languages and exchange protocols. IGD's own components can be reimplemented using novel informatics technology (network and interprocess communication or data storage).

Our strategy in building the IGD modules is to reuse or modify existing software, provided it is not merely functionally appropriate and reliable but also publicly available and portable. Currently the only proprietary software is the Sybase relational DBMS for the central data repository. Whereas at the moment IGD is developed for the UNIX operating system and X11 graphical windowing environment (public domain), it has been designed so that the front-end is portable to IBM and Macintosh PCs.

The IGD front-end (FRED) is a set of programs that users will be running on their computers. These programs communicate with each other and also with the remote parts of IGD. The network communication is asynchronous so that the user is not blocked waiting for answers to his/her queries. FRED assists the user in composing queries in a high level object query language which will be optionally translated by IGD into the language of the target database, retrieves the data from the outside world, stores them in a local database, displays and manipulates the local data, and enables the user to call services which might be distributed over the network.

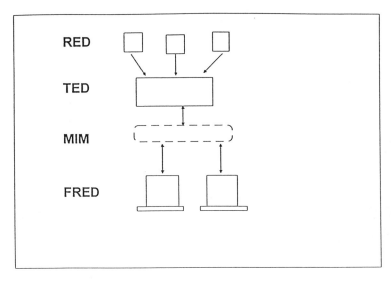

The system is subdivided into four functional levels:

Resource End Database	RED:	existing databases which contribute data
Target End Database	TED:	the integrated database management system
Middle Manager	MIM:	the network communication level
Front End	FRED:	the front-end interface level

Figure 6
Distributed implementation of IGD

It is important that the user can store private data together with the retrieved public data. Data models can be locally extended, that means that new attributes for experimental data can be added to object models. The resulting hybrid data sets can be consistently maintained and updated. FRED stores proper data and metadata in the local database. The database for proper data is based on the ACEDB software which is an efficient object oriented database system with a powerful graphical display. Complex objects like genetic and physical maps of chromosome, DNA and protein sequences, hybridisation filter grids and scanned images are displayed graphically and the user can browse through and manipulate them in a very intuitive and friendly fashion, just pointing and clicking the mouse device (see Figure 7 for an example of this procedure).

The first prototype version of IGD was ready in June 1992. It comprised of sequence and mapping data and the bibliography, but not as a fully detailed model. By May 1993, the FRED module had become functional and the TED was populated with all the important databases mentioned before. It is available in ACEDB and SYBASE versions, respectively. For the SYBASE version, the queries can be formulated with the help of the graphical query specification tool of V. Markowitz (LBL). During the first half of 1993, the FRED of IGD has been adapted for use as a data collection, verification and visualisation tool for single chromosome workshops on chromosomes 3, 7, and 21. In addition, the CEPH YAC data on chromosome 21 have been integrated in IGD.

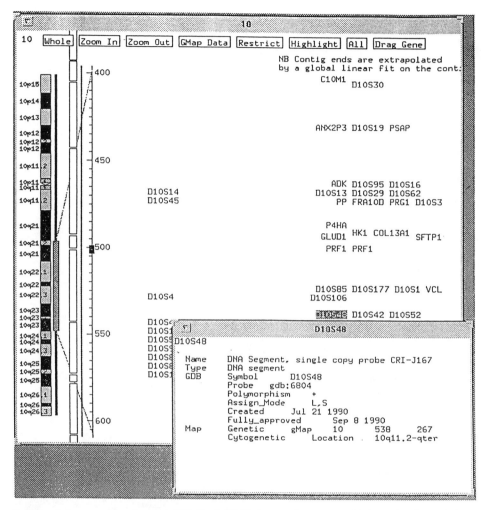

Snapshot from a user's session with IGD Fred: Within human chromosome 10 the region from 10q21 to 10q23 is visible. By pointing the mouse at locus D 10S48 a new window showing details is opened. This process can be interated: e.g. clicking on the probe entry in the locus window would display the related probe information from GDB.

Figure 7
Graphical user interface of the FRED

From the technical point of view, a graphical command line builder for X-Windows has been implemented for easier use of command line driven programs like HUSAR. Procedures for automatically generating GDB submission forms, filled with data entered into an IGD front-end, have also been developed. This will turn FRED into a user-friendly data submission tool for GDB. The data translation from ACEDB to SYBASE can now handle inherited types in IGD: a new object oriented feature available. An OPM (Object Protocol Model) editor has also been implemented and the IGD-ACEDB model has been translated to OPM, providing constructs for modelling experimental protocols. This enables IGD to store relationships between experimental objects in a natural way.

2.5 Training and support of the user community

Since the official foundation of the Data Resource (June 1, 1991) about 650 new user accounts have been installed on its SUN 470 and CONVEX 210 computers (leading to a total number of about 850 users in July 1993). According to the results of our polls, 2.2 scientists work with each account on the average. This means that in these days about 2000 scientists make regular use of the Data Resource computing facilities. On the other hand, the number of registered users is continually increasing but at present, no saturation can be observed. (For comparison, on its two other CONVEX computers, models 3440 and 220, respectively, DKFZ serves about 600 local users with biocomputing applications).

One of the most important activities of the Data Resource was the organisation of training and development workshops in the field of genome computing. Several one-week training workshops provided a comprehensive introduction to several important aspects of computer aided genome analysis including theoretical and hands-on training in UNIX, OMIM, GDB, sequence databases and networking. Besides interactive computer training, several scientific lectures on different aspects of genome research have been given by outstanding experts. Participants have been invited to these workshops from several European countries including Denmark, Germany, Greece, Ireland, Italy, Portugal, Spain and the UK. All the participant expenses were covered by the Data Resource. Most of the workshops took place at the location of EDR at DKFZ, but extra mural workshops were also organised (twice at EMBL, once in Lisbon, Stuttgart and Jena, respectively). Several further on-site workshops are being planned which will be held outside of Heidelberg, at institutions where a larger number of scientists can be expected as potential users.

A one week workshop for genome database developers on July 1 - 7, 1991 in Heidelberg (funded completely by the *Data Resource*) opened a series of technical meetings with the aim to co-ordinate the European effort to develop the Integrated Genomic Database (IGD). Twelve scientists of several institutions participated in this workshop in Heidelberg and put forward the first design scheme of the IGD. Four subsequent meetings of the same group took place afterwards (alternatively in London and Heidelberg) to discuss IGD matters and especially its networking aspects. In August 1991 and August 1992, the *Data Resource* co-organised a one-week EMBO Course on Genome Computing in Heidelberg and made a full-day presentation of its software, hardware and communication facilities to the participants of the course.

On July 1 - 4, 1992 an international conference on Computational Methods in Genome Research was organised by the *Data Resource*. Twenty-four invited lecturers and twenty-seven posters provided a comprehensive overview of the recent situation in genome informatics for about 280 participants. Scientific lectures and posters given by co-workers of the *Data Resource* presented the Heidelberg activities in this field and on several workstations an interactive demonstration of our services and developments have been available.

Manuals for HUSAR, OMIM and GDB will be provided for all training workshop participants. The same tools are sent to registered users by mail. An on-line phone advisory service has been implemented to answer questions related to databases, analysis programs or network connection. A booklet containing introductory information on the *Data Resource's* services has been sent to about 800 scientists in Europe whom we regard as potential users of our facilities. Several advertisements in Nature helped to make the service known in the science community.

Contract number: GENO-CT91-0008
Contractual period: 1 June 1991 to 31 July 1993

Coordinator
Dr. Suhai
European Data Resource for Human Genome Research
German Cancer Research Center (DKFZ)
Im Neuenheimer Feld 280
D - 69120 Heidelberg
Germany
Tel: 49 6221 422 369
Fax: 49 6221 422 333

Human Genome Analysis Programme
M. Hallen and A. Klepsch (Eds.)
IOS Press, 1995

UPGRADING OF THE COPENHAGEN FAMILY BANK

J. Mohr
University of Copenhagen, Denmark

The tasks and results during the passed period of the grant, up to April 1993, have been as follows:

(1) Work towards immortalization of lymphocytes from, ideally, all the approximately 6,000 individuals in the bank (to make sure that DNA would be available ad libitum in the future),

(2) Work towards complete typing of all the 6,000 individuals in the bank for each of a large number (at least 200) of highly polymorphic DNA marker systems well spread over the genome.

This testing for polymorphic systems has greatly supplemented the earlier marker testing in the bank, which at the beginning of the current project had already been fully typed for most classical marker systems including blood type systems, serum types, enzyme systems, HLA-system, i.e. a total of about 70 marker systems. In addition, physiological genetic variants concerning such traits as PTC taste sensitivity, hair and eye colour have been recorded.

The general purpose is to use the bank - with increasing efficiency as a marker grid grows larger - as an instrument for analysis of such complex traits and disease dispositions that are sufficiently frequent for segregating in a number of families within the bank. This is being accomplished through genetic linkage analysis, testing the trait or the disease disposition against the full array of markers.

(3) Further, to exploit the laboratory facilities and methodological routines that are being established for marker testing, in material collected from families with certain Mendelian and chromosomal conditions.

Ad 1): We have, at the present stage, immortalized some 100 families (with at least 5 individuals per family), the transformation being effected by exposure of lymphocytes to Epstein-Barr virus. The transformed cells have been cultured to a quantity sufficient to supply ample DNA also for distribution to collaborating groups.

Ad 2): There has, since the original planning of the project, been a shift of emphasis from RFLP systems to the far more labour economic PCR based marker systems, and we are now set for a larger scale testing for a considerable number of these (as originally planned, we wanted to wait for more efficient techniques before the large scale testing for PCR based polymorphisms, and then include only highly informative systems - such as the recently established so called Weissenbach set).

Ad (3): As a corrolary to these (1 & 2) tasks, exploiting techniques established during the upgrading, we have pursued a number of special studies:

Certain complicated features like hair colour, hair curling, and eye colour have been considered. Following an indication of linkage between a category of green eye colour and the Luther-Secretor marker complex (lod score + 4.3), we have found apparent linkage/non-association relationships between brown hair colour and green eye colour (lod score + 12), as well as between hair curling and red hair (lod score + 3.5). A linkage study of smell sensitivity to various substances (in particular: androstenone) has been initiated (in cooperation with a group in Philadelphia and one in Bruxelles, the latter representing a molecular genetics approach).

In other material - exploiting the same techniques established during the upgrading, we have pursued linkage studies with Mendelian (or apparently Mendelian) diseases. We discovered linkage of Groenouw's disease with markers on chromosome region 5q (lod score over + 19). Further, in a large Danish kindred with an apparently Mendelian distribution of manio-depressive disease, a suggestion of linkage with the enzyme marker PGP and accordingly tentative assignment of a locus for this kind of MD to chromosome 16 (Lod score + 2,2). In a study of Marner's cataract (CAM) it was shown that CAM is localized between the markers D16S4 and the haptoglobin locus on the long arm of chromosome 16. In further mapping with PCR based markers we are developing a more precise map of the CAM region. A study towards cloning the CAM-gene has been initiated.

We have (1991-92) mapped some 40 RFLP systems located on the short arm of chromosome 5 in patients with the Cri-du-Chat syndrome, including deviant clinical forms.

Contract number: GENO CT91 - 0009
Contractual period: 1 December 1991 to 30 November 1993

Coordinator
Professor J. Mohr
University of Copenhagen
Panum Institute
Institute of Medical Genetics
Blegdamsvej 3B
DK - 2200 Copenhagen
Denmark
Tel: 45 313 57900 Ext. 2479
Fax: 45 428 02363

Participants
Hans Eiberg
Erik Niebuhr
Marie Luise Bisgaard and
Ida Berendt
Genome Group
IMBG, Panum Institute
University of Copenhagen
Blegdamsvej 36
DK-2200 Copenhagen
Denmark
Tel: 45 353 27819
Fax: 45 313 93373

SINGLE CHROMOSOME WORKSHOPS:
CONCERTATION BY HUGO

M.A. Ferguson-Smith
HUGO Europe, London, United Kingdom

1. General objectives

Single chromosome workshops (SCWs) are an important, relatively new development in the global endeavour to map the human genome. They involve a small number of active researchers on a particular chromosome who meet approximately once a year; their purposes are the agreeing of the map to date, the entry of data into the Genome Database (GDB), the planning of future strategies to promote closure of the map, and, if appropriate, the sharing of biological materials such as YAC library of the chromosome in question.

The broad goals of the concertation action were:
- to improve the organisation of single chromosome workshops (SCWs);
- to provide a centralised mechanism for the efficient channelling of the European contribution, inclusive of support from CEC, for SCWs;
- to provide effective liaison between SCW organisers, participants, and funding agencies;
- to produce guidelines for the organisation of SCWs, and to update them from time to time.

2. Methodology

Human gene mappers used to meet every one or two years at Human Gene Mapping (HGM) workshops, in order to collate work on assigning genes to chromosomes and to construct genetic maps. The increasing volume of work led to the development of a computerised database (GDB) and to the updating of GDB in a continuous fashion rather than once a year. The tasks of the HGM workshops have been taken over by SCWs, which now provide the best means for the international genome community to construct consensus genetic and physical maps of the human genome. This is achieved by individual research groups presenting their recent data, resolving inconsistencies and collaborating in future research by sharing results and making genetic material, new technology etc. available to each other. The emphasis is on collation and validation of genome data and not on the biology of the genes being mapped.

The importance of SCWs was recognised by the conclusion of a "concordat" between funding agencies of those countries (or supra-national bodies) which have established genome projects (notably US, UK, France, Netherlands, Canada, Japan, Australia, Russia and the EC). This concordat calls for each agency to support the travel of all its residents who will make a substantial contribution to a workshop, whatever its location. The host country provides support for the local arrangements.

HUGO, after consultation with the genome community and with funding agencies, drew up a set of guidelines for the organisation of SCWs. These have been reviewed, and adapted, in the light of experience.

HUGO has managed the EC funding for SCWs in accordance with the requirements of the inter-agency concordat and the objective of optimising European participation in the workshops.

3. Results and conclusions

During the period of the contract, there were 24 SCWs, held in nine different countries. For all these workshops, HUGO made sure that adequate funding was provided for EC participants travelling to SCWs held outside Europe; for those held in the EC, "core" funding was provided. The SCW co-ordinator (or other HUGO staff) attended virtually all workshops, in order to advise on organisational matters, such as the presentation of reports, the submission of data to GDB, and the selection of dates and venues for future meetings.

The achievements of SCWs were reviewed by HUGO staff at the Chromosome Coordinating Meeting (CCM92) in Baltimore in November 1992. Following discussion with the genome mapping community at the meeting, and consultation with funding agencies, the HUGO guidelines were revised to take account of various concerns. In particular, it was agreed that:
- all intending participants must not only be willing to share data, but must have deposited it in GDB prior to the workshop; all data presented at an SCW are considered to be in the public domain;
- SCW reports should be submitted for publication not later than one month after the meeting and funding (at least in part) will be contingent on this;
- much more detailed guidance should be provided on data presentation at the workshops.

Nearly all the SCWs in 1992-93 met their objectives, i.e. production of a consensus map and (eventual) publication of a report. It has, however, been noticeable that the 8 SCWs held *after* the HUGO review at CCM92 have all complied with the revised guidelines about sharing and deposition of data, and the timely submission of a report. By enabling HUGO attendance at SCWs, and hence the production of the CCM92 review, this contract has improved the effectiveness of SCWs. It has also enabled a significant number of European scientists to attend SCWs in the US, Canada, Australia and Japan and made possible the organisation of others within the EC.

Contract number: GENO-91-0048
Contractual period: 1 February 1992 to 31 January 1993

Coordinator
Professor M.A. Ferguson-Smith
HUGO Europe
One Park Square West
UK - London NW1 4LJ
United Kingdom
Tel: 44 71 935 8085
Fax: 44 71 935 8341

Part 2

Transnational Research Projects

Human Genome Analysis Programme
M. Hallen and A. Klepsch (Eds.)
IOS Press, 1995

CONSTRUCTION OF ORDERED CLONE LIBRARIES COVERING THE XQ27.3 TO XQTER REGION OF THE HUMAN X CHROMOSOME

A. Poustka
DKFZ, Heidelberg, Germany

1. Background information

Xq27.3-qter has, for a long time, been of special interest for human genetics, due to the large number of disease genes located in this area. As a step in the molecular analysis of the as yet uncloned disease genes, and as a test for the detailed analysis of larger regions of the genome, we have constructed YAC and cosmid clone contigs covering the 9 megabase region between FRAXA to the telomere on the long arm of the human X chromosome. The cloned region is expected to contain yet unidentified genes for at least ten genetic diseases. The construction of ordered YAC and cosmid clone contigs of Xq27.3-qter represents an important step in the molecular identification of these genes, and the further analysis of one of the genetically most interesting regions of the human genome.

Key words: Ordered clone libraries; Xq28; genetic desease; integrated mapping.

2. Objectives and primary approaches

Ordered clone libraries have to be constructed to allow a molecular analysis of the genes in the region, and to provide a high resolution map of the entire region. This map provides the link between the genetic and physical maps, is required to identify single genes, and is an essential step in the determination of the DNA sequence of Xq27.3-Xqter, which will provide the ultimate (single base pair resolution) map of this region. We have, in our work, especially emphasised the integration of many different sources of information, especially the integration of information from YAC and cosmid cloning systems, allowing us to combine the increased ease of establishing long range contigs of YAC clones, with the simplified analysis and increased resolution possible with the bacterial cloning systems. Contigs have been positioned, and in most cases oriented on the physical map serving as a high resolution mapping system for the region, allowing the exact localization of newly isolated genes.

3. Results and discussion

As a first step towards the construction of ordered clone libraries in the Xq28 region and the identification of genes located in this area, we have constructed a cosmid library of 1 million clones (12 fold coverage of the hamster genome) from Q1Z, a cell hybrid containing the Xq28 region in a hamster background. Human clones were identified by hybridization with an Alu repeat sequence, picked into microtiter plates and spotted with a robotic device to give high density filter grids. As an additional tool to correlate contig maps and to establish anchor markers on the physical map of the region a NotI

Linking clone library (also in cosmid vectors) was established from the same cell hybrid, human clones were isolated as described above and used to construct high density filter grids. As another source for cosmid clones a flow sorted human X chromosome library constructed in the laboratory of H. Lehrach was used. As a source for clones propagated in different vector system a large number of high density filter grids containig YAC and P1 clones were distributed to us by our coworkers at ICRF.

These filters carrying different types of clones were hybridized with different types of probes (single copy probes, oligonucleotides, cosmid clones, inserts from YAC clones, PCR products of PFG-gel slices) to establish a contig coverage of the region. Since cosmid contigs offer a much more appropriate system for the detailed molecular analysis required to e.g. localize large numbers of transcripts of the region we have concentrated on the construction of cosmid contigs using YAC clones to initiate contig formation.

3.1 Isolation of human clones and construction of high density filter grids

Cosmid libraries were constructed from high molecular weight DNA isolated from cells of the cell line Q1Z (Warren et al., 1991, PNAs) containing the telomere to the position of the fragile X gene at Xq27.3 in a hamster background, using Lawrist7 as vector system. One million clones were plated at a density of approximately 10.000 clones per 22x22 Nunc plate, transferred to nylon membranes. To identify human clones, filters were hybridized with cloned Alu repeat sequences labelled by oligo priming with P32dCTP at a total concentration of 1 million counts per ml. To allow easier identification of the colonies, all colonies were visualized by including S35 labelled cosmid vector in the hybridizations. A total of 4000 candidate colonies hybridizing to the Alu probe were picked into micro titer plates, spotted onto filters, and rescreened with Alu and labelled hamster DNA. 1500 clones were found to be hybridizing more strongly with the Alu probe. These clones were then repicked into microtiter plates, and used to construct high density filter grids using a robotic device at the ICRF (London). Since 1 million clones correspond to 12 fold coverage of the (diploid) hamster genome, this should correspond to 6 fold coverage of the Xq28 region, in agreement with the number expected for a 9 megabase segment in a diploid hamster genome. NotI Linking clones were constructed in the same vector (containing a NotI restriction site) and 200 human clones (20 fold coverage) were picked from this library. Both libraries were brought to the ICRF and a total number of 400 high density filters were spotted using the ICRF robots.

3.2 Characterisation of libraries

As a first probe to characterise these clones total human and total hamster DNA was hybridized to the grids. 30% of the total number of clones in the library, were identified as containing hamster DNA and 500 clones did not hybridize strongly with probes made from radiolabelled total human or hamster DNA, caused by possible deletions, errors in rescreening or not containing repeats. To verify the effective depth of the library, to identify loci for genetically identified markers, and to initiate contigs at known locations, single copy probes used previously in the establishment of the physical map of the region (Poustka et al., PNAs, 1991) were used as hybridization probes to screen cosmid filter grids. On the average, two to ten clones per probe (20 probes used) were recovered, verifying the approximate extent of the coverage. From the NotI Linking clone library 12 unique NotI site containing clones were isolated, and placed on the PFG as well as on the cosmid contig map.

3.3 YAC contigs (isolation and characterisation)

To establish YAC contigs to be used as hybridization probes on cosmid grids and also as an alternative cloning system to elevate the chance of getting an as complete clone map as possible for the following transcript and sequence analysis, over 50 YAC clones isolated from different YAC libraries, were characterised and analysed as Xq28 specific. Initially YAC clones were isolated from a primary plated YAC library constructed and screened by T. Monaco (Oxford), later high density grids of this library as well as the CEPH and the ICI library were screened. YACs were isolated using unique cloned markers from the region, cloned in our or other laboratories, as well as cosmid clones and cDNA clones identified by us. YAC clones were analysed by fingerprinting, ends of clones were isolated and again used to screen different clone libraries. This work results in YAC contigs comprising over 90% of the terminal 10 Megabase of the long arm of the X chromosome containing at least 10 genetic deseases which have not been isolated yet (Rogner et al. submitted).

3.4 Construction of overlapping cosmid contigs

To construct contigs of overlapping cosmid clones covering most of Xq27.3-Xqter, a number of different hybridization strategies were used. Hybridization probes used included probes of known position to localise contigs relative to the genetic and physical map of the region, the use of YAC clone hybridizations to localize cosmids to subregions, the use of cosmids or ends of cosmids to close remaining gaps, as well as the use of Alu-PCR products from different sources.

In the first stage of the contig construction, 42 DNA probes were used to identify cosmids corresponding to previously identified markers. In most cases these contigs were very short, between 40 and 60 kb of average size. Only in regions with a very high density of probes, contigs with an average size of 200 - 300 kb could be constructed.

14 NotI linking clones from a Xq27.3 - Xqter specific NotI linking cosmid library were hybridized to cosmid grids to establish clone contigs throughout the NotI sites previously shown in the PFG data (Poustka et al., PNAS 1991).

In parallel with the establishment of a YAC contig of Xq27.3-qter (Rogner et al., submitted), cosmid clones were assigned to subregions of Xq27.3-qter based on the results of hybridizations of DNA from YAC clones to the cosmid filter grids. Three different protocols for YAC-probe generation have been used, to identify most or all cosmids underlying a YAC clone. Alu and LINE PCR products of YAC clones as well as YAC inserts excised from PFG have been used as hybridization probes. Routinely we have however used labeling of entire yeast containing YAC blocks with excellent results. Results of these hybridizations contributed not only to the localization of the cosmid clones, but they also verified postulated overlaps of YAC clones, and helped to detect major rearrangements or deletions in YACs.

Cosmid contigs were elongated by using the end cosmids of previously established contigs as hybridization probes (contig walking). In parallel 150 cosmid clones not identified by previous hybridizations were used as probes in a sampling-without-replacement-strategy (Hoheisel et al., Cell, 1993).

4. Results of analysis

The contig analysis by hybridization has now reached the end of a first stage in which all cosmid clones in this library hybridizing to human DNA have been identified by one or more other cosmid clones or single copy probes and has, in combination with the YAC insert hybridizations, allowed the establishment of 39 cosmid contigs with sizes up to 800 Kilobases throughout the Xq28 region. Out of the 39 contigs ,34 cosmid contigs could be physically assigned according to the PFG map while 5 cosmid contigs remain physically unassigned, together comprising 7 Megabase (80 %) of the DNA of the region. The combined clone map (YACs and cosmid clones) currently consists of 8.5 MB Xq27.3-qter DNA (see attached figure). In the last, and still ongoing, phase of the contig building process, remaining gaps, usually due to the relative low coverage of the library, are being closed by hybridizing cosmids from the ends of existing contigs to high density filter grids of cosmid libraries constructed from human X chromosomes isolated by fluorescence activated chromosome sorts as well as to high density filter grids carrying clones from a P1 library containing the entire genome and libraries constructed from subcloning of YACS.

We have, in our work, especially emphasised the integration of many different sources of information, as well as especially also the integration of information from YAC and cosmid cloning systems, allowing us to combine the increased ease of establishing long range contigs with YAC clones, with the simplified analysis and increased resolution possible with the bacterial cloning systems. Ordered clone libraries offer a number of attractive features, since they can serve as an efficient, high resolution, complete mapping system, able to integrate information on clones with genetic, transcriptional and sequence information and provide immediate access to the relevant genomic sequence.

The detailed molecular analysis of Xq27.3-qter made possible by the construction of ordered clone libraries will simplify the identification of genes for the as yet unidentified genetic diseases, provides an overview over a long region of the human X chromosome, and will serve as a test for the analysis of larger regions of the human genome.

5. Major scientific breakthroughs

During the course of this work the cloned material has been used to establish new technology for the isolation of transcribed and conserved sequences. These techniques have been used to establish transcription maps, resulting in the isolation of over 40 new genes. As a further result of the systematic molecular analysis of Xq27.3-qter we have cloned the gene for X-chromosomal adrenoleukodystrophy in collaboration with two french groups. By molecular analysis of patients with MASA syndrome, we have identified a deletion in a large family and point mutations in two further families located in the L1CAM gene. In addition the material established here has been helpful in the identification of a number of deletions in fragile X patients. Finally a new polymorphic microsatellite marker has been isolated and used to delineate the Myotubular Myopathy gene.

6. Major cooperative links

Throughout this work information as well as existing cosmid and YAC contigs have been distributed to other laboratories in Europe and the USA, resulting in a number of publications.

Jean Louis Mandel (Strasbourg, France), Patrick Willems (Leuven, Belgium), Horst Hameister (Ulm, Germany), Ben Oostra (Rotterdam, The Netherlands), Andre Rosenthal (Jena, Germany), John Sulston (Cambridge, United Kingdom), Daniela Toniolo (Pavia, Italy).

References

- Poustka, A., Dietrich, A., Langenstein, G., Toniolo, D., Warren, S.T, Lehrach, H. (1991) Physical Map of Human Xq27-qter Localizing the Region of the Fragile X Mutation. PNAS, 88, 8302-8306.
- Poustka, A. and Kioschis, P. (1992) Analysis of psychiatric disease by molecular genetics. In Genetic Research in Psychiatry, (Ed: H. Hippius and J. Mendlewiecz) Springer Verlag, 117-125.
- Dietrich, A., Korn, B. and Poustka, A. (1992) Completion of the physical map of Xq28: the location of the gene for L1CAM on the human X chromosome. Mammalian Genome, 3, 186-172.
- Van den Ouweland, A. M. W., Kioschis P., Verdijk M., Tamanini F., Toniolo D., Ropers H., Poustka A. and van Oost B. A. (1992) Identification and Characterisation of a new gene in the human Xq28 region. Hum. Mol. Gen.,1, 4, 269-275.
- Wöhrle D., Kotzot D., Hirst M., Manca A., Korn B., Schmidt A., Barbi G., Rott H., Poustka A., Davies K.E. and Steinbach P. (1992) A microdeletion of less than 250 kb, including the proximal part of the FMR-1 gene and the fragile X site, in a male with the clinical phenotype of fragile X syndrome. Am. J. Hum. Gen. 51, 299-306.
- Gedeon, A.K., Baker, E., Robinson, H., Partington, M., Gross, B., Manca, A., Korn, B., Poustka, A., Yu, S., Sutherland, G.R. and Mulley, J.C. (1992) Fragile X Syndrome without CCG amplification. Nature Genetics 1, 5, 341-345.
- Maestrini, E., Kioschis, P., Tamanini, F., Gimbo, E., Marinelli, P., Tribioli, C., D'Urso, M., Schlessinger, D., Palmieri, G., Poustka, A. and Toniolo, D. (1992) An archipelago of CpG islands in Xq28: identification and fine mapping of 20 new genes of the human X chromosome. Hum. Mol. Gen. 1, 4, 275-281.
- Korn, B., Sedlacek, Z., Manca, A., Kioschis, P., Konecki, D. and Poustka, A. (1992) A strategy for selection of transcribed sequences in the Xq28 region. Hum. Mol.Gen. 1, 4, 235-243.
- Poustka, A. (1992) Fragile X syndrome; the molecular analysis reveals a new mechanism of mutation in human genetic desease. Annals of Medicine, Vol.24, 6, 453-456.
- Bächner, D., Manca, A., Steinbach, P., Wöhrle, D., Just, W., Vogel, W., Hameister, H. and Poustka, A. (1993) Enhanced Fmr-1 expression in testis. Nature Genetics, 4, 115-116.
- Mosser, J., Douar, A.M., Sarde, C., Kioschis, P., Feil, R., Moser, H., Poustka, A., Mandel, J.L. and Aubourg, P. (1993) The putative X linked Adrenoleukodystrophy gene shows unexpected homology to "ABC" superfamily of transporters. Nature, 726-730.
- Verkerk, A., Graaff, E., Konecki, D., Manca, A., de Boulle, K., Reyniers, E., Willems, PJ., Poustka, A., Nelson, D., Oostra, B. (1993) Alternative splicing in the fragile X (FMR-1) gene. Hum. Mol. Gen., 399-405.
- Sedlacek, Z., Konecki, D., Kioschis, P., Siebenhaar, R. and Poustka, A. (1993) Direct selection of DNA sequences conserved between species. NAR, 21, 3419-3425.
- Bächner, D., Manca, A., Steinbach, P., Wöhrle, D., Just, W., Vogel, W., Hameister, H. and Poustka, A. (1993) Enhanced expression of the murine Fmr-1 gene during germ cell proliferation suggests a special function in both the male and the female gonad. Hum. Mol. Gen.; 2, 2043-2051
- Bione, S., Tamanini, F., Maestrini, E., Tribioli, C., Rivella, S., Torri, G., Poustka, A. and Toniolo, D. (1993) Transcriptional organization of a 450-kb region of the human X chromosome in Xq28. PNAS, 90, 10977-10981.
- Sedlacek, Z., Korn, B., Coy, J., Kioschis, P., Siebenhaar, R., Konecki, D. and Poustka, A. (1993) Construction of a transcription map of a 300 kb region surrounding the human G6PD locus by direct cDNA selection. Hum. Mol. Gen. 2, 1856-1871.
- Van den Ouweland, A.M.W., Verdijk, M., Kioschis, P., Poustka, A. and van Oost, B.A. (1993) The human renin-binding protein gene (RnBP) maps in Xq28. Genomics, 21, 279-281.
- Coy, J., Kioschis, P., Sedlacek, Z. and Poustka, A. (1994) Identification of tissue specific expressed sequences in Xq27.3 to Xqter. Mammalian Genome, 5, 131-137.
- Gong, W., Kioschis, P., Monaco, A. and Poustka, A (1994) Identification of region-specific cosmid clones by hybridization with Alu-LINE PCR products of YAC clones. Meth. in Mol. Cell Biol., 4, 269-272.
- Chatterjee, A, Faust, C.J., Molinari-Storey, L., Kioschis, P., Poustka, A., and Herman, G.E. (1993) A 2.3 Mb yeast artificial chromosome contig spanning from Gabra3 to G6PD on the mouse X chromosome. Genomics, 21, 49-57.
- Trottier, Y., Imbert, G., Fryns, J.P., Poustka, A. and Mandel, J.L. (1993) A male fragile X phenotype is deleted for part of the FMR1 gene and for about 100 kb of upstream region. Am. J. Med. Genet., in press.
- Sarde, C.O., Mosser, J., Kioschis, P., Kretz, C., Vicaire, S., Aubourg, P., Poustka, A., Mandel, J.L. (1993) Genomic Organization of the Adrenoleukodystrophy Gene. Hum. Mol. Genet., in press.

- Viets, L., can Camp, G., Coucke, P., Fransen, E., de Boulle, K., Reyniers, E., Korn, B., Poustka, A., Wilson, G., Schrander-Stumpel, C., Winter, R.M., Schwart, C. and Willems, P.J. (1994) MASA syndrome is due to mutations in the neuronal cell adhesion gene L1CAM. Nature Genetics, in press.
- Dahl, N., Samson, F., Thomas, N.S.T., Hu, L.J., Gong, W., Herman, G., Laporte, j., Kioschis, P., Poustka, A., Mandel, J.L. (1994) X-linked myotubular myophathy (MTM1) mapped between DXS304-DXS305, closely linked to the DXS455 VNTR and a new, highly informative microsatellite marker (DXS1684). J. Med. Genet., in press.
- Gong, W., Hu, L.J., Kioschis, P., Poustka, A., Dahl, N. (1994) A polymorphic dinucleotide repeat at the DXS1684 locus. Hum. Mol. Gen., in press.
- Sedlacek, Z., Konecki, D.S., Korn, B., Klauck, S.M., Poustka, A. (1994) Evolutionary conservation and genomic organisation of XAP-4, an Xq28 located gene coding for a novel human rab GDP-dissociation inhibitor (GDI). Mammalian Genome, in press.
- Rogner, U., Kioschis, P., Wilke, K., Gong, W., Pick, E., Dietrich, A., Zechner, U., Hameister, H., Pragliola, A., Herman, G.E., Yates, J.R.W., Lehrach, H., Poustka, A (1994) A YAC clone map spanning the human chromosomal band Xq28. Nature Genetics, submitted.
- Kioschis, P., Gong, W., Rogner, U., Zehetner, G., Lehrach, H., Poustka, A. (1994) Construction of cosmid contigs covering 7 Megabase of Xq27.3-qter, in preparation.
- Gong, W., Kioschis, P., Wilke, K., Rogner, U., Korn, B., Klauck, S., Poustka, A. (1994) A 1.7 Mb cosmid contig containing a α3-subunit of the human τ-aminobutyric receptor (GABRA3) gene and 6 new human genes in Xq28, in preparation.

Contract number: GENO-CT91-0010 (SSMA)
Contractual period: 1 December 1991 to 29 February 1994

Coordinator
Dr. A. Poustka
Angewandte Tumorvirologie
Deutsches Krebsforschungszentrum
Im Neuenheimer Feld 280
D-6921 Heidelberg
Germany
Tel: 49 62 21 424 742
Fax: 49 62 21 423 454

Participants
Dr. H. Lehrach
Imperial Cancer Research Fund
44 Lincoln's Inn Fields
London WC2A 3 PX
United Kingdom
Tel: 44 71 269 3308
Fax: 44 71 269 3068

Dr. A.P. Monaco
Imperial Cancer Research Fund
Institute of Molecular Medicine
John Radcliffe Hospital
Headington
Oxford OX3 9DU
United Kingdom
Tel: 44 865 222 371
Fax: 44 865 222 431

Human Genome Analysis Programme
M. Hallen and A. Klepsch (Eds.)
IOS Press, 1995

A DELETION RESTRICTION SITE AND OVERLAPPING CLONE MAP OF THE HUMAN Y CHROMOSOME

N.A. Affara
University of Cambridge, United Kingdom

1. Background information

The human Y chromosome is, on average, 50 megabase pairs (Mb) long, the difference in size between individuals being due to variation in the length of the heterochromatic repeats (without any apparent clinical consequences) which compose the distal half of the Y long arm. The euchromatic part of the chromosome is invariant in size at 29 Mb. This is the active part of the chromosome which contains all the genetic functions which have so far been assigned to the Y (see figure 1, appendix). At 50 Mb in size, the Y is one of the smallest chromosomes in the human genome and thus is amenable to a complpete molecular analysis with the current cloning and sequencing technology. It is, therefore, an attractive target for detailed physical mapping and sequence analysis.

Traditionally, the mapping of human chromosomes has proceeded through conventional genetic analysis and the construction of genetic linkage maps upon which physical maps are then elaborated. This is only possible for the small segment of the Y known as the pseudoautosomal region which pairs with the X chromosome during meiosis and where recombination can occur between the sex chromosomes. This covers some 3 Mb and thus repesents only one tenth of the euchromatin. This has meant that the vast majority of the Y chromosome has necessarily been analysed by physical means. The first approach has been through deletion analysis using patients with aberrant Y chromosomes to order cloned DNA markers into a series of intervals along the chromosome. Thus XX male and XY female patients which arise from illegitimate X-Y interchange, X:Y and Y:autosomal translocations and various Y rearrangements have been invaluable in providing deletion panels to refine the deletion map of the Y. These studies not only divide the chromosome into ordered intervals and a series of ordered markers, but also permit karyotype / phenotype correlations to be made and thus genetic functions can be assigned to particular segments of the chromosome. These include sex-determination, Turner's stigmata, linear growth, spermatogenesis, the male-specific HY antigen and the development of gonadoblastoma (see figure 1). It has therefore been possible to assemble a model of the Y based on deletion analysis upon which further more detailed molecular study using modern genome analysis techniques can be prdicated. The deletion map has been used to drive higher levels of analysis.

The interest in mapping and cloning the Y stems from several perspectives. (1) It is important to clone the genes for genetic functions that have been assigned through karyotype / phenotype correlations. For example, what is the nature of the genes which underlie growth and other aspects of the Turner phenotype? What is the nature of the gene(s) involved in germ cell maturation that are known to lie on the Y long arm? (2) What are the structures of key functional chromosome elements such as the telomeres and centromeres and what is essential for their function? Isolation of these elements from a small chromosome such as the Y offers a means for their detailed study. (3) What is the coding potential of the Y? Is it largely devoid of genes as a result of becoming the genetically isolated, specialized sex-determining chromosome? Or is the number of functional genes greater than suggested by crude karyotype / phenotype correlations. Isolation of large segments of the chromosome will permit direct resolution of this issue by the application of gene searching methodologies. (4) The study of the evolution of the Y will be aided by the isolation of further genes and polymorphic DNA segments. More detailed coverage of the chromosome will permit a fine analysis of the relationship between the sex chromosomes and autosomes during mammalian evolution.

Key words: Y-Chromosome; deletion map; YAC / cosmid overlapping maps.

2. Objectives and primary approaches

The overall objective of this project was to construct an overlapping clone map (based on YAC and cosmid clones) for the Y chromosome in order to provide the reagent base for the kinds of studies outlined above. The development of this map fell into three stages which could be achieved through the pooling of resources and expertise available to each of the collaborating groups.

The first, short term, objective was the creation of a unitary deletion map based on the patients and markers possessed by the collaborating groups. Southern blots carrying all the patient DNA samples from the collaborating groups were prepared in Paris and distributed to each group to probe with their particular series of DNA markers. In this way, all the patients were typed with all the DNA markers held in common and this has resulted in the creation of a very detailed deletion map (see below).

The second, medium term, objective was the assembly of an overlapping YAC clone map of the Y euchromatin using primarily the CEPH series of YAC libraries (mainly the megaYAC library). This task was divided as follows between the groups:

Paris: The Yp pseudoautosomal region.
Oxford: The Y centromeric region and the Yq pseudoautosomal region.
Cambridge: The remaining Y euchromatin.

The London group has focussed on the analysis of cosmid clones as a means of underpinning YAC contigs developed by the other groups. The main approach used to develop YAC contigs of the Y was through the use of the STS (sequence tagged sites) content analysis of YAC clones. This proceeds through several steps.

1. The conversion of markers ordered by deletion analysis into STSs by generating limited DNA sequence from each marker clone.

2. The DNA sequence is then used to design primers for Polymerase Chain Reaction (PCR) analysis. In this way, rather than molecular hybridization being used to demonstrate the presence of a specific Y markers, PCR with primers specific to that marker is used to generate a DNA fragment from the target sequence. This not only allows rapid analysis of DNA clones and patient DNA, but also provides a very rapid means of screening YAC libraries arrayed for PCR screening. The synthesis of PCR primers for about 70 of our own markers and some 170 published by Foote et al. (1992) and Vollrath et al. (1992) was shared by the Cambridge and Paris laboratories and provided a large number of STSs with which to isolate YAC clones.

3. Screening of YAC libraries with STS markers to isolate at least a three-fold depth of coverage of the euchromatin.

4. Assessment of overlaps between YAC clones through extensive STS content analysis. This is simply the determination of whether an STS is carried on a YAC by subjecting it to PCR analysis with STS markers that surround the cognate STS used to isolate the YAC in the first instance. This defines the limits of the YAC (in terms of

STSs) and from the STS content shared by different YAC clones it is possible to derive the overlaps between adjacent clones. The analysis can be complicated by the presence of repetitive STSs and rearrangements within YAC clones. Nevertheless, it is a very rapid means of deriving a first generation overlapping clone map which can be subjected to further refinement. The maps produced by this project and the one published by Foote et al. (1992) using a different Y chromosome, when combined provide a very comprehensive coverage of the chromosome.

The third, long term objective, was to begin to underpin the YAC clone map with a more detailed cosmid contig map and to construct long-range restriction maps of overlapping clones. The basic strategy being used to achieve cosmid contigs is through Hinf I finger-printing of large numbers of chromosome Y-specific cosmid clones. Hinf I cuts frequently in genomic DNA and will generate a fragment pattern that is unique to a given cosmid clone. If cosmid clones overlap sufficiently, they will share a proportion of their fragment pattern and thus indicating they are adjacent to one another. With sufficiently large numbers of cosmids subjected to this analysis, the clones will begin to fall into small contigs that gradually merge to form larger ones. Marker probes used in deletion analysis and in the isolation of YAC clones to form YAC contigs can then be used to assign the growing cosmid contigs against the YAC and deletion map framework. Two libraries have served as the source of cosmid clones; a cosmid library (constructed by the London group) from the 3E7 Y-only somatic cell hybrid and a flow-sorted Y-specific cosmid library obtained from the Lawrence Livermore National Laboratory.

3. Results and Discussion

3.1 Unitary Deletion Map

Genomic DNA from all the patients within the collaboration was used to create Southern blot panels for analysis with Y-specific DNA clones which had already been mapped on less comprehensive panels. By integrating both patients and DNA markers into a unitary map, it was hoped to integrate all our Y markers and refine their order by defining a greater number of deletion intervals. Each DNA sample was digested with EcoR1, Hind III and Taq I to create three different panels. Each group analysed these panels with their Y DNA probes. From the pattern of hybridization of the probes to the various patient DNA samples, it is possible to derive a consensus deletion map in which the Y DNA probes are odered into a series of deletion intervals; this is shown in figures 2A (Yp) and B (Yq). The map contains 94 DNA probes and it has been possible to divide the Y chromosome into 72 deletion intervals which now provide the basis for more careful assignment of clinical phenotype to regions of the Y. This map compares favourably with the 43 interval map derived by Vollrath et al. (1992) who used an almost completely different group of patients and makers. By typing our patients with some of the markers used by Vollrath et al. (1992) it will be possible to integrate the two maps and maximize the number of deletion intervals on the Y.

3.2 YAC Contigs of the Y

YAC clones from seven different libraries were isolated primarily by a PCR based screening strategy. The libraries were: (1) The earlier CEPH YAC library and the CEPH MegaYAC library made from a normal XY individual (2) The small Cambridge YAC library made from an XYY individual (3) The Oxford YAC library made from the

Oxen 4Y cell line (4) The St. Louis YAC library made from an XY individual (5) The
ICRF Oxen 4Y library and (6) The Oxen library made by Foote et al. for a small
number of clones in the centromeric region. Approximately 70 of the DNA probes
ordered by deletion mapping were sequenced and used to derive STS primers. These
markers were added to those published by Foote et al., (1992) and used to select YAC
clones by PCR. Once a clone had been identified it was subjected to STS content
analysis by markers in the vicinity of the cognate STS. Each clone was tested with STS
markers until at least three markers on either side proved to be negative. This was
taken as defining the limits of the YAC clone. The marker content of some YAC clones
was determined by molecular hybridization of labelled probes. Figures 3A, 3B and 3C
summarise the overall YAC map derived for most of the human Y chromosome and
figure 4 summarises the principle of STS content analysis as illustrated by the data
drawn from a region of the Y contig. In total, over 100 YAC clones have been used to
assemble the YAC map with over 250 STS markers.

We have gone for as much depth of coverage of the chromosome as possible to
ensure that any given region of the chromosome is represented by several YACs. This
is important to achieve a consensus map at any point since YAC clones can be
rearranged or deleted internally. If there are several YACs covering a given region then
it is unlikely that all of them will be rearranged. The major problem with assessing
overlaps by STS content is the existence of Y-specific repeat sequences. This will tend
to lead to the detection of false overlaps. To minimise this effect we have concentrated
on the use of unique Y specific markers to construct the main overlap framework.
Coligated YAC clones do not present a major problem in obtaining coverage of the
chromosome by STS content analysis. However, it is important to know which clones
are coligated when the physical restriction map is constructed (see below). The
coligation status of many of the YAC clones has been checked by fluorescence in situ
hybridization. Some of the internal deletions in YAC clones may be more apparent than
real in that they may reflect uncertainty of the exact marker order in that region of the
chromosome and once this is established in fine detail many of these gaps will be
resolved. The centromere remains the least well covered segment of the chromosome
as many of the clones from this region are unstable due to the presence of alphoid
repeats (see below for more detailed analysis). The second region which is not
represented is the Yq heterochromatin which consists largely of two repeat sequences.
Coverage of the Yq pseudoautosonmal region has been achieved by combination of
YAC, cosmid and lambda genomic DNA clones (see below).

3.3 Physical Maps of YAC Contigs and Y Genomic DNA

The physical mapping of these YAC contigs has focussed, to begin with, on three
regions. (1) The distal Yp block of X-Y homology; (2) The proximal Yp block of X-Y
homology; (4) The centromeric region; (5) The Yq pseudoatosomal region. In general,
the physical maps of large DNA clones have been assembled by the use of probes
specific for either vector arm combined with partial digestion of insert DNA. In this
way, the ladder of fragments detected by vector probes from each side of the insert
marks the location of restriction enzyme sites. Through the use of a range of different
restriction enzymes, a map can be elaborated for the entire clone. Analysis of digested
clones with markers that are known to be carried on the inserts allows their location
in the insert to be established. For the most part, rare cutting restriction enzyme sites
have been used to produce these maps as these will enable the identification of CpG
islands and, hence, the location of potential genes. The development of these physical
maps, will provide detailed validation of the clone overlaps determined by STS content
analysis.

3.4 Distal and Proximal Yp X-Y Homology and the Centromeric Region

Figures 5, 6, 7 and 8 summarise the map information derived from a number of YAC clones studied by the Cambridge group that form contigs in the X-Y homologous blocks of distal and proximal Yp respectively. The distal block of X-Y homology covers the region believed to carry a gene or genes which are involved in the Turner phenotype (figures 5, 6 and 7). The figures show the maps derived for three different YAC clones. Thus definition of the location of any CpG islands would assist in the identification of potential gene candidates for this syndrome, although not all genes are associated with such structures. Figure 8 summarises the map derived from several clones which cover the proximal block of X-Y homology around the amelogenin gene. A more extensive analysis of the proximal region of Yp extending across the centromere has been undertaken by the Oxford group. Figure 9 gives a summary of the YAC contigs and regions examined (including the centromere) and figures 10 through to 14 summarise the mapping data for each of these contigs. The detailed organisation of sequences in the centromere has been determined from a combination of YAC and genomic DNA analysis (not shown). The combined analysis of YAC clones and pulsed-field gel electrophoresis of genomic DNA has led to a map which covers almost 10 Mb around the centromere.

3.5 The Yq Pseudoautosomal Region

A low frequency of genetic exchange between the Yq and Xq telomeres has been reported by Freije et al. (1992), implying the existence of a second psuedoautosomal region. Detailed physical analysis of both the Xq and Yq telomeric regions has confirmed the existence of a strictly homologous region which contains the markers DXYS64 and DXYS61. The order is Cen - DXYS64 - DXYS61 - Tel. The Oxford group has performed a detailed analysis of the terminal 400 kb of both sex chromosomes which have been isolated in overlapping YAC, cosmid and lambda clones. Several new X-Y homologous probes have been placed on to these contigs and are shown on the map for the Yq and Xq telomeres illustrated in figure 15. The physical analysis of these contigs has defined the extent of strict X-Y homology as extending to a position 320 Kb from the long arm telomeres of the sex chromosomes. Sequence analysis of the point of breakdown in homology has shown that the boundary is defined by a member of the LINE repeat sequence family. Proximal to this point are X and Y specific sequences. The data suggest that the Yq PAR is of recent evolutionary origin and may have arisen as a consequence of a recombination event between LINE sequences leading to transfer of the region of Xq distal to the LINE sequence on to the Y.

3.6 Cosmid Contigs of the Y

The London group has developed detailed underpinning of YAC clones through the assembly of cosmid contigs by memans of finger-print analysis. The technique requires that the cosmids overlap by 50% of their inserts before the computer identifies them as significantly similar. This has the advantage that the level of detail of the map is very high but it suffers from the obvious disadvantage that it breaks down whenever a contig includes a repeat sequence which is either itself of a length comparable to about half the length of a cosmid insert or which by tandem repetition exceeds this value. Nevertheless, the approach produces very detailed mapping information scattered over the entire chromosome which can be aligned against the YAC framework using the probes ordered by deletion and YAC STS content analysis.

3300 cosmids have been entered into the cosmid database and the analysis has been completed for 3091 clones. There are 322 contigs of which 312 appear to represent single copy regions of the genome. Figure 16 summarises the progress and shows a steady increase in the number of contigs built. At the 2200 clone stage, the number of two clone contigs began to fall and the number of three clone contigs may also be diminishing. At present, the number of clones in each contig ranges from 27 clones to 2 clones (see figure 17), the largest contig spanning 240 Kb across the amelogenin region in proximal Yp. Of the repetitive contigs, several groups have been identified. (1) 77 clones fall into a contig representing DYZ1. Two other contigs contain clones which resemble closely, but are not identical to, the fingerprints of the DYZ1 contig clones. The repetitive sequences DYZ2 and DYZ3 do not label in the Hinf I finger-printing scheme and are therefore not observed. (2) The finger-prints of several singleton clones contain low molecular weight intense bands which are indicative of short tandem repeats. (3) Many clones fall into the DYZ5 (TSPY) category (a 20 Kb direct repeat) and form one major (70 clones) and three related groups (each about 15 clones). At present it is not possible to separate these into locus specific contigs or to stretch out the clones of the contigs to represent the large region of proximal Yp which must be covered by this repeat. In addition, at least eight different interspersed repeats (each at least half a cosmid insert ~20 Kb long) have been observed. One of these repeats is estimated to be >50 Kb long.

In general, the frequency of Y-specific repeat elements is high and an indication of this is given by the fact that 10% of the ends of single copy contigs are bounded by a repeat. As with the assembly of YAC contigs, this can make contig assembly very difficult in repeat rich areas where there is a dearth of single-copy sequences to act as reference points to assess overlaps. At the present stage of the analysis, 8% of newly analysed clones will hit a singleton clone in the database to form a new contig, 3% will join together two existing contigs and 48% will fall within or extend and existing contig. It is estimated that at this point in the analysis, 69% of the chromosome is covered by these cosmid clones.

This is an extensive source of partially charcterised cosmids that, with the aid of markers ordered along the chromosome by deletion mapping and YAC STS content analysis, can be aligned against the deletion interval and YAC framework. Such clones will provide the basis for detailed analysis of novel Y-linked genes.

4. Summary

This project has been successful in exploiting the resources that the collaborating groups were able to bring to bare on the development of a more detailed map of the Y. Four areas have been developed to higher levels of resolution. (1) The deletion maps of both the short and long arms of the Y. The detail will be increased further as more patients and markers are contributed to the analysis. (2) The YAC map which gives a high level of overlapping coverage of the Y euchromatin. This coverage is further increased by combination with the YAC clones characterised by Foote et al. Detailed verification of the YAC contigs defined by STS content analysis is underway by developing restriction maps of individual clones and by Alu fingerprint analysis. (3) The detailed restriction analysis of YACs covering selected regions of the map. This is being extended to the rest of the euchromatin. (4) The development of cosmid contigs by Hinf I finger-print analysis which are estimated to cover 69% of the Y chromosome.

5. References

- Foote S., Vollrath D., Hilton A. and Page D.C.: The human Y chromosome: overlapping DNA clones spanning the euchromatic region. Science 258: 60-66 (1992).
- Freije D., Helms C., Watson M.S. and Donis-Keller H.: Identification of a second pseudoautosomal region near the Xq and Yq telomeres. Science 258: 1784-1787 (1992).
- Vollrath D., Foote S., Hilton A., Brown L.G., Beer-Romero P., Bogan J.S., and Page D.: The human Y chromosome: a 43 interval map based on naturally occurring deletions. Science 258: 52-59 (1992).

6. Publications

Cambridge

- Bailey D.M.D., Affara N.A. and Ferguson-Smith M.A.: The XY Homologous Gene Amelogenin Maps to the Short Arms of Both the X and Y Chromosomes and Is Highly Conserved in Primates. Genomics 14: 203-205 (1992).
- O'Reilly A.J., Affara N.A., Simpson E., Chandler P., Goulmy E. and Ferguson-Smith M.A.: A Molecular Deletion Map of the Y Chromosome Long Arm Defining X and Autosomal Homologous Regions and the Localisation of the HYA Locus to the Proximal Region of the Yq Euchromatin. Human Molecular Genetics 1: 379-385 (1992).
- Lambson, B., Affara, N.A., Mitchell, M. and FergusonSmith, M.A. (1992). Evolution of DNA Sequence Homologies Between the Sex Chromosomes in Primate Species. Genomics 14: 1032-1040 (1992).
- Affara N.A., Chalmers I.J. and Ferguson-Smith M.A.: Analysis of the SRY Gene in 22 Sex-Reversed XY Females Identifies 4 New Muatations in the Conserved DNA Binding Domain. Human Molecular Genetics 2: 784-789 (1993).
- Jones M.H., Khwaja O., Briggs H., Walker E., Lambson B., Davey P., Chalmers I.J., Zhou C.-Y., Walker E.M., Zheng Y., Todd C., Ferguson-Smith M.A. and Affara N.A.: A Set of Ninety-Seven Overlapping Yeast Artificial Chromosome Clones Spanning the Human Y Chromosome Euchromatin. Genomics, submitted (1994).

Oxford

- Cooper K.F., Fisher R.B. and Tyler-Smith C.: Structure of the sequences adjacent to the centromeric alphoid satellite DNA array on the human Y chromosome. J. Mol. Biol. 230: 787-789 (1993).
- Cooper K.F., Fisher R.B. and Tyler-Smith C.: The major centromeric array of alphoid satellite DNA on the human Y chromosome is non-palindromic. Hum. Mol. Genet. 2: 1267-1270 (1993).
- Kvaloy K., Galvagni F. and Brown W.R.A.: The sequence organisation of the long arm pseudoautosomal region of the human sex chromosomes. Hum. Mol. Genet. 3: 771-778 (1994).
- Tyler-Smith C., Oakey, R.J., Larin Z., Fisher R.B., Crocker M., Affara N.A., Ferguson-Smith M.A., Muenke M., Zuffardi O. and Jobling M.A. Localization of DNA sequences required for human centromere funiction through an analysis of rearranged Y chromosomes. Nature Genetics 5: 368-375 (1993).

Paris

- Slim R., Le Paslier D., Compain S., Levilliers J., Ougen P., Billault A., Conohue S.J., Klein D.C., Mintz L., Bernheim A., Cohen D., Weissenbach J. and Petit C.: Construction of a yeast artificial chromosome contig spanning the pseudoautosomal region and isolation of 25 new sequenc-tagged sites. Genomics 16: 691-697 (1993).

Contract Number: GENO-CT91-0012
Contractual period: 1 May 1992 to 31 May 1994

Coordinator
Dr. N.A. Affara
University of Cambridge Department of Pathology
Tennis Court Road
Cambridge CB2 1QP
United Kingdom
Tel: 44 223 333700
Fax: 44 223 333346

Participants
Dr. Jonathan Wolfe
Department of Genetics and Biometry
The Galton Laboratory
4 Stephenson Way
University College London
United Kingdom
Tel: 44 71 380 7417
Fax: 44 71 387 3496

Dr. Jean Weissenbach
Institut Pasteur
25 Rue du Docteur Roux
75724 Paris CEDEX
France
Tel: 33 1 45 688850
Fax: 33 1 45 688790

Drs. Christopher Tyler-Smith
and William Brown
University of Oxford
Department of Biochemistry
South Parks Road
Oxford OX1
United Kingdom
Tel: 44 865 275222
Fax: 44 865 275283

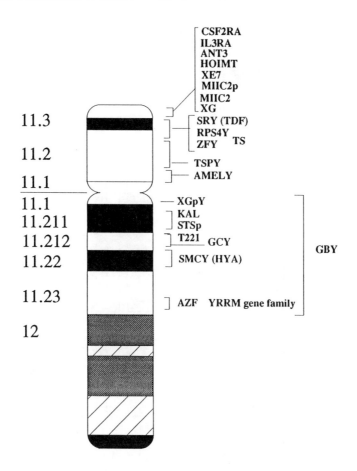

Human Y

Figure 1
Schematic representation of the human Y chromosome showing the location of assigned genes and genetic functions.

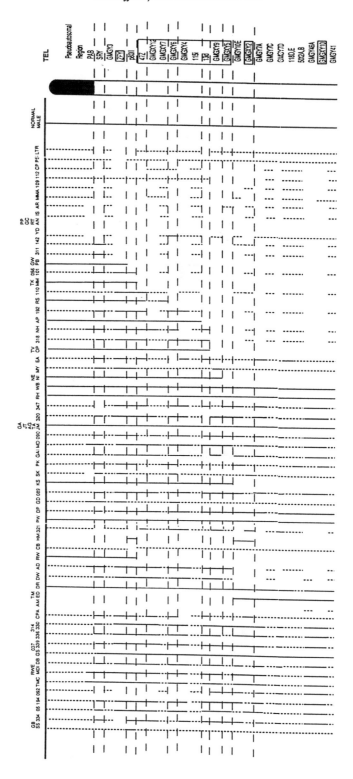

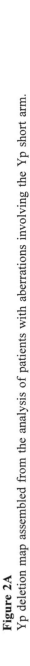

Figure 2A

Yp deletion map assembled from the analysis of patients with aberrations involving the Yp short arm.

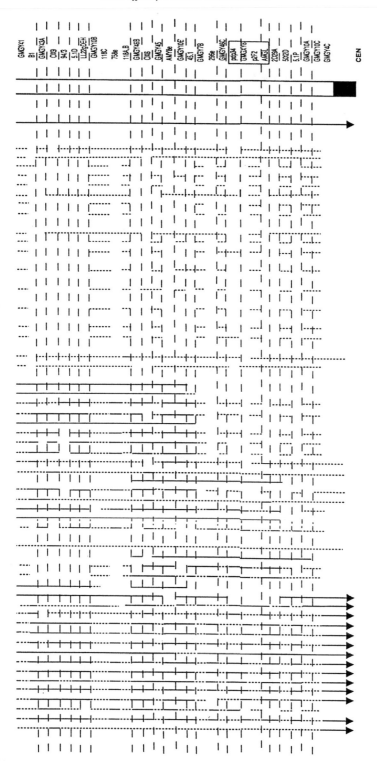

Figure 2A (continued)

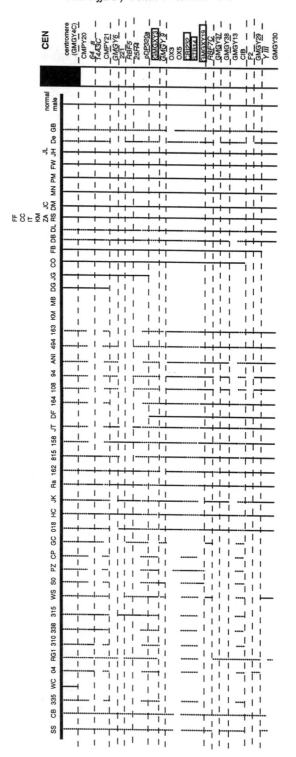

Figure 2B

Yq deletion map assembled from the analysis of patients with aberrations involving the Y long arm. The solid lines indicate the markers present in each patient, the blanks the markers absent from the DNA of the patient and the dashed lines the markers which remain to be tested.

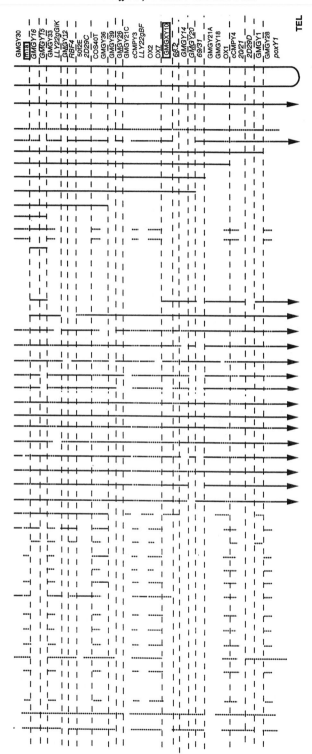

Figure 2B (continued)

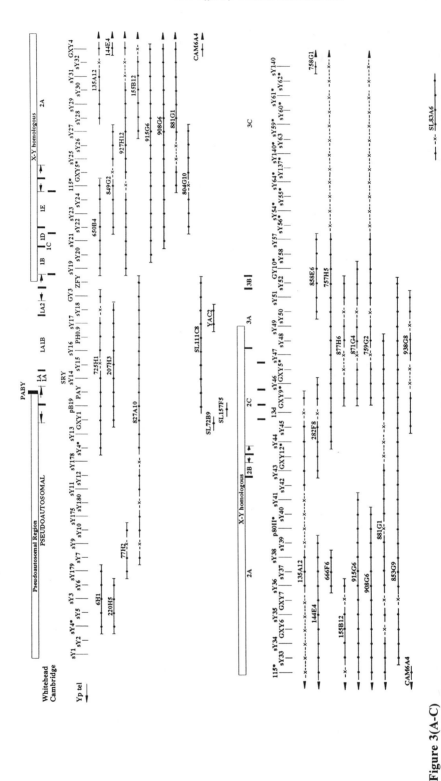

Figure 3(A-C)
Figures A, B and C summarise the STS content analysis of the YAC clones isolated with various Y markers and their assembly into contigs based on this data. A dot represents the presence of an STS in a YAC clone and a cross its absence. Figure 3A covers most of Yp, 3B the centromeric region and 3C the Yq euchromatin. The intervals marked above the contigs summarise the deletion maps derived by Vollrath et al. (1992) and the maps elaborated by the Cambridge group.

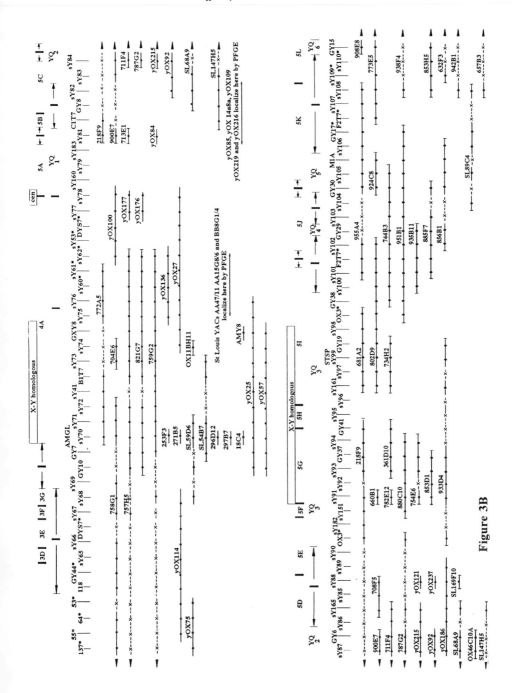

Figure 3B

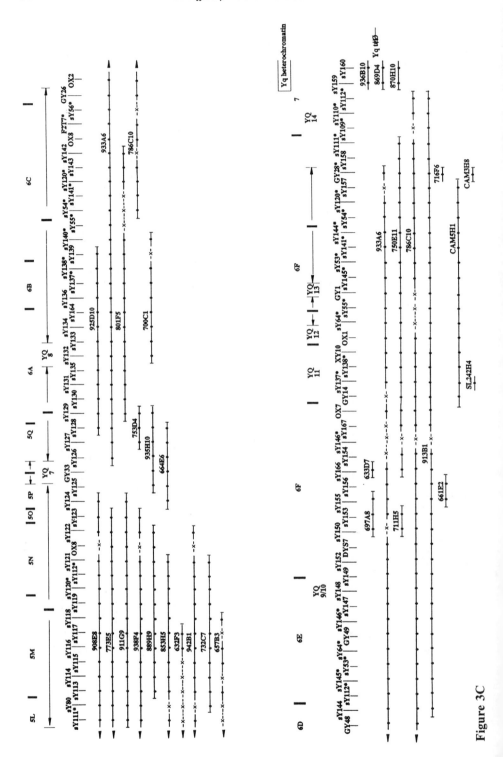

Figure 3C

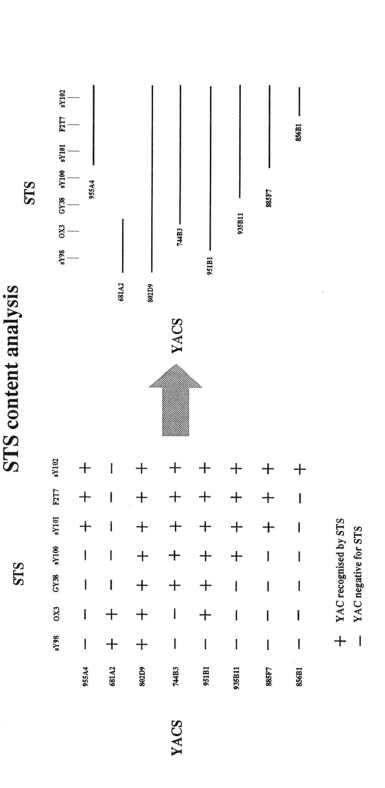

Figure 4

The figure illustrates STS content analysis for a series of YAC clones and the manner in which the overlaps are evaluated.

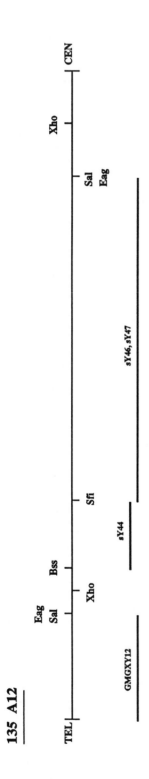

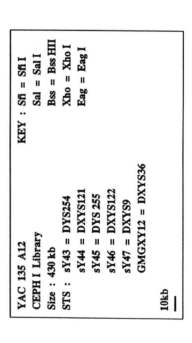

Figure 5
Restriction map of YAC clone mapping to the distal block of X-Y homology on Yp.

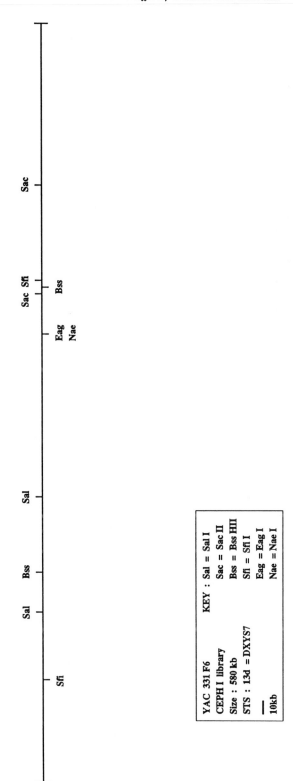

Figure 6
Restriction map of YAC clone mapping to the distal block of X_Y homology on Yp.

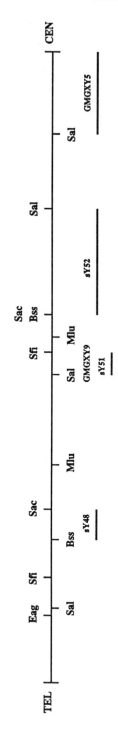

Figure 7
Restriction map of YAC clone mapping to the distal block of X-Y homology on Yp.

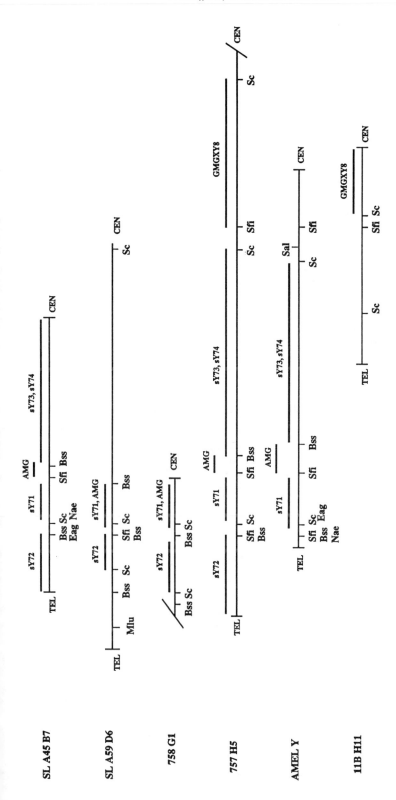

Figure 8
Restriction maps of a series of overlapping YAC clones which cover the proximal block of X-Y homology on Yp.

Summary of YAC contigs

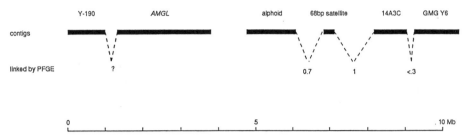

Figure 9

A summary of YAC contigs across the Y centromeric region which have been subjected
to physical restriction analysis presented in figures 10 -14.

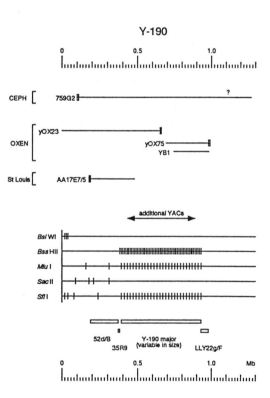

Figure 10

The restriction map of YAC clones in the Y-190 region.

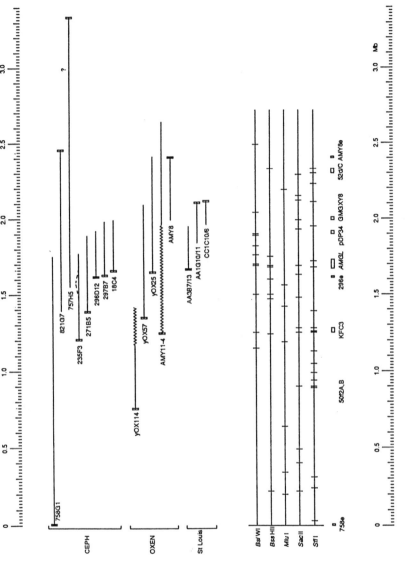

Figure 11
The restriction map of YAC clones in the amelogenin region.

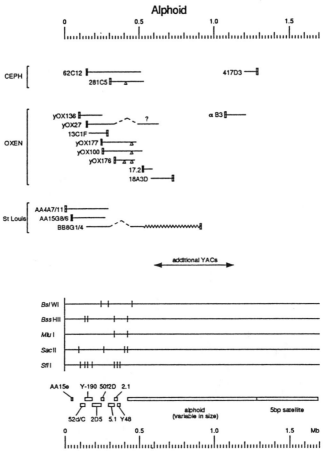

Figure 12
The restriction map of YAC clones which cover the alphoid sequences in the Y
centromere.

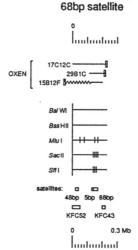

Figure 13
The restriction map of YAC clones in the centromeric region containing 68 bp satellite
DNA.

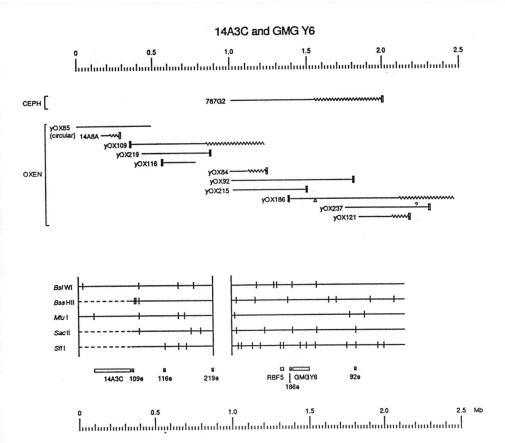

Figure 14

The restriction map of YAC clones located in the Yq centromeric region.

In figures 10 - 14 the zig-zag portion of some YAC clones represents co-ligated segments which are not of Y origin.

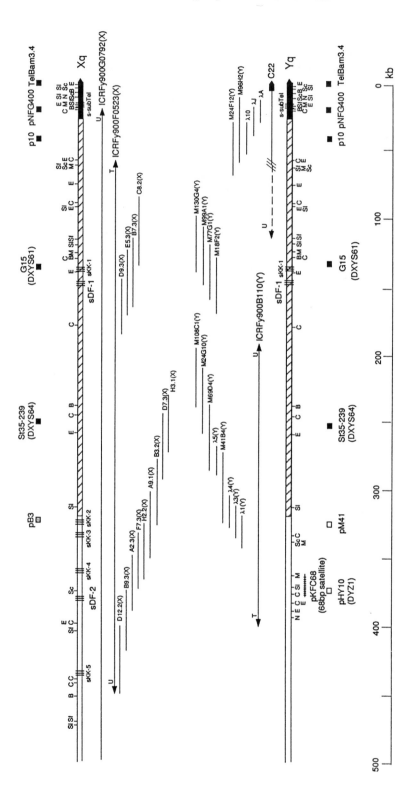

Figure 15

The figure summarises contigs and restriction maps of the Yq and Xq pseudoautosomal regions, the hatched segment representing the extent of strict X-Y homology.

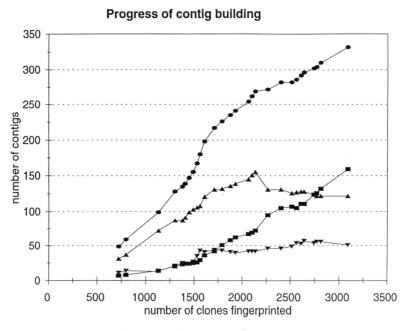

Figure 16
The figure summarises the progress in contig construction from cosmid clones by means of Hinf I finger-print analysis.

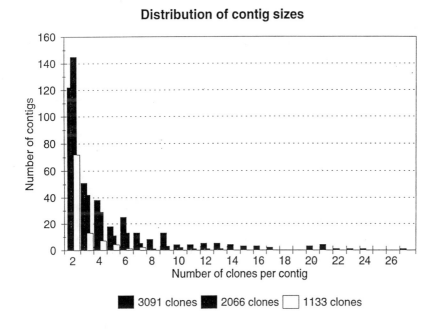

Figure 17
The figure summarises the number of clones in contigs of different size.

Human Genome Analysis Programme
M. Hallen and A. Klepsch (Eds.)
IOS Press, 1995

PHYSICAL, GENETIC AND TRANSCRIPT MAP OF THE JUXTACENTROMERIC REGION OF THE HUMAN X CHROMOSOME LONG ARM (XCEN-XQ21)

A.P. Monaco,
Imperial Cancer Research Fund Laboratories, Oxford, United Kingdom

1. Background information

The goal of the Human Genome Project is to sequence the complete human genome and to identify all the genes, including those responsible for inherited diseases and cancer. This project involves several stages of which the first stage is to construct physical and genetics maps of human chromosomes.

The physical maps are being generated using human DNA fragments cloned in yeast artificial chromosomes (YACs). Contiguous overlapping YAC clones that correspond to megabasepairs (Mb) of DNA are called contigs. The genetic map requires large numbers of highly polymorphic markers that are called microsatellites. The next stage of the project is to isolate new genes from the cloned DNA and to search these genes for mutations which give rise to human inherited diseases and cancers. This process is called positional cloning and has great potential once the gene is isolated for diagnosis and better understanding of the disease and potential therapies.

2. Objectives and primary approaches

The primary objectives of this project were to construct physical, genetic and transcript maps for the juxtacentromeric region of the human X chromosome. The physical maps were generated using YAC clones and the genetic map was generated by isolating new microsatellite polymorphisms from the cloned DNA. The transcript map was constructed using several approaches to isolate new genes from cloned DNA.

Key Words: yeast artificial chromosome (YAC); physical map; genetic map; transcript map; positional cloning.

3. Results and discussion

In the two years of this EC funded project, substantial progress has been made towards the goal of an integrated physical, genetic and transcript map of Xcen-Xq13.3 and this is outlined in Figure 1. The results will be divided into three parts describing the physcial, genetic and transcript maps generated in this project.

3.1. Physical Map

The physical map is based mostly on yeast artificial chromosome (YAC) clones from the ICRF and CEPH libraries. It also involved a close collaboration between the ICRF laboratory and the laboratory of Dr. Hunt Willard (Cleveland, Ohio). The YAC libraries were screened and isolated YACs were subsequently tested by both

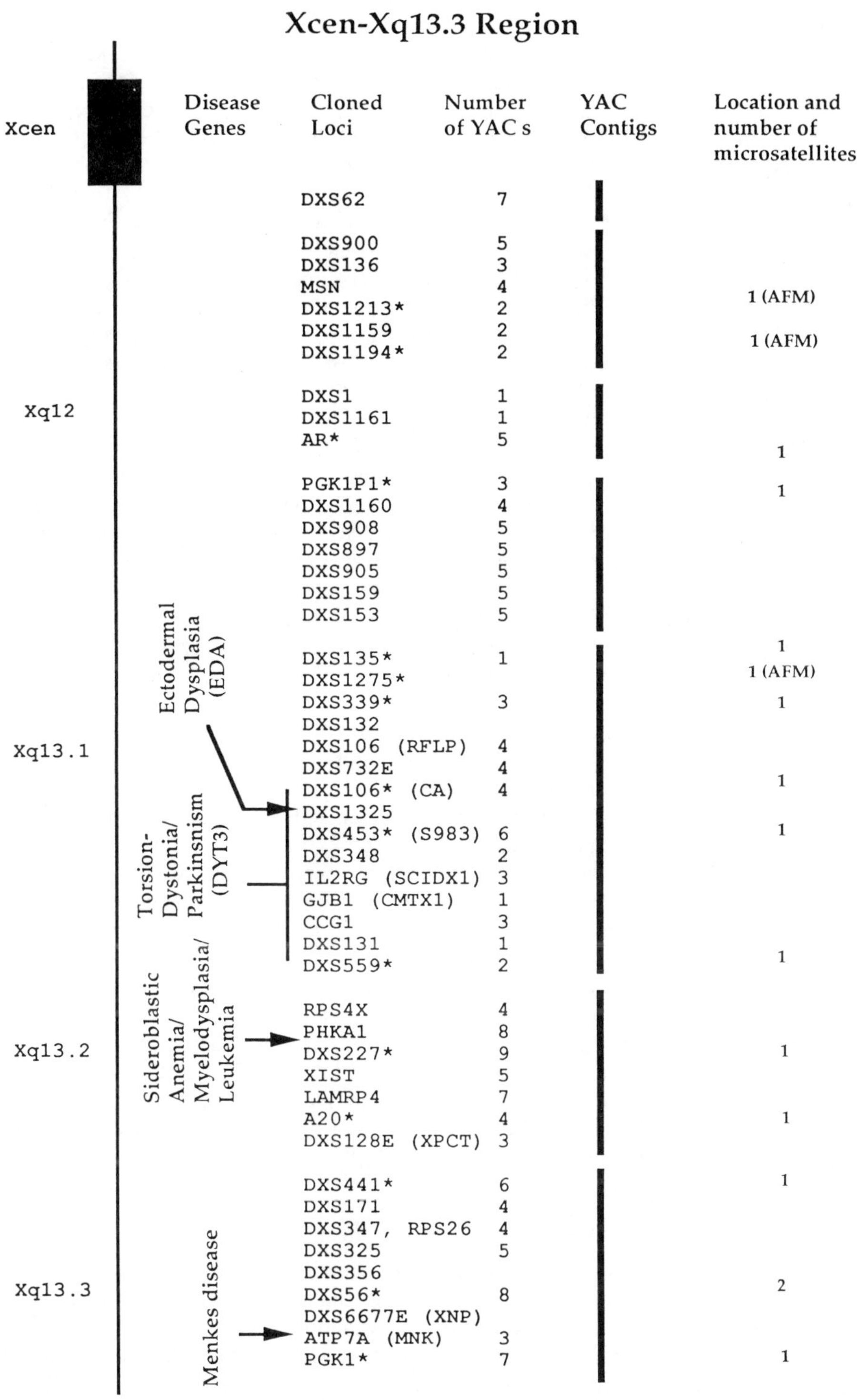

Xcen-Xq13.3 Region

Xcen	Disease Genes	Cloned Loci	Number of YACs	YAC Contigs	Location and number of microsatellites
		DXS62	7		
		DXS900	5		
		DXS136	3		
		MSN	4		1 (AFM)
		DXS1213*	2		
		DXS1159	2		1 (AFM)
		DXS1194*	2		
Xq12		DXS1	1		
		DXS1161	1		
		AR*	5		1
		PGK1P1*	3		1
		DXS1160	4		
		DXS908	5		
		DXS897	5		
		DXS905	5		
		DXS159	5		
		DXS153	5		
	Ectodermal Dysplasia (EDA)				1
		DXS135*	1		1 (AFM)
		DXS1275*			
		DXS339*	3		1
		DXS132			
Xq13.1		DXS106 (RFLP)	4		
		DXS732E	4		
		DXS106* (CA)	4		1
		DXS1325			
	Torsion-Dystonia/ Parkinsnism (DYT3)	DXS453* (S983)	6		1
		DXS348	2		
		IL2RG (SCIDX1)	3		
		GJB1 (CMTX1)	1		
		CCG1	3		
		DXS131	1		
		DXS559*	2		1
	Sideroblastic Anemia/ Myelodysplasia/ Leukemia	RPS4X	4		
		PHKA1	8		
Xq13.2		DXS227*	9		1
		XIST	5		
		LAMRP4	7		
		A20*	4		1
		DXS128E (XPCT)	3		
		DXS441*	6		1
		DXS171	4		
		DXS347, RPS26	4		
		DXS325	5		
Xq13.3	Menkes disease	DXS356			
		DXS56*	8		2
		DXS6677E (XNP)			
		ATP7A (MNK)	3		
		PGK1*	7		1

Figure 1

hybridization and PCR by the ICRF and INSERM labs with 48 available probes from the Xcen-Xq13.3 region. Figure 1 shows the 48 DNA probes and genes used to isolate these YACs and the extent of overlapping YACs forming contigs. Most distally, the ICRF and CEPH YAC libraries produced an approximately 2.1 megabasepair (Mb) contig from PGK1 to DXS441 which is currently submitted for publication (Villard et al., 1994). More proximally, the ICRF, CEPH and St. Louis YAC libraries produced an approximately 3 Mb YAC contig from DXS128E to RPS4X which was a collaborative effort between the ICRF lab and the lab of Hunt Willard (Cleveland, Ohio) and was published (Lafreniere et al., 1992). More proximally, there is a large 4.0 Mb contig covering DXS559 to DXS135 that includes 15 DNA and gene loci. In collaboration with the Willard laboratory, a series of smaller contigs of approximately 1-2 Mb each were isolated for the most proximal loci, DXS159 to DXS62. We estimate that approximately 85% of the region is currently isolated in this set of YAC contigs and there are 6 gaps remaining.

To close the gaps in the present YAC contigs we have used several methods to isolate end fragments from individual YACs to be used to rescreen the ICRF and CEPH YAC libraries. One method is to isolate the YAC from a pulsed field gel, and radioactively label the insert DNA and hybridise this to the ICRF flow-sorted chromosome X cosmid libraries. This has been done successfully for 8 YACs. The cosmids have then been used to define end fragments, to develop genetic markers (Section 2) and to find transcripts using exon amplification (Section 3). The second method was to construct partial digest genomic phage libraries from the total yeast DNA containing the YACs and to screen these with left and right YAC vector arm probes to define end fragments. This has been done successfully for 6 YACs. The resulting phage libraries can also be used to isolate new genetic markers (Section 2) and to find transcripts (Section 3). The final method used was an adapter mediated PCR method called vectorette PCR to develop small PCR products from the ends of YACs. This method worked in about 60% of YACs tested and these small end fragments could be sequenced directly to develop primers for rescreening the YAC library or to screen the ICRF X specific cosmid library to define cosmids near the YAC ends. Although the EC funded project is now completed we will continue to produce end fragments and rescreen the YAC libraries as well as continue to screen the libraries with any new probes which are produced in other labs. We hope to be able to close the remaining gaps in the next year to cover the complete Xcen-Xq13.3 region in overlapping YAC clones.

Many of the YAC clones in the contigs have been mapped by rare cutting restriction enzymes to help define the position of CpG islands and to position the YACs relative to each other in both the ICRF and INSERM laboratories. Nick Fairweather from the Aberdeen lab has spent two years in the ICRF lab mapping YACs in the proximal contigs. Ron Lafreniere in Hunt Willard's lab has made restriction maps of the DXS128E to RPS4X contig and the INSERM and ICRF labs have made maps of the YACs in the distal contig from PGK1 to DXS441.

3.2. Genetic Map

We have used two approaches to develop and map microsatellite polymorphisms in the Xcen-Xq13.3 region (see Figure 1). The first and simplest method was to localise microsatellite markers that had been previously mapped to the general region of Xcen-Xq13.3 or that were recently identified in other labs in the YAC contigs by PCR. These included eleven microsatellites for DXS1213, DXS1194, AR, PGK1P1, DXS135, DXS1275, DXS339, DXS453, DXS559, A20, and DXS441. The recent CEPH marker DXS983 identified the same YACs as the microsatellite marker DXS453. Sue Rider in the ICRF lab has showed that they both identify the same CA repeat by mixing the primers in PCR reactions and hybridizing the products with internal primers (Rider and Monaco, 1993).

The second method was to develop new CA repeat polymorphisms using the YAC clones as the DNA source. Using cosmid or phage clones derived from or identified with the YAC we have developed 5 new CA repeats from this region (Graeber et al, 1992; Fairweather et al., 1993). This included YACs from DXS106, DXS227, DXS56 and PGK1.

All the microsatellite markers that were fine mapped using the YACs or newly derived from the YACs, have been used by the Aberdeen lab to perform genetic linkage analysis in families with X-linked dominant Charcot-Marie-Tooth disease (CMTX1). This analysis as well as data from a large international consortium using these microsatellites has localized CMTX1 to the interval between DXS106 and DXS559 (Cochrane et al., 1994; Pericak-Vance et al., 1994). These same microsatellites have been used by other collaborating labs to further define the localisation of Torsion Dystonia with Parkinsonism (DYT3; Müller et al., 1994) and X-linked severe combined immunodeficiency disease (SCIDX1; Markiewicz et al., 1993). At present, there is fairly good microsatellite coverage of the Xcen-Xq13.3 region. We are currently trying to identify several more highly informative microsatellites in the region between DXS453 and DXS227 to fine map the DYT3 locus.

3.3. Transcript Map

Two methods for identifying transcription units in genomic DNA have greatly aided our progress in this region. The ICRF lab has mostly used exon amplification protocols (Buckler et al., 1991) while the INSERM lab has used a modification of the cDNA selection protocols (Parimoo et al., 1991). We have also used more conventional techniques such as searching for CpG islands and conserved DNA fragments across species. The ICRF lab has isolated the gene responsible for Menkes syndrome (MNK) located between DXS56 and PGK1 (Chelly et al., 1993). This gene is transcribed in all tissues except liver and encodes for a copper transporting ATPase (ATP7A). Closely flanking microsatellite markers are being used by the Aberdeen group to study the inheritance of a family segregating Menkes disease to define those individuals who are at risk of carrying the disease gene.

From this same YAC contig, the INSERM lab has used cDNA selection to isolate four new genes besides MNK and PGK1 and is currently obtaining full length cDNA clones for DNA sequencing (Gecz et al., 1993). One of these genes, XNP, has also been isolated from the mouse and encodes for a potential nuclear transcription factor, mainly expressed in brain and skeletal muscle (Gecz et al., 1994). They have extended the transcriptional map more proximally and have isolated two new genes and one cDNA that encodes for a known ribosomal protein (RPS26, Villard et al., submitted). The INSERM laboratory have used a novel method of cDNA selection using as templates Alu-PCR products generated from YAC clones.

In the central 3 Mb YAC contig from DXS128E to RPS4X, the Willard lab has identified one new gene near DXS128E that extends over 125 Kb that encodes for a PEST domain containing transporter (XCPT). The ICRF lab is currently searching for transcripts near the DXS227 locus in this contig. In this region they have mapped, in collaboration with Veronica Buckle's lab, two isodicentric chromosome breakpoints associated with acute myleoid leukemia with ringed sideroblasts (Rack et al., 1994). Sue Rider in the ICRF lab has constructed a cosmid contig across 400 kb of this region where there are several CpG islands and she is currently searching for new genes.

In the proximal YAC contigs near DXS106 and DXS453 the ICRF lab has identified the translocation breakpoint in a female with hypohydrotic ectodernal dysplasia (EDA) in collaboration with Nick Thomas and Jonathan Zonana (Thomas et al., 1993). We are currently searching for new genes in cosmids from this breakpoint region using exon amplification and cDNA selection. The gene seems to map over 150 kb when the location of translocations and deletions in EDA patients are analysed relative to the cloned DNA in YACs and cosmids.

The Aberdeen group and the ICRF group have collaborated on the identification of the gene responsible for X-linked dominant Charcot-Marie-Tooth neuropathy (CMTX1). They have used twelve highly polymorphic markers in the Xcen-Xq21 region to study a set of families segregating CMTX1.

From the recombination events they could limit the gene between DXS106 and DXS559 (Cochrane et al., 1994). In this region the gene for connexin 32 (GJB1), had been mapped in the YAC contig. This gene encodes a possible gap junction protein which is known to be expressed at high levels in liver and a wide range of other mammalian tissues. They have sequenced the coding region of exon 2 of the GJB1 gene from affected individuals in twelve families with CMTX1 and have found point mutations which segregate with the disease in eleven of these families (Fairweather et al., 1994). The mutations detected include missence point mutations at codons 15, 40, 56, 60, 63, 208, and 215, a nonsense mutation at codon 220, deletions of one base in codon 72/73 producing a stop codon 12 codons downstream and a three base pair deletion which can be predicted to result in the loss of a single amino acid. These findings are consistent with the disease CMTX1 being the result of mutations affecting the gene connexin 32 (GJB1). The multiplicity of mutations detected in this gene in CMTX1 patients are consistent with the hypothesis that individual new mutations have occurred to account for the various families. In addition, the mutations detected are spread around the gene and include amino acid substitutions in the membrane spanning regions, in the extracellular domain and in the carboxy terminal region in the intracellular domain. While it is hypothesised that connexin 32 is a component of a gap junction protein, others have suggested that it may in fact be a membrane adhesion molecule with another gene Ductin coding for the gap junction protein. It is possible that the finding of mutations in this gene in CMTX1 may help to resolve this debate.

Both the ICRF and INSERM labs will continue to search for new genes in the Xcen-Xq13.3 region using exon amplification and cDNA selection. This continued development of the transcription map of this region should be important for the large number of X-linked mental retardation loci that have been mapped to the region.

4. Summary

We have made substantial progress to construct an integrated physical, genetic and transcript map of the Xcen-Xq13.3 region. Approximately 85% of the region is covered in existing YAC clones and end fragments are being rescreened on the ICRF and CEPH YAC libraries to close the six remaining gaps. There are 16 microsatellites in the region, 5 of which were newly derived and 11 of which were fine mapped using the YAC clones. These new genetic markers and refined localizations are being used by the X chromosome community to make a high resolution genetic map and to define the position of several disease genes such as X-linked mental retardation and DYT3. The transcript map was initially focused on chromosome breakpoints giving rise to Menkes disease (MNK), EDA and AML with sideroblasts. We have now identified many new genes in the region using more comprehensive methods such as exon amplification and cDNA selection. The integrated map that has been developed in this project will continue to be useful in the mapping of new genes in the region that are identified in other labs.

5. Major Scientific breakthroughs and/or industrial applications

The major breakthroughs of the project were the construction of YAC contigs for 85% of the region, the generation of a dense microsatellite genetic map, the identification of 8 new genes, the precise mapping of 6 disease loci and the isolation by positional cloning of the genes for Menkes disease and Charcot-Marie-Tooth neuropathy.

6. Major Cooperative links

The major links were:
1) The frequent exchange (monthly to bimonthly) of mapping data between the ICRF, INSERM and Aberdeen laboratories to develop the integrated map.
2) The training of a student, Nicholas Fairweather, from the Aberdeen laboratory for two years in the ICRF laboratory on physical mapping and positional cloning techniques.
3) The productive collaboration with Dr. Hunt Willard's laboratory (Cleveland, Ohio) in the construction of the physical map.
4) Many collaborations of all three participants with other laboratories to use the genetic, physical and transcript map developed from this project in the search for disease genes; these include Dr. U. Müller, Giessen for torsion dystonia-Parkinsonism (DYT3), Dr. G. de Saint-Basile, Paris for severe combined immunodeficiency disease (SCIDX1), Dr. V. Buckle, Oxford for AML/sideroblastic anemia, Drs J. Zonana, Portland and N. Thomas, Cardiff for ectodermal dysplasia (EDA), Dr. N. Horn, Glostrup, Denmark and Dr. G. Romeo, Genoa, Italy for Menkes disease (MNK) and Drs. C. Schwartz, North Carolina and C Moraine, Tours for X-linked mental retardation.

References

- Tümer Z., Chelly J., Tommerup N., Ishikawa-Brush Y., Tønnesen T., Monaco A.P., Horn N. Characterization of a 1.0 Mb YAC contig spanning two chromosome breakpoints related to Menkes disease. Hum. Mol. Genet. 1992; 1:483-489.
- Chelly J., Tymer Z., Tønnesen T., Petterson A., Ishikawa-Brush Y., Tommerup N., Horn N., Monaco A.P. Isolation of a candidate gene for Menkes disease which encodes for a potential heavy metal binding protein. Nature Genet. 1993; 3:14-19.
- Fairweather N., Chelly J., Monaco A.P. Dinucleotide repeat polymorphisms from DXS106 and DXS227 YACs using a two stage approach. Hum. Mol. Genet. 1993; 2:607-608.
- Markiewicz S., DiSanto J.P., Chelly J., Fairweather N., Le Marec B., Griscelli C., Graeber M.B., Myller U., Fischer A., Monaco A.P., de Saint Basile G. Fine mapping of the human SCIDX1 locus at Xq12-13. Hum. Mol. Genet. 1993; 2: 651-654.
- Lafreniére R.G., Brown C.J., Rider S., Chelly J., Taillon-Miller P., Chinault A.C., Monaco A.P., Willard H.F. 2.6 Mb YAC contig of the human X inactivation center region in Xq13: Physical linkage of the RPS4X, PHKA1, XIST and DXS128E genes. Hum. Mol. Genet. 1993; 2:1105-1115.
- Rider S.H. and Monaco A.P. Primers for the dinucleotide repeat at the DXS453 locus also recognizes the DXS983 locus. Hum. Mol. Genet. 1993; 2:1510.

- Thomas N.S.T., Chelly J., Zonana J., Davies K.J.P., Morgan S., Gault J., Rack K., Buckle V., Brockdorff N., Clarke A., Monaco A.P. Characterization of molecular DNA rearrangements within the Xq12-q13.1 region, in three patients with X-linked hypohidrotic ectodermal dysplasia (EDA). Hum. Mol. Genet. 1993; 2:1679-1686.
- Reed V., Rider S., Maslen G.L., Hatchwell E., Blair H.J., Uwechue I.C., Craig I.W., Laval S.H., Monaco A.P., Boyd Y. A 2Mb YAC contig encompassing three loci (DXF34, DXS14 and DXS390) which lie between Xp11.2 translocation breakpoints associated with incontinentia pigmenti type1. Genomics 1994; 20:341-346.
- Cochrane S., Bergoffen J., Fairweather N.D., Müller E., Mostaccuiolo M., Monaco A.P., Fischbeck K.H., Haites N.E. X-linked Charcot-Marie-Tooth disease (CMTX1): a study of 15 families with 12 highly informative polymorphisms. J. Med. Genet. 1994; 31:193-196.
- Rack K.A., Chelly J., Gibbons R.J., Rider S., Benjamin D., Lafreniére R.G,. Oscier D., Hendricks R.W., Craig I.W., Willard H.F., Monaco A.P., Buckle V.J. Lack of XIST expression from late-replicating isodicentric X chromosomes. Hum. Mol. Genet. 1994; 3:1053-105.
- Müller U., Haberhausen G., Wagner T., Fairweather N.D., Chelly J. and Monaco A.P., DXS106 and DXS559 flank the X-linked dystonia-parkinsonism syndrome (XDP) locus. Genomics 1994; 23:114-117.
- George A.M., Reed V., Glenister P., Chelly J., Tymer Z., Horn N., Monaco A.P., Boyd Y. Analysis of Mnk, the murine homologue of Menkes' disease in normal and mottled mice. Genomics 1994; 22:27-35.
- Fairweather N., Bell C., Cochrane S., Chelly J., Wang S.-P., Mostaccuiolo M.L., Monaco A.P., Haites N.E. Mutations in the connexin 32 gene in X-linked dominant Charcot-Marie-Tooth disease (CMTX1). Hum. Mol. Genet. 1994; 3:29-34.
- Pericak-Vance M.A., Barker D.F., Bergoffen J., Chance P., Cochrane S., Dahl N., Exler M.-C., Fain P.R., Fairweather N.D., Fischbeck K., Gal A., Haites N., Ionasescu R., Ionasescu V.V., Kennerson M.L., Monaco A.P., Mostaccuiolo M., Nicholson G.A., Sillén A., Haines J.L. Consortium fine localisation of X-linked Charcot-Marie-Tooth disease (CMTX1): Additional support that connexin is the defect in CMTX1. Human Heredity 1994; (in press).
- Stafford A.N., Rider S.H., Hopkins J.M., Cookson W.O., Monaco A.P. A 2.8 Mb YAC contig in 11q12-q13 localizes candidate genes for atopy: FcER1§ and CD20. Hum. Mol. Genet. 1994; 3:779-785.
- Consalez G., Gecz J., Stayton C.L., Dabovic B., Pasini B., Pezzolo A., Bicocchi P., Fontes M., Romeo G. Characterization and subcloning of a 400 Kb region spanning the translocation breakpoint associated with Menkes syndrome in a female patient. Genomics 1992; 14:562-567.
- Gecz J., Villard L., Lossi A.M., Millasseau P., Djabali M., Fontes. Physical mapping and transcriptional mapping of DXS56-PGK1 1 Mb region:identification of three new transcripts. Hum. Mol. Genet. 1993; 2:1389-1396.
- Villard L., Gecz J., Lossi A.M., Fontes M. Progress toward the construction of a YAC contig covering the whole Xq13.3 sub-band. Cytogenet. Cell Genet. 1993; 64:177.
- Gecz J., Villard L., Lossi A.M., Fontes M. Construction of a transcriptional map of the DXS56-PGK1 1Mbp region via direct cDNA selection approach. Cytogenet. Cell Genet. 1993; 64:178.
- Gecz J., Villard L., Lossi A.M., Fontes M. Direct cDNA selection using human and mouse cDNAs: application to Xq13.3 chromosomal region. Proceedings of the 3rd International Workshop on the Identification of Transcribed Sequences, Plenum Press 1994.
- Gecz J., Polard H., Consalez G., Villard L., Stayton C., Millasseau P., Khrestchatisky M., Fontes M. Cloning and expression of a murine homologue of a human X-linked nuclear protein gene close to PGK1 (Xq13.3). Hum. Mol. Genet. 1994; 3:39-44.
- Villard L., Gecz J., Colleaux L., Lossi A.M., Chelly J., Ishikawa-Brush Y., Monaco AP, Fontes M. Construction of an Xq13.3 physical and transcriptional map using Alu-PCR products for cDNA selection. 1994; (submitted).

Contract number: GENO-CT91-0017
Contractual period: 1 January 1991 to 31 December 1993

Coordinator
Dr. Anthony P. Monaco
Imperial Cancer Research Fund Laboratories
Institute of Molecular Medicine
John Radcliffe Hospital
Headington, Oxford OX3 9DU
United Kingdom
Tel: 44 865 222 371
Fax: 44 865 222 431

Participants
Dr. Michel Fontes
INSERM Unit 242
Faculté de Médecin
27 Boulevard Jean Moulin
13385 Marseille Cedex 5
France
Tel: 33 9178 4477
Fax: 33 9180 4319

Dr. Neva Haites
Medical Genetics Laboratories
Department of Molecular and Cell Biology
Medical School Building
University of Aberdeen
Foresterhill
Aberdeen AB9 2ZD
United Kingdom
Tel: 44 224 681 818 ext 53008
Fax: 44 224 685 157

Human Genome Analysis Programme
M. Hallen and A. Klepsch (Eds.)
IOS Press, 1995

PHYSICAL MAPPING OF THE LONG ARM OF CHROMOSOME 22

G. Thomas
Institut Curie, Paris, France

1. Background information

Chromosome 22 is the second smallest chromosome. Its long arm amounts to approximately 1.5% of the whole human genome (35 to 40 Megabase pairs). Possibly because of its high content in R-bands which are known to be rich in coding sequences, this chromosome segment is involved in many pathologies. Inherited diseases with no known cytogenetic anomalies include enzymopathies and predisposition to neuronal tumor development. Diseases associated with cytogenetically visible chromosome 22 alterations are frequent and comprise both constitutional anomalies and aberrations acquired by neoplastic cells during tumorigenesis. They include interstitial deletions such as those almost always found in the proximal part in DiGeorge syndrome patients. Chromosome 22 is also frequently altered in the tumorigenic process being subjected to balanced translocation in the Ewing's family of tumors (i.e.: Ewing's sarcoma, peripheral neuroepithelioma, Askin's tumors..) or to deletions in a large variety of tumors, primarily meningiomas and schwannomas. When the project was initiated none of the genes involved in these processes were known. Thus a physical map of this comparatively small part of the genome was expected not only to contribute to the knowledge of the structure of a whole chromosome arm but also to lead rapidly to the isolation of a number of presently unknown genes involved in human pathologies.

2. Objectives and primary approaches

The overall aim of the project was to create large contiguous arrays of genomic clones on chromosome 22, through a collaboration including 3 European laboratories. Two laboratories (London, Paris) were directly funded by the EC, while the third (Stockholm) was funded through the Swedish medical research council. A strategy for the generation of ordered arrays of overlapping clones covering the chromosome 22 long arm was to be developed based on the use of a common set of chromosome 22 specific cosmids, a panel of somatic cell hybrids which distinguishes 30 different subregions on the long arm of chromosome 22 and a large number of single copy probes. In this process, genes involved in chromosome alterations associated with human pathologies were to be identified by positional cloning.

3. Results and discussion

3.1 Mapping Loci and Expansion into Cosmids4

Single copy, small insert clones were obtained from several sources. In the London group, 55 clones from the proximal third of the long arm of chromosome 22 were mapped by somatic cell hybrid analysis. Some probes detected more than one locus on

22, especially when low stringency hybridizations were used. This work, and fluorescent in situ hybridization (FISH) studies indicated that many clones thought to detect "single copy" loci do, in fact, cross hybridise with low-copy-repeat sequences distributed throughout 22q11. This remarkable feature of 22q11 has implications for genome stability in the region. For this reason, several clones map into more than one subregion defined by the panel of somatic cell hybrids. In Paris two groups of mapping experiments have been performed using the panel of somatic cell hybrids. First using the conventional Southern technique, 150 new single copy probes have been localized precisely within one of 30 different subregions of chromosome 22. An additional 45 loci containing Not1 restriction fragment (linking clones) have been mapped in collaboration with the group of Dr. G. Rouleau (Montreal). Second the development of a PCR technology on DNAs extracted from somatic cell hybrids has enabled the mapping of 13 highly polymorphic probes previously mapped to chromosome 22 by cosegregation studies in CEPH pedigrees. FISH experiments were developed and enabled a precise and independent mapping of many of these loci.

A gridded array of cosmids in microtiter well dishes was obtained from the Lawrence Livermore laboratories in California. In the three collaborating laboratories, a Biomeck 1000 robot was used to create filters representing the library. These filters were used to isolate cosmids from the small insert clones previously studied. In London, cosmid coordinate sets corresponding to 54 clones have been identified, some of these including low-copy-repeat members. In Paris a total of 17 independent small single copy probes were successfully used to screen the gridded libraries. In each case, overlapping cosmids were retrieved and their location were verified by FISH.

3.2 Physical mapping

A physical map of the chromosome 22q12 region was constructed by the Stockholm group using pulsed-field gel electrophoresis, fluorescence *in situ* suppression hybridization and somatic cell hybrids. This map spans five megabase-pairs of genomic DNA and includes 26 previously isolated markers and genes including VIIIF2, Ewing's sarcoma translocation breakpoint, NEFH, LIF, OSM and SCH/NF2 genes. The map contains one discontinuity dividing the restriction map into two separate fragments.

3.3 Genomic clone walking

In Paris, 9 cloned loci that had been identified in the region flanked by D22S1 and D22S15 were progressively expanded by the recurrent isolation of overlapping cosmids from the gridded libraries. In this process several contigs were connected so that a total of 7 large cosmid contigs was finally obtained. Four of them were in close proximity. Isolation of yeast artificial chromosomes and/or Southern analysis of total human DNA provided an estimate of the sizes of the gaps between these 4 contigs. They were 0.5 kb, 10 kb and 100 kb. The distance between the two flanking markers for the neuro-fibromatosis type 2 gene, D22S212 and D22S32, could be estimated and was shown to be about one million base pairs. Thus in the D22S1-S22S15 region a total of close to 1.7 megabase was cloned into cosmid contigs.

In Stockholm, a combined cosmid and YAC contig was constructed spanning part of the 22q12 physical map. The contig consists of 6 YAC's and two separate cosmid contigs of 40 continuous steps. The total cosmid contigs encompass more than 900 kb. Similar contigs and PFGE maps have been constructed in more telomeric regions of the chromosome.

In London, the initial intention was to proceed entirely by cosmid walking. However, because of the problems of low-copy-repeat units cosmid contigs in the proximal region of 22q were small. However, the availability of YAC libraries changed the overall strategy slightly. The work in YACs was undertaken in collaboration with J. Collins, I. Dunham and D. Bentley at the Sanger Center, Cambridge. Some large contigs were constructed e.g. around approximately 4 Mb encompassing the IGL region as far proximally as D22S264 (in the DiGeorge critical region). The DiGeorge syndrome critical region or DGCR, was shown based on FISH studies to be at least 2Mb in length. In this region three contigs covering 1.6Mb were constructed. However, this region has proved difficult to clone in standard vectors and therefore cosmids and P1 clones have been employed. In the latest attempt to fill the gaps, PAC and BAC libraries were screened and the positives clones are presently being characterized. Within the YAC contigs, there are three large cosmid contigs ranging in size from 150 to 200 Kb. In addition, cosmid pools have been developed from some YACs e.g.: IGL YACs, which should enable construction of a whole cosmid contigs in the future.

3.4 Gene identification

The large 1.5 megabase contig constructed in the D22S1/D22S15 region was shown to contain three genes previously known to reside on chromosome 22.: the neurofilament heavy chain gene (NFH), the leukaemia inhibiting factor (LIF) and the oncostatin M gene (ONM). In addition, two new genes that are relevant to human pathology were identified in this region. First, a gene located in the proximal region of the contig and termed EWS was shown to be recurrently involved in chromosome translocations in Ewing's sarcoma, peripheral neuroepithelioma and related tumours. More recently EWS was also shown to be systematically altered in Malignant Melanoma of Soft Parts. The second gene, termed SCH, was identified in collaboration with the group of Dr. Rouleau (Montreal). Alterations in this gene were shown to be associated with neurofibromatosis type 2, a genetic disease which predisposes to the development of tumours from the nervous system. This gene is inactivated by a two hit process in schwannomas and meningiomas suggesting that it is a tumor suppressor gene. In Stockholm, using exon amplification, a new expressed gene (pK12.3) with a cDNA of 2.7 kb was isolated in the same region. The gene has no marked homologies with previously sequenced genes and encompasses an open reading frame coding for a protein of predicted molecular weight 78.5 kD.

In the proximal region, several coding sequences have been identified and isolated from the genomic clone. The genes T10 and TUPLE1 lie in the region recurrently deleted in DiGeorge syndrome patients. The latter is a candidate gene to take part in the expression of the disease phenotype. A further four transcribed sequences are being characterized.

3.5 Major scientific breakthroughs

This work has contributed to our basic understanding of human carcinogenesis by enabling the isolation of two genes of major importance. The EWS gene which is systematically altered in the family of Ewing tumors and in malignant melanoma of soft parts. EWS has recently been shown by others to be also recurrently altered in desmoplastic tumors. These alterations are believed to be instrumental in the development of these aggressive cancers, by generating aberrant transcription factors. The SCH/NF2 gene when altered causes neurofibromatosis. This gene encodes a product likely to play a role in connecting membrane proteins and cytoskeletal components.

The work has also provided reagents of diagnostic interests which have been distributed to many research and diagnostic laboratories. These reagents include

1. cosmids that flank the Ewing's sarcoma breakpoint and which are of major interest in the diagnosis of Ewing's sarcoma, a tumor well known to be a difficult diagnosis to the pathologist.
2. cosmids useful in the cytogenetic demonstration of chromosome 22 alterations in germline or tumours using the FISH technology. These cosmids allow in many instances precise diagnosis of De George syndrome.

On a more fundamental ground, the physical maps that have been constructed should lead, in the near future, to the isolation of the genes that are responsible for the DiGeorge syndrome.

Finally, the numerous cloned DNA fragments that have been precisely mapped on the long arm of chromosome 22 by the 3 cooperating laboratories are a valuable source of reagents to physical mapping, positional cloning and characterization of chromosome 22 rearrangements at the constitutional or tumor level.

4. Major cooperative links

The cooperation has been mainly performed through the sharing of common reagents. The three groups have used a common set of somatic cell hybrids, common chromosome 22 specific libraries and many common chromosome 22 specific probes. The sharing of this material and informations generated from it has speeded up the physical mapping of large regions of the long arm of chromosome 22. More specifically, it has provided a decisive advantage in the isolation of genomic regions implicated in human diseases. The number of joint publications testifies the usefulness of this cooperation.

Joint/individual publications

1992

1. Individual publications

Paris group

1. Aubry M., Marineau C., Zhang F., Zahed L., Figlewicz D., Delattre O., Thomas G., De Jong P., Julien J.P. and Rouleau G. Cloning of six new genes with zinc finger motifs mapping to the short and long arms of human acrocentric chromosome 22 (p and q11.2). Genomics 13:641-643, 1992.
2. Delattre O., Zucman J., Plougastel B., Desmaze C., Melot T., Peter M., Kovar H., Joubert I., De Jong P., Rouleau G., Aurias A. and Thomas G. Gene fusion with an ETS domain caused by chromosome translocation in human tumours. Nature 359:162-165, 1992.
3. Desmaze C., Zucman J., Delattre O., Thomas G. and Aurias A. In situ hybridization of PCR amplified inter-Alu sequences from a hybrid cell line. Hum Genet 88:541-544, 1992.
4. Desmaze C., Zucman J., Delattre O., Thomas G. and Aurias A. Unicolor and bicolor in situ hybridization in the diagnosis of peripheral neuroepithelioma and related tumors. Gene Chromosome Cancer 5:30-34, 1992.
5. Levy A., Zucman J., Delattre O., Mattei M-G., Rio M-C. and Basset P. Assignment of the human stromelysin-36 gene to the q11.2 region of chromosome 22. Genomics 13:881-883, 1992.
6. Zucman J., Delattre O., Desmaze C., Azambuja C.J., Rouleau G., De Jong P., Aurias A. and Thomas G. Rapid isolation of cosmids from defined subregions by differential Alu-PCR hybridization on chromosome 22 specific library. Genomics 13:395-401, 1992.
7. Zucman J., Delattre O., Desmaze C., Plougastel B., Joubert I., Melot T., Peter M., De Jong P., Rouleau G., Aurias A. and Thomas G. Cloning and characterization of the Ewing's sarcoma and

peripheral neuroepithelioma t(11;22) translocation breakpoints. Genes Chromosome Cancer 5:271-277, 1992.

London group

1. Carey A.H., Claussen U., Ludecke H-J., Horsthemke B., Ellis D., Oakey H., Wilson D., Burn J., Williamson R. and Scambler P.J. Interstitial deletions in DiGeorge syndrome detected with microclones from 22q11. Mammalian Genome, 3:101-105, 1992.
2. Sharkey A.M., McLaren L., Carroll M., Fantes J., Green D., Wilson D., Scambler P.J. and Evans H.J. Isolation of anonymous DNA markers for human chromosome 22q11 from a flow sorted library, and mapping using hybrids from patients with DiGeorge syndrome. Hum Genet, 89: 73-78, 1992.

Stockholm group

1. Stenman G., Sahlin P., Dumanski J.P., Hagiwara K., Ishikawa F., Miyazono K., Collins V.P., Helding C.H. Regional localization of the human platelet-derived endothelial cell growth factor (ECGF1) gene to chromosome 22q13. Cytogent Cell Genet, 59:22-3, 1992.

2. Joint publications

1. Carey A.H., Kelly D., Halford S., Wadey R., Wilson D., Goodship J., Burn J., Paul T., Sharkey A., Dumanski J., Nordenskjold M., Williamson R. and Scambler P.J. Molecular genetic study of the frequency of monosomy 22q11 in DiGeorge syndrome. Am J Hum Genet 51:964-970, 1992.

1993

1. Individual publications

Paris group

1. Desmaze C., Prieur M., Amblard F., Aïkem M., Ledeist F., Demszuk S., Zucman J., Plougastel B., Delattre O., Croquette M.F., Brevière G.M., Huon C., Le Merrer M., Mathieu M., Sidi D., Stephan J.L. and Aurias A. Physical mapping by FISH of the DiGeorge critical region (DGCR): involvement of the region in familial cases. Am J Hum Genet 53:1239-1249, 1993.
2. Figlewicz D.A., Delattre O., Guellaen G., Krizus A., Thomas G., Zucman J. and Rouleau G. Mapping of human gamma-glutamyl transpeptidase genes on chromosome 22 and other human autosomes. Genomics 17:299-305, 1993.
3. Lamour V., Levy N., Desmaze C., Baud V., Lecluse Y., Delattre O., Berheim, A., Thomas G., Aurias A. and Lipinski M. Isolation of cosmids and fetal brain cDNAs from the proximal long arm of human chromosome 22. Hum Mol Genet 2:535-540, 1993.
4. Marineau C., Baron C., Delattre O., Zucman J., Thomas G. and Rouleau G. Dinucleotide repeat polymorphism at the D22S268 locus. Hum Mol Genet 3:336-336, 1993.
5. Sanson M., Marineau C., Desmaze C., Luchtman M., Baron C., Narod S., Delattre O., Lenoir G., Thomas G., Aurias A. and Rouleau G. Germ-line deletion in a neurofibromatosis type 2 kindred inactivates the NF2 gene and a candidate meningioma locus. . Hum Mol Genet 2:1215-1220, 1993.
6. Sanson M., Zhang F., Demczuk S., Delattre O., De Jong P., Aurias A., Thomas G. and Rouleau G. Isolation and mapping of 45 Not 1 linking clones to chromosome 22. Genomics 17:776-779, 1993.
7. Zucman J., Delattre O., Desmaze C., Epstein A.L., Stenman G., Speleman F., Fletchers C., Aurias A. and Thomas G. EWS and ATF-1 gene fusion induced by t(12;22) translocation in malignant melanoma of soft parts. Nature Genetics 4:341-345, 1993.
8. Zucman J., Melot T., Desmaze C., Ghysdael J., Plougastel B., Peter M., Zucker J.M., Triche T., Sheer D., Turc-Carel C., Ambros P., Combaret V., Lenoir G., Aurias A., Thomas G. and Delattre O. Combinatorial generation of variable fusion proteins in the Ewing family of tumours. EMBO J 12:4481-4487, 1993.

London group

1. Halford S., Lindsay E., Nayudu M., Carey A.H., Baldini A., Scambler P.J. Low-copy-rpeat sequences flank the DiGeorge/velo-cardio-facial syndrome loci at 22q11. Hum Mol Genet 2: 191-196, 1993.
2. Halford S., Wadey R., Roberts C., Daw S.C.M., Whiting J.A., O'Donnell H., Dunham I., Bentley D., Lindsay E., Baldini A., Francis F., Lehrach H., Williamson R. Wilson D.I., Goodship J., Cross I., Burn J. and Scambler P.J. Isolation of a putative transcriptional regulator from the region of 22q11 deleted in DiGeorge syndrome, Shprintzen syndrome and familial congenital heart disease. Hum Molec Genet 2:2099-2107, 1993.
3. Halford S., Wilson D.I., Daw S.C.M., Roberts C., Wadey R., Kamath S., Wickremasinghe A., Burn J., Goodship J., Mattei M-G., Moorman A.F.M. and Scambler P.J. Isolation of a gene expressed during early embryogenesis from the region of 22q11 commonly deleted in DiGeorge syndrome. Hum Molec Genet 2:1577-1582, 1993.
4. Lindsay E.A., Halford S., Wadey R., Scambler P.J., Baldini A.: Molecular cytogenetic characterisation of the DiGeorge syndrome region using fluorescence in situ hybridisation. Genomics, 17:403-7, 1993.
5. Wadey R., Daw S., Wickremasinghe A., Roberts C., Wilson D., Goodship J., Burn J., Halford S. and Scambler P.J. Isolation of a new marker and conserved sequences close to the DiGeorge syndrome marker HP500 (D22S134). J Med Genet, 30:818-21, 1993.

Stockholm group

1. Ruttledge M.H., Narod S.A., Dumanski J.D., Parry D.M., Eldridge M.D, Weterlecki W., Parboosingh J., Faucher M.C., Lenoir D.V.M., Collins V.P., Nordenskjöl M.and Rouleau G.A. Pre-symptomatic diagnosis for neurofibromatosis 2 with chromosome 22 markers. Neurology, 43:1753-60, 1993.
2. Xie L-G., Han F-Y , Peyrard M., Ruttledge M., Fransson M., DeJong P., Collins V.P., Duham I., Nordenskjöl M. Dumanski J.P. Cloning of a novel, anonymous gene from a megabase-range YAC and cosmid contig in the neurofibromatosis type 2/meningioma region on human chromosome 22q12. Human Mol Genet, 2:1361-8, 1993.

2. Joint publications

1. Bijlsma E., Delattre O., Juyn J.A., Melot T., Westerveld A., Dumanski J., Thomas G. and Hulsebos T.J.M. Regional fine mapping of the beta crystallin genes on chromosome 22 excludes these genes as physically linked markers for neurofibromatosis type 2. Genes Chromosome Cancer 8:112-118, 1993.
2. Desmaze C., Scambler P., Prieur M., Halford S., Sidi D., Ledeist F. and Aurias A. Routine diagnosis of DiGeorge syndrome by fluorescent in situ hybridization. Hum Genet 90:663-665, 1993.
3. Rose T.M., Lagrou M.J., Fransson I., Werelius B., Delattre O., Thomas G., De Jong P., Torado G.J. and Dumanski J. The genes for onconstantin M (OSM) and leukemia inhibitory factor (LIF) are tightly linked on human chromosome 22. Genomics 17:136-140, 1993.
4. Rouleau G., Merel P., Lutchman M., Sanson M., Zucman J., Marineau C., Hoang-Xuan K., Demczuk S., Desmaze C., Plougastel B., Pulst S., Lenoir G., Bijlsma E., Fashold R., Dumanski J., De Jong P., Parry D., Eldrige R., Aurias A., Delattre O. and Thomas G. Alteration in a new gene encoding a putative membrane-organizing protein causes neuro-fibromatosis type 2. Nature 363:515-521, 1993.

1994

1. Individual publications

Paris group

1. Bailly R.A., Bosselut R., Zucman J., Cormier F., Delattre O., Roussel M., Thomas G. and Ghysdael J. DNA binding and transcriptional activation properties of the EWS/FLI-1 protein resulting from the t(11;22) translocation in Ewing' s sarcoma. Mol Cell Biol 14:3230-3241, 1994.
2. Bijlsma E., Merel P., Bosch D.A., Westerveld A., Delattre O., Thomas G. and Hulsebos T.J.M. Analysis of mutations in the SCH gene in schwannomas. Genes Chromosome Cancer 1994.(In Press)
3. Delattre O., Zucman J., Melot T., Sastre X., Zucker J.M., Lenoir G., Ambros P., Sheer D., Turc-Carel C., Triche T., Aurias A. and Thomas G. The Ewing family of tumours: a subgroup of small round cell tumours defined by specific chimeric transcripts. New Engl J Med 1994.(In Press)
4. Demczuk S., Desmaze C., Aikem M., Prieur M., Ledeist F., Sanson M., Rouleau G., Thomas G. and Aurias A. Molecular cytogenetic analysis of a series of 23 DiGeorge syndrome patients by fluorescence

in situ hybridization. Ann Genet Paris 1994.(In Press)
5. Desmaze C., Zucman J., Delattre O., Melot T., Thomas G. and Aurias A. Interphase molecular cytogenetics of Ewing's sarcoma and peripheral neuroepithelioma t(11;22) translocation with flanking and overlapping cosmid probes. Cancer Genet Cytogenet 1994. (In Press)

London group

1. Fisher E.M.C. and Scambler P.J. Human haploinsufficiency: One for sorrow, two for joy. Nature Genetics 7:5-7, 1994.
2. Franke U.C., Scambler P.J., Loffler C., Lons P. Hanefeld F., Zoll B. and Hansmann I. Interstitial deletion of 22q11 in DiGeorge syndrome detected by high resolution and molecular analysis. Clin Genet 46:187-192, 1994.
3. Lindsay E.A. Greenberg F., Shaffer L.G., Shapira S.K. Scambler P.J. and Baldini A. Submicroscopic deletions at 22q11.2: variability of the clinical picture and delineation of a commonly deleted region. Am J Med 1994. (In Press)
4. Mattei M-G., Halford S. and Scambler P.J. Mapping of the Tuple1 gene to mouse chromosome 16A-B1. Genomics 1994. (In Press)
5. Scambler P.J. DiGeorge syndrome and related birth defects. Seminars in Developmental Biology 1994. (In Press)
6. Scambler P.J. Report of the fourth international workshop on the mapping of the chromosome 22. Cytogenet Cell Genet 1994. (In Press)

Stockholm group

1. Kurahashi H., Akagi K., Karakawa K., Nakamura T., Dumanski J.P., Sano T., Okada S., Takai S. and Nishisho I. Isolation and mapping of cosmid markers on human chromosome 22, including one within the submicroscopically deleted region of DiGeorge syndrome. Hum Genet 93:248-54, 1994.
2. Nesslinger N.J., Gorski J.L., Kurczynski T.W., Shapira S.K., Siegel-Bartelt J., Dumanski J.P., Cullen R.F. Jr, French B.N. and McDermid H.E. Clinical, cytogenetic, and molecular characterization of seven patients with deletions of chromosme 22q13.3. Am J Hum genet, 54:464-72, 1994.
3. Lindblom A., Ruttledge M., Collins V.P., Nordenskjold M. and Dumanski J.P. Chromosomal deletions in anaplastic meningiomas suggest multiple regions outside chromosome 22 as important in tumor progression. Int J Cancer, 56:354-57, 1994.

2. Joint publications

1. Bijlsma E., Delattre O., Juyn J.A., Melot T., Westerveld A., Dumanski J., Thomas G. and Hulsebos T. Regional fine mapping of the beta crystallin genes on chromosome 22 excludes these genes as physically linked markers for neurofibromatosis type 2. Gene Chromosome Cancer 1994.(In Press)
2. Ruttledge M.H., Sarrazin J., Rangaratnam S., Phelan C.M., Twist E., Merel P., Delattre O., Thomas G., Nordenskjold M., Collins V.P., Dumanski J. and Rouleau G. Evidence for the complete inactivation of the neurofibromatosis type 2 gene in the majority of sporadic meningiomas. Nature Genetics 6:180-184, 1994.
3. Ruttledge M.H., Xie Y-G., Han F-Y., Giovannini M., Janson M., Fransson I., Werelius B., Delattre O., Thomas G., Evans G. and Dumanski J.P. Physical mapping of the NF2/meningioma region on human chromosome 22q12. Genomics 19:52-59, 1994.

Contract number: GENO-CT91-0018
Contractual period: 1 April 1992 to 31 March 1994

Coordinator
Dr. G. Thomas
Institut Curie
Section de Biologie
Laboratoire de Génétique des Tumeurs
26, rue d'Ulm
75231 Paris Cedex 05
France
Tel: 33 1 40 516 679
Fax: 33 1 40 516 630

Participants
Dr. P.J. Scambler
Molecular Medicine Unit
Division of Biochemistry and Genetics
Institute of Child Health
University of London
30 Guilford street,
London WC1N 1EN
United Kingdom
Tel: 44 71 242 9789 (ext 2635)
Fax: 44 71 831 0488

Prof. M. Nordenskjöld
Department of Clinical Genetics
Karolinska Institutet
P.O. Box 60500
10401 Stockholm
Sweden
Tel: 46 8729 3928
Fax: 46 8327 734

Human Genome Analysis Programme
M. Hallen and A. Klepsch (Eds.)
IOS Press, 1995

SEQUENCE TAGGED SITE MAP OF THE XQ24 - QTER REGION

P. Vezzoni
Istituto di Tecnologie Biomediche Avanzate, Milano, Italy

1. Summary of aims

The main aim of our scientific proposal was to utilize the YAC technology to establish the physical map of portions of the chromosomal region Xq24-qter.

We report here our preliminary results obtained in the two years of work under our CEE grant.

This report is *confidential*, as most of the data have not yet been published.

The main effort of the Milan group in these two years has been directed towards mapping the Xq27 band. Our findings are summarized in Fig 1. Our work in this region has been quite successful, since we have now assembled 246 YACs in a single contig spanning approximately 12 Mb including the whole Xq27 band. This region joins a contig across Xq26 (Little et al., 1992) at the centromeric side and is merged with the IDS contig in the proximal portion of Xq28 (Palmieri et al.,1992) at the telomeric side.

The London group has consolidated and extended YAC contigs from FRAX (A) to U6.2 in Xq27.3-q28.1 (Flomen et al., manuscript in preparation), and is currently trying to close the last gap. The remainder of the effort has been focussed in the lesser mapped Xq24-25 region. As a result of extensive YAC library screening, over 500 YACs have been identified which map to this region, some of which have been assembled into contigs of up to 3 Mb (Coffey et al., unpublished work).

Key words: X chromosome; YAC; STS map.

2. Source of clones

The principal source of YACs for the Milan group was a YAC library constructed in the lab of David Schlessinger starting from the X3000.11 cell line, a human/hamster hybrid containing the Xq24-qter region as the only human component (described in Abidi et al., 1990). A supplementary collection of 266 YAC clones was made from the same hybrid using a telomere capture vector as in Reithman et al. (1990). An additional group of clones from Xpter-q27.3 was developed from a different hybrid cell line by Lee et al. (1992). Supplementary clones were found in two libraries made from total human DNA: the CGM library (Brownstein et al.,1989) and the GM06061B library constructed from the 49 XXXXX cell line according to published procedures (Imai and Olson, 1990). Finally, 7 additional YAC clones spanning the fragile X region were provided by Dr AM Poustka, in the framework of the EC grant.

The sources of YACs in Guy's were initially the CGM library and the ICRF library made from the cell line GM1416B (48, XXXX) (Larin et al., 1991). Later, YACs from the ICI library (Anand et al., 1990) and more recently the CEPH megaYAC library (Cohen et al., 1993) were also incorporated into the study. Between the two collaborating centres, therefore, all the current YAC resources were available for the study.

3. Strategy

3.1. Strategy of the Milan Group

Mapping proceeded in two phases: In the first, contigs were seeded with YACs from the Xq24-qter ("X3000") library and extended with walking steps based on hybridization techniques, and clone overlaps were identified with additional sources of information. In a second phase, based on PCR techniques, attempts were made to close gaps between contigs that had reached a limit where YACs were no longer found in the Xq24-qter clone collections: STS primer pairs from contig ends were generated in order to screen different libraries to close the gaps. The course of the studies is outlined, with emphasis on some special features of the region around the Fragile X locus.

Phase I: Growth and verification of contigs

Contigs were seeded in several ways:
1. Screening with known probes. The collection of YACs from the Xq24-q28 (x3000.11 hybrid) were screened for cognate clones with a series of probes (Abidi et al.., 1990). The final map in Figure 1 includes the results obtained with 33 hybridization probes, of which 25 were reported in Klinger et al. (1989) and 8 in Zucchi and Schlessinger (1992). These include the probes for DXS loci and the genes listed in Table 1 section A, as well as pTR5 and LF1 probes (Zucchi and Schlessinger, 1992). All the single copy probes had been roughly mapped to the Xq26-q28 region in the literature, and some had been further localized (see below). Five additional probes were found to be of particular interest, since they had been localized by hybrid panel studies and by genetic linkage analysis of Fragile X region (see especially Suthers et al., 1991; 1992), in the following order from the centromere to the telomere: PRN1(for locus DXS369) and VK23 (for locus DXS297); VK16 (DXS293, the probe nearest to the Fragile X site by linkage analysis); VK21 (DXS296) and VK18 (DXS295) which are telomeric to the X fragile site.
    2. Fingerprinting with the moderately repetitive sequences pTR5 and LF1, and with the highly repetitive sequences Alu and L1 as described (Zucchi and Schlessinger, 1992; Porta et al., 1993).
    3. Assignment to the Xq27 region by *in situ* hybridization of 12 YACs larger than 300 kb from the Xq24-qter collection (Montanaro et al., 1991); these YACs were used as hybridization probes against the entire collection (YAC cross-hybridization; Wada et al., 1990);
    4. Generation of end-clones and use as probes for walking by hybridization; 13 end probes were produced from appropriate YACs at the end of growing contigs.
    5. 397 Alu/Alu PCR-generated internal probes were produced for additional confirmation.
    6. 76 STSs were generated to screen additional libraries with the aim of closing the remaining gaps.

Phase II. Gap closure

When an end-clone from a YAC was used to screen the collections and no further YACs were identified, that position was noted as a "gap" in the collection. Many such regions are missing from any particular YAC collection for statistical reasons (Schlessinger et al., 1991). Rescreening additional collections of YACs is the first

Xq27 YAC Contig

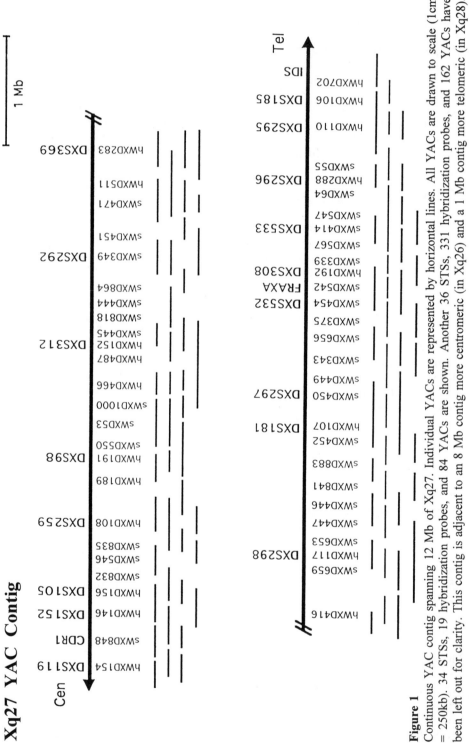

Figure 1

Continuous YAC contig spanning 12 Mb of Xq27. Individual YACs are drawn to scale (1cm = 250kb). 34 STSs, 19 hybridization probes, and 84 YACs are shown. Another 36 STSs, 331 hybridization probes, and 162 YACs have been left out for clarity. This contig is adjacent to an 8 Mb contig more centromeric (in Xq26) and a 1 Mb contig more telomeric (in Xq28).

A- HGM PROBES-

PROBE		LOCUS	YACs PICKED
hWXD154	780	DXS119	yWXD533-536-438-310-681
" 150	pCDR13	CDR 1	yWXD468-156-369-586
" 146	cX33.2	DXS152	yWXD637-720-268-490-505-596
" 156	cX55.7	DXS105	yWXD564-720-268-490-842-628
" 108	MJ013/19	DXS259	yWXD477-433-204-742-320-551
" 191	4D-8	DXS98	yWXD1-228
" 145	pD9	---	yWXD414-902-903
" 152	pX135f	DXS312	yWXD229-151-496-874
" 98	VK14	DXS292	yWXD340-247-1786-1674-1676-1677
" 283	pRN1	DXS369	yWXD1080-1081-925-926-927-2022-4347
" 117	VK24	DXS298	yWXD351-691-860-1799-1800
" 107	p76	DXS181	yWXD497-673
" 197	VK23/B	DXS297	yWXD497-686-436-202
---	AFM224ZG11	DXS998	yWXD1789-1791-1792-1097
"	759M	DXS532	yWXD1097-1798
" 279	35.677	---	yWXD2134-530-965-966
" 193	Do33	DXS465	yWXD2026-120-965-966
" 287	pVK16-B1	DXS293	yWXD2026-965-966
" 192	VK47	DXS308	yWXD2026-965-966
" 159	yBP1(L)		yWXD2026-965-966
" 606	749M	DXS533	yWXD291-1073-1074-1075
" 288	VK21	DXS296	yWXD539-961
" 110	VK18 A	DXS295	yWXD512-412-861
" 106	p188	DXS185	yWXD153-441
" 161	pc2S15	IDS	yWXD341-571-873-395-776

B- pTR5/LF1 PROBES-

hWXD1035	pTR5-5.8	tWXD22-5.8	yWXD637-720-268-490
" 1125	LF1-5.4	tWXD116-5.4	yWXD156-573-310
" 1036	pTR5-6.8-2.6	tWXD23-6.8	yWXD532-602-551
" 1127	LF1-5.0	tWXD117-5.0	yWXD471-758-775-454
" 1129	LF1-2.5	tWXD119-2.5	yWXD300-558-430- 891
" 1042	pTR5-03	tWXD28- 0.3	yWXD497-686-436-847
" 1044	pTR5-5.8	tWXD30-5.8	yWXD2134-530-965-966
" 1046	pTR532-4.2	tWXD32-4.2	yWXD141-661-724-873

Table 1

HGM Probes

approach to gap closure. Such closure activities were initiated at selected points during contig growth. Systematic applications of this approach found the additional 155 clones in other libraries. These clones have now allowed us to establish a single contig spanning approximately 12 Mb covering the whole Xq27 band, joining the previously described Xq26 contig (Little et al., 1992) on one side and the small contig containing the IDS gene in the proximal Xq28 on the other side (Palmieri et al., 1992).

3.2. Strategy of the London Group

The strategy for contig assembly taken by the Guy's group was broadly similar to that taken by Milan. However, more emphasis was placed on the use of hybridisation techniques using high density gridded colony filters of all the available YAC libraries (Bentley et al., 1992).

1. Probes used in this part of the study were:
a) Clones from a library of DNA microdissected from the Xq27 region (kindly provided by M Hirst and KE Davies).
b) 130 human DNA-specific cosmids constructed from DNA of the X 3000.11 cell line, identified by prior hybridisation to a total human cDNA probe.
c) 25 EagI/EcoRI subclones of DNA from the X 3000.11 cell line. (Human clones identified by the same approach used in 2 above).

Probes were hybridised either singly or in pools of up to 30 to filter sets. Individual clones were picked off and in most cases streaked to purify single colonies before rescreening. Individual clones were deposited in new microtitre plates and gridded on a single small filter (polygrid).

2. In addition, a number of STSs were prepared from a variety of sources:
a) Known markers in the Xq27.3-q28.1 region and the Xq24-q25 region.
b) A panel of clones from the Xq27 microdissection library.
c) Ends of YAc clone inserts isolated by a modified version of the vectorette PCR procedure.

All STSs were used to screen the YAC libraries in a 3-tier screening scheme. Confirmed positive clones were added to the polygrid.

3. Contigs were overlapped by a combination of the following approaches:
a) Hybridisation of vectorette ends to the polygrid;
b) Alu-PCR fingerprinting (Coffey et al., 1992; and manuscript in preparation) and analysis using the CONTIG 9 software;
c) Hybridisation and Alu-PCR products from individuals YACs to the polygrid;
d) Probes which failed to detect positive clones in the polygrid were then used to rescreen the libraries.

4. Results

4.1. The Xq27.1-q28.1 region (Milan group)

Based on this strategy, and in collaboration with Dr Schlessinger lab in St Louis, we have assembled, oriented and formatted a single contig from 246 YACs covering the whole chromosomal Xq27 band extending for approximately 12 Mb. It joins an 8 Mb contig in Xq26 assembled in Schlessinger's lab (Little et al., 1992) at the centromeric side and a smaller contig assembled in Xq28.1 in the region of the IDS gene (Palmieri

et al, 1992). Cognate YACs were found for every probe tested, and two discrepancies between reported locations of probes and their positions in the current contig were resolved. Several zones were, however, under-represented in YACs. In some regions screening of 10 equivalents of Xq DNA did not recover any YACs, or recovered only unstable clones. The most problematic area was in the vicinity of the Fragile X site; in particular the coverage was relatively poor in an initial YAC collection derived from a Fragile X patient. YAC libraries from unaffected individuals, however, finally yielded clones that provide coverage of the region [as described in Hirst et al., 1991).
It is therefore possible that clonability is affected by the special character of the DNA around the Fragile X locus.

Quality of the map

Xq27 is now one of the best characterized regions, since its self-consistence is strongly validated by independent criteria, such as the localization of probes in hybrid panels, linkage analysis and in situ hybridization.
Since many of the probes isolated in the course of these efforts were used, the content and order of probes in the contigs can be directly compared to the cytogenetic and genetic data. In one approach, probes were hybridized to DNA from each of a series of somatic cell hybrids containing portions of the X chromosome. In a literature review of the results obtained with hybrid panels, the order of the probes from the centromere to the telomere was: F9; cX55.7; 4D8; VK14; RN1 and VK24; VK47; VK23; VK16; VK18, VK21, and IDS. In general, the long-range probe contents and relative order inferred from hybrid panels is mirrored in the contigs.
In several cases, however, particularly in the contig containing VK23 and RN1, some probes were placed discordantly. For example, probe VK47, reported to be centromeric to the Fragile X site between probes VK23 and RN1, was instead mapped just telomeric to the Fragile X site in the contigs. This discrepancy was resolved by the subsequent findings of Sutherland's group that, when tested by *in situ* hybridization to metaphase chromosomes expressing the Fragile X site, VK47 indeed lies distal to the Fragile X site (G. Sutherland, personal communication). There are many possible reasons for the original misassignment, ranging from data entry error to DNA rearrangements in one or more hybrid cell lines of a panel; but the case both underlines the importance of independent verification of map orders, and supports the general accuracy of the physical map obtained with overlapping YACs.
The final map is shown in Fig 1. It is beyond the aims of the present report to list in detail the results obtained and all the efforts that have been made in achieving this result. However we want to briefly summarize the work performed on the Fragile X site in order to emphasize some of the difficulties that can be found in assembling contigs in regions of relatively difficult clonability.

Contig encompassing the Fragile X lesion

YACs were first selected by screening the library with VK16, VK21, Do33 (DXS465), 35.677, and VK47 and the cognate YACs were identified. However, in contrast to the average of three YACs for each probe sought in Xq26.1-q27.1 (Little et al., 1992) and the rest of Xq27, the original X3000 library yielded no clones for VK16, one for 35.677, one containing both Do33 and VK47, one for DXS295, and one for DXS296. Moreover, these clones were all relatively small, and the region proved impossible to cover without screening several other YAC libraries for additional clones. In the first phase of the work, screening of the additional telomere capture clones detected yWXD2026 with both an end-clone from yWXD530 and probe VK16. Independent work in several other laboratories supported this order by assembling these YACs in contigs across the same region (Hirst et al., 1991); and yWXD2026 proved to cover the Fragile X lesion by in situ and structural analysis (Kremer et al., 1991).

The borderline of poor recovery seems relatively defined: yWXD 454 on the centromeric side of the Fragile X region was part of a group of 6 YACs, while DXS181 and DXS295 in the telomeric direction identified 2 and 3 YACs, respectively, in the collection. These numbers are consistent with findings from the total library, in which a total of 300 probes over a region of 25 Mb identified an average of 3.2 YACs (Schlessinger et al., 1991).

Clones have been recovered from other YAC libraries, however, that cover much of the region and are often much larger. For example, two clones reported by Heitz et al. (kindly provided by Dr. J.L. Mandel) and a clone from the CGM library (provided in repurified form by Dr. M. Hirst) easily covered a region of about 500 kb in the vicinity of the Fragile X site.

STS Map

Relevant to the present report is the construction of an STS map of the Xq27 region. One interesting point of our analysis is the formatization of our YAC map and the establishment of 76 STSs evenly distributed about every 100 kb.

STSs are characterized by unique primer pairs and the length of the amplification product. They are highly informative tools that can be used for genome analysis. About half of them were derived from contig ends in order to close gaps, while the other half was developed with the purpose of contig verification. The 76 STSs listed in Table 2 provide an average resolution map of approximately 150 kb.

4.2. FRAX(A)-Xq28.1 (London group)

While the Milan group concentrated initially on the more proximal region, the London group focussed its efforts on linking contigs containing the FRAX(A) locus and the IDS gene to U6.2 (DXS304).

In the course of this work it became apparent that the DXS29 and its associated clones were originally misplaced in Xq28.1 (Palmieri et al., 1992). In the more distal section, different isolates of probe 2A1 (DXS497) revealed different patterns of hybridisation, suggesting more than one location for this sequence within Xq28.1. Furthermore, comparison of our data with that of our collaborators indicated an inconsistency in an order of 2A1 and U6.2. Accordingly, our strategy has been to consolidate the FRAX(A)/IDS contig and to extend it by walking. In parallel, a contig was constructed using U6.2 and additional STSs derived from microclones or from sub-cloned Alu-PCR products derived from radiation-reduced somatic cell hybrids (Cole et al., 1991). The contig was then extended in both directions by walking in an attempt to join it with the IDS contig. To resolve the uncertainty of orientation of the U6.2 contig, two-colour fluorescent analysis was carried out using cosmids that were positive for selected landmarks within the contig. A conclusive order was obtained using cosmids that tested positive for STS3/40 (Cole et al., 1991) and U6.2 respectively. The results showed that 3/40 and hence 2A1 were distal to U6.2.

STS name	YAC end fragment	STS- size bp	STS name	YAC end fragment	STS- size bp
sWXD 2	A65B8L	125	sWXD 549	1077R	97
sWXD 3	564R	162	sWXD 550	D73C11R	91
sWXD 53	414R	131	sWXD 574	F2A6L	157
sWXD 54	436R	177	sWXD 575	370R	72
sWXD 55	539R	250	sWXD 576	291L	147
sWXD 57	813R	251	sWXD 583	786R	74
sWXD 64	539L	270	sWXD 586	E9G9L	65
sWXD 275	F6D2R	63	sWXD 587	1077L	69
sWXD 282	E3H10L	60	sWXD 612	1078L	91
sWXD 339	595R	129	sWXD 621	F6A7R	88
sWXD 340	699R	127	sWXD 639	141R	500
sWXD 341	815R	122	sWXD 652	233L	99
sWXD342	269R	87	sWXD 653	351L	108
sWXD 343	454R	88	sWXD 654	433L	63
sWXD 344	137R	75	sWXD 655	477L	63
sWXD 345	305L	116	sWXD 656	758R	93
sWXD 346	340R	72	sWXD 657	881R	108
sWXD 347	1078R	118	sWXD 658	758L	129
sWXD 348	F2A6R	121	sWXD 659	860R	85
sWXD 351	847L	73	sWXD 660	753R	145
sWXD 404	F6E6R	147	sWXD 661	433R	78
sWXD 413	F23G9R	78	sWXD 662	775R	106
sWXD 444	756R	96	sWXD 748	247L	92
sWXD 445	151R	125	sWXD 749	E115A10R	93
sWXD 447	631R	69	sWXD 750	E141B11L	134
sWXD 448	710R	105	sWXD 751	F21A6L	67
sWXD 449	497L	112	sWXD 752	F6C2L	92
sWXD 451	854R	164	sWXD 753	247R	75
sWXD 452	497R	80	sWXD 818	F7F11L	65
sWXD 453	767L	103	sWXD 826	370R	95
sWXD 455	200R	77	sWXD 827	870L	117
sWXD 456	377R	83	sWXD 828	710L	111
sWXD 457	822L	65	sWXD 829	1674L	70
sWXD 458	E150H3R	112	sWXD 831	1675L	151
sWXD 471	854L	90	sWXD 832	E74C12R	96
sWXD 545	E150H3L	99	sWXD 833	1666L	127
sWXD 546	F6C2R	69	sWXD 834	1666LB	93
sWXD 547	584L	97	sWXD 835	E74C12L	65

Table 2

Xq27 - STS Probes

4.3. Xq25 region (Milan group)

Whereas the contig assembly and orientation in Xq 27.1-q28 is complete, the map of the Xq24-25 region is still incomplete, due in part to a lack of polymorphic markers in this region. One contributory approach has been to use sets of overlapping somatic cell hybrids containing defined translocations or deletions to localize contigs in intervals. In one case, a group of five hybrids was used to localize contigs in a region estimated to be 3cM in Xq25, and to define the corresponding breakpoints in the DNA of one of these hybrids. Probes were obtained as inter-Alu and Alu-vector fragments from a series of YACs selected from a number of contigs.

With this approach, a 2 Mb contig was localized between DXS79 and DXS100, which was assembled around a probe for DXS 172 that previously had had an ambiguous localization.

4.4. Xq24-25 (London group)

The London group also focussed some attention on the poorly mapped Xq24-q25 region. Our strategy was to use a series of landmarks as starting points to isolate YAcs from available libraries, and particular attention was paid to the use of two classes of probes: (1) A set of X3000-derived cosmids. These were hybridised to the ICRF YAC library in pools of 5-10 cosmids each. 130 cosmids (which correspond to an average density of 1 per 250 kb) were successfully hybridised, identifying 300 YACs. Some of these YACs were also positive for other probes in Xq. (2) The set of EagI/Ecori subclones derived from the same hybrid cell line (isolated by D. Toniolo). Clones within this subset were mapped to the Xq24-q25 region by hybridisation to somatic cell hybrid panel (by D. Toniolo) and then used to screen the available YAc libraries. Approximately 240 YACs were isolated. Seed contigs were constructed using these probes, and a series of additional landmarks were used to consolidate these contigs. These landmarks consisted of YACs from D. Nelson et al. (1991) which had previously been mapped to the region; and STSs or probes which were specific known markers. A series of new probes were isolated by vectorette PCR from selected YACs. These were used to further extend the contigs. A subset of the probes were also re-tested across the panel of somatic cell hybrids (by D. Toniolo) to refine their location.

4.5. Xq28 region (Milan group)

A contig of about 200 kb has been established in the Xq28 band, in the region of the L1CAM gene. Within this contig we established physical linkage between L1CAM and the type 2 vasopressin receptor (V2R) gene, responsible for the nephrogenic diabetes insipidus. STSs for V2R have been developed (Frattini et al., 1993). In addition we have identified a new gene mapping several kb proximal to V2R gene and have established STSs for this gene as well.

A cosmid contig has been established in the region of R/GCV genes containing the Filamin gene (Maestrini et al., 1993). This region has been thoroughly characterized by mapping and sequencing (Patrosso et al., 1994), since Filamin was a good candidate for Emery Dreifuss Muscular Distrophy (EDMD). Several STSs for this gene spanning approximately 35 Kb have been implemented.

4.6. Gene associated STSs (Milan group)

CpG islands containing fragments from a phage library (EagI-EcoRI total digestion) from the Xq24-qter have been mapped to specific chromosomal bands and sequenced at their ends. Analysis of the obtained sequences and the methylation status allowed us to define real undermethylated C+G rich fragments and separate them from EagI containing repetitive sequences. We also demonstrated that this discrimination can be simply obtained by the sequencing of the EagI site. This sequence data can be the basis for primer design of gene associated STSs. We have also defined other gene-oriented STSs, two of which map to the already published 8 Mb contig in Xq26 (ZNF75 and gp39).

References

1. Abidi F.E. et al. Genomics 7:363, 1990.
2. Anand R.A. et al. Nucleic Acid Res 18:1951-1956,1990.
3. Brownstein B.H. et al. Science 244:1348, 1989.
4. Cohen D. et al. Nature 366:698-701,1993.
5. Cole C.G. et al. Genomics 10:816-826,1991.
6. Heitz et al. Science 251:1236-1239,1991.
7. Frattini A. et al. Biochem Biophys Res Commun 193:864-871,1993.
8. Hirst M. et al. Nucl. Acids Res. 19:3283-3288.
9. Imai T. and Olson M.V. Genomics 8:297,1990.
10. Kere J. et al. Nucleic Acid Res 19:2755, 1991.
11. Klinger K. et al. Human Gene Mapping 1992.
12. Kremer E.J. et al. Science 252:1711-1714,1991.
13. Larin Z. et al. Proc Natl Avcad Sci USA 88:4123-4127,1991.
14. Lee J.T. et al. Genomics 12:526,1992.
15. Little R.D., et al. Proc Natl Acad Sci USA 89:177-181,1992.
16. Maestrini et al. Hum Mol Gen 2:761-766,1993.
17. Montanaro et al. Am J Hum Genet 48:183-194,1991.
18. Mueller P.R. et al. Science 246:780, 1989.
19. Nelson D.L. et al. Proc Natl Acad Sci USA 88:6157-6161, 1991.
20. Palmieri G. et al Genomics 12:52-57,1992.
21. Patrosso M.C. et al, Genomics, in press.
22. Porta G. et al. Genomics, 16:417-425,1993.
23. Riethman H.C. et al. Proc Natl Acad Sci USA 87:1213,1989.
24. Schlessinger et al. Genomics 11:783-793,1991.
25. Suthers G.K. et al. Am. J. Hum. Genet. 47:187-195,1990.
26. Suthers G.K. et al. Am. J. Hum. Genet. 48:460-467,1991.
27. Wada et al. Am J Hum Genet 46:95-106,1990.
28. Zucchi and Schlessinger. Genomics 12:264-275,1992.

Papers published under EC grant

1. A. Frattini, I. Zucchi, A. Villa, C. Patrosso, M. Repetto, L. Susani, D. Strina, E. Redolfi, P. Vezzoni, Giovanna Romano, Giuseppe Palmieri, Teresa Esposito and Michele d'Urso.
    "Vasopressin Receptor Gene, the Gene Responsible for Nephrogenic Diabetes Insipidus, Maps to Xq28 Close to the Licam Gene" (Biochem., Biophys. Res. Commun. 193: 864-871, 1993).

2. Anna Villa, Ileana Zucchi, Giuseppe Pilia, Dario Strina, Lucia Susani, Federica Morali, Cristina Patrosso, Annalisa Frattini, Franco Lucchini, Monica Repetto, Maria Grazia Sacco, Monica Zoppè and Paolo Vezzoni.
    "ZNF75: Isolation of a cDNA Clone of the KRAB Zinc Finger Gene Subfamily Mapped in YACS 1Mb Telomeric of HRPT" (Genomics 18: 223-229, 1993).

3. A. Frattini, S. Faranda, E. Redolfi, I. Zucchi, A. Villa, M.C. Patrosso, D. Strina, L. Susani and Paolo Vezzoni.
    "Genomic Organization of the HUman VP16 Acessory Protein (HCF1), a Housekeeping Gene Mapping to Xq28" (Genomic, in press).

Contract number: GENO-CT91-0019
Contractual period: 1 January 1992 to 31 December 1993

Coordinator
Dr. Paolo Vezzoni
Consorzio Milano Ricerche
Consiglio Nationale delle Ricerche
Istituto di Tecnologie Biomediche Avanzate
Dipartimento di Biotechnologie
Via Ampere 56
I - 20131 Milano
Italy
Tel: 39 2 7064 3380
Fax: 39 2 266 3030

Participants
Dr. Francesco Gianelli
Pediatric Research Unit
Guy's Hospital
London Bridge
London SE1 9RT
United Kingdom
Tel: 44 71 955 4450
Fax: 44 71 955 4644

Dr. Ileana Zucchi
CNR ITBA
Via Ampère 56
20131 Milan
Italy
Tel: 39 2 706 43384
Fax: 39 2 266 3030

Dr. David Bentley
Pediatric Research Unit
Guy's Hospital
London Bridge
London SE1 9RT
United Kingdom
Tel: 44 71 955 5000
Fax: 44 71 955 4644

Human Genome Analysis Programme
M. Hallen and A. Klepsch (Eds.)
IOS Press, 1995

CONSTRUCTION OF AN INTEGRATED OVERLAP, PHYSICAL, GENETIC AND TRANSCRIPTIONAL MAP OF THE CHROMOSOME 21

J.M. Delabar
Hôpital Necker, Paris, France

1. Background Information

The project GENO-0024 was funded by the Human Genome Analysis Programme of the European Economic Community. It started at the beginning of the year 1992.

During 92-93 the collaborative effort of the seven participants of the Chromosome 21 Consortium has brought important advances in the different aspects of chromosome 21 analysis. The data produced by these collaborations have been presented at internal meetings, at international workshops and in 44 publications.As it was proposed in the work programme, the participants have developed several approaches in the five domains of chromosome analysis:
- linkage map
- physical map of the genomic DNA
- cloning of YACs and cosmids, contigs mapping
- mapping and analysis of diseases related to chromosome 21
- cDNA identification and mapping

State of the chromosome 21 maps at the beginning of the project:
genetic map: resolution less than 5cM
Physical map: partial physical map mainly obtained by hybrids mapping

2. Results

2.1 Linkage map

The first task was to isolate new polymorphic markers. The main set of new markers was developed by P7 (Ref I 1, I 2, I 4), in collaboration with P1 for one centromeric marker D21S258 (Ref I 5), and in collaboration with P2 for a marker located within intron 1 of the APP gene (I 6). The linkage map of these markers was realized by P6 who has placed 12 restriction fragment length polymorphisms and 18 microsatellites on the chromosome 21 map. P2, P6, and P7 have also participated, together with other institutions, to the construction of a map of 43 PCR markers with an average heterozygocity of 61 % and with an average distance between adjacent markers of 2.5cM (I 3).

The map of HSA21 represents now a highly informative and dense meiotic linkage map.

2.2 Physical map of the genomic DNA

P1 has developed and used a slot blot method to assess the copy number of 30 markers in the DNA of 11 patients with rearranged chromosome 21 and to determine their physical order (II 2). FISH was also developed, with one or two colors labelling on metaphasic and interphasic chromosomes; this technic was used to locate a collection of cosmids around the centromere, and YACs and cosmids in the Down Syndrome Chromosome Region (DCR). A partial restriction map of 26 markers has also been established by PFGE (II 1) using a set of improved experimental conditions (CrØtØ et al. Biotechniques 11, 711-717, 1991). Using an original cloning technique from PFGE purified fragment, P1 has isolated 14 new markers in the band q22 (II 6). PFGE was used to construct genomic maps around specific loci: around the oncogene ETS2 (II 6) and around the t(8;21) breakpoint (IV 20).

Hybrid mapping of unique probes, FISH of phages and YACs have identified a 135-500kb region of homology on the long arm of chromosome 21 (III 3).

Four physical linkage groups have been established by PFGE:
- including the region CRYA1 - BCEI and spanning 1200kb (II 1)
- including the region ETS2 - D21S65 and spanning 5000kb (III 1, III 2)
- including the region APP - D21S12 and spanning 1450kb (II 5)
- including the pericentromeric region D21S52- D21Z1 and spanning 6500kb (II 4, II 5).

These macrorestriction maps cover 1/3 of the 21q arm.

2.3 Cloning of YACs and cosmids, contigs mapping

P5 has generated a chromosome 21 specific enriched YAC library of 4 genome equivalents (III 7). This library has been screened by other members of the consortium. A collection of 1.5 genome equivalent of YAC clones generated by P4 from a hybrid cell line containing a chromosome 21 has been added to this library (III 6). By using YAC ends isolation ,ALU PCR probes, radiation hybrids and other specific markers, these collections and part of the CEPH CHR21 YAC library have been used to construct a *YAC overlap spanning 90% of the chromosome* (III 4, III 5).

YAC detailed restriction maps, comparison with genomic maps and FISH analysis have permitted to P1 to select a set of YACs spanning *ETS2-ERG (1200kb) (III 1) and a set of YACs spanning D21S55-D21S65 (3600kb) (III 2)*. YACs containing the region of homology on the long arm of chromosome 21 have also been isolated from the P4 and P5 libraries. FISH analysis of these YACs confirm the existence of this homology.

Direct screening of the CHR21 cosmid library with YACs was performed by P5 for the whole q arm and by P1 for the D21S55-CBR region . These screenings identified *6000 cosmids organized in 145 cosmids pockets (III 5).*

2.4 Mapping and analysis of diseases related to chromosome 21

Down syndrome

Using the slot blot method of gene dosage to study two patients with partial trisomy 21, P1 was the first laboratory to identify with accuracy a critical region for the pathogenesis of Down syndrome (Rahmani et al. P.N.A.S. (USA) 86,5958,1989). This result was developed and confirmed by analysing 8 other patients (IV 9), and permitted to assign 13/24 phenotypic features to the duplication of ETS2-D21S17 region including hypotonia, short stature and mental retardation, 6/24 to the duplication of the

MX1-D21S17 region including facial and dermatoglyphic anomalies, and heart defects (DS type) to the duplication of the CRYA1- D21S17 region.

P3 has selected DS patients with congenital heart defects and has identified new polymorphisms in the COL6A1-COL6A2 gene cluster (IV 8). A study of meiotic crossovers in the family of these patients suggest that each non disjoined CHR21 pair has been involved in at least one crossover event (IV 14). P6 has studied the meiotic stage of nondisjunction in 200 families and the origin of the nondisjoined chromosome 21 in 68 families (IV 1, IV 15). A study of the paternal nondisjunction in trisomy 21 revealed another interesting feature: the excess of male patients (IV 16). P6 has also reported a uniparental isodisomy due to duplication of CHR21 occurring in somatic cells monosomic for chromosome 21 (IV 17).

Monosomy 21

P1 has studied 5 patients with partial monosomy 21 and has defined a minimal region (SOD1-APP) the deletion of which is associated to characteristic features of monosomy 21: arthrogryposis, hypertonia and mental retardation.

Acute myelogenous leukemia

A PFGE study of the DNA of 11 patients with acute myelogenous leukemia with an (8;21) translocation has permitted to P1 to localize the breakpoints in a 100 kb region encompassing the AML1 gene (IV 20).

Presenile dementia and cerebral amyloid angiopathy

P7 has identified a mutation of the APP gene (in exon 17 at position 2075 resulting in amino acid substitution of alanine into glycine at codon 692 of APP751) which cosegregates in one family with presenile dementia and cerebral haemorrhage due to cerebral amyloid angiopathy. These results suggest that the clinically distinct entities, presenile dementia and cerebral amyloid angiopathy, can be caused by the same mutation in the APP gene (IV 12).

2.5 cDNA identification and mapping

Known genes have been localized accurately on chromosome 21: BCEI, CRYA1, CBS, ERG, ETS2, CBR, APP (II 1,II 2, III 1, III 2, II 5). P4 has assigned the human glutamate receptor gene GluR5 to 21q22 by screening a chromosome 21 YAC library (V 2). P3 has observed the conservation of the SON gene which maps on 21q22.1 (V 1).

P5 has applied the exon trapping method developed on cosmid clones to the amplification of exons contained in a YAC spanning part of the ERG gene (V 3, V 4).

3. Technological Improvements and New Resources

Technological improvements:
- Genomic cDNA mapping with vertical pulsed field gel electrophoresis: P1
- Exon trapping on YACs and cosmid pools: P5

New resources:
- Construction of a chromosome 21 specific YAC library: P5
- Construction of a chromosome 21 specific YAC library: P4
- Construction of a chromosome 21 specific cosmid library: P5
- Construction of cDNA libraries: P5

4. Integration of the Data

A collaboration with Dr O. Ritter from DKFZ and Dr J. Thierry Mieg from CNRS has permitted to create a chromosome 21 data base using the model of the Caenorhabditis data base ACEDB.This data base integrates genetic maps, genomic maps, YAC maps , transcriptional data and locus informations coming from the Genome Data Base (Baltimore) and from the data collected at the 4th International Workshop on chromosome 21 (Paris) which included data from the participants of this consortium. Informations necessary to get this data base can be obtained from Dr O. Ritter (E mail: oritter@dkfz-heidelberg.de).

5. Interaction and Collaboration between Participants

Exchanges between participants have occurred at four levels:
Exchange of clones: during this year there has been an intensive exchange of plasmids, cosmids phages and YACs between participants in order to improve the genetic and physical map.
Exchange of libraries: P5 has produced a gridded CHR21 YAC library and a gridded CHR21 cosmid library. P5 has also gridded the YACs from a CHR21 specific YAC library constructed by P4. These libraries have been used by P1, P2, P3, P4 and P7.
Exchange of technics: exchange of mapping technics with the transfer of the vectorette technic from P4 to P1 and P7 and the transfer of hybrid mapping technics from P7 to P4; transfer of exon trapping from P5 to P1.
Exchange of informations: informations have circulated informally among the participants during small meetings and by phone or E Mail.
Every 6 months a full day meeting was organized in the country of one of the participant. These meetings allowed each participant to present the recent advances on chromosome 21 and permitted to define the next step to be accomplished and the future collaborations. (October 91, Antwerpen; June 92, Elsinore; November 92, Paris; April 93, Paris; October 93, Roma).

Publications of the members of the chromosome 21 consortium (92-93)
(EEC grant N°GENO-CT91-0024)

N° of joint/individual publications:
  joint   14
  individual   30

1. Linkage map

1. M. Cruts, H. Backhovens, C. van Broeckhoven (1992) Dinucleotide repeat polymorphism at the D21S16 locus. Nucleic Acids Research 20, 1159.
2. M. Cruts, H. Backhovens, C. Van Broeckhoven (1992) Dinucleotide repeat polymorphism at the D21S145 locus. Nucleic Acids Research 20, 1159.

3. G. McInnis, A. Chakravarti, J. Blaschak, M.B. Petersen, V. Sharma, D. Avramopoulos, J.L. Blouin, U. Konig, C. Brahe, T. Cox, A.C. Warren, C.C. Talbot Jr, C. Van Broekchoven, M. Litt, S.E. Antonarakis.(1993) A linkage map of human chromosome 21: 43 PCR markers at average interval of 2.5 cM. Genomics, 16, 562-571.

4. A.C. Warren, M.B. Petersen, W. van Hul, M.G. McInnis, C. van Broeckhoven, T.K. Cox, A. Chakravarti, S.E. Antonarakis (1992) D21S215 is a (GT)n polymorphic marker close to centromeric alphoid sequences on chromosome 21. Gnomics 13, 1365-1367.

5. A. Wehnert, M. Cruts, H. Backhovens, J.M. Delabar, G. Thomas, C. van Broeckhoven (1992) Dinucleotide repeat polymorphism at the D21S258 locus. Hum. Molec. Genet. 1, 449.

6. S. Zappata, M.B. Petersen, U. Konig, J. Blaschak, A. Chakravarti, F. Tassone, A. Serra, S.E. Antonarakis, C. Brahe (1994) Highly polymorphic repeat marker within the B-amyloid precursor protein gene. Human Genetics, 93, 85-86.

2. Physical map of the genomic DNA

1. N. Crete, J.M. Delabar, Z. Rahmani, M.L. Yaspo, J. Kraus, A. Marks, P.M. Sinet, N. Creau-Goldberg (1993) Partial physical map of human chromosome 21 from fibroblast and lymphocyte DNA. Hum. Genet. 91, 245-253.

2. J.M. Delabar, Z. Chettouh, Z. Rahmani, D. Theophile, J.L. Blouin, R. Bono, J. Kraus, J. Barton, D. Patterson, P.M. Sinet (1992) Gene dosage mapping of 30 DNA markers on chromosome 21. Genomics 13, 887-889.

3. G. van Camp, M. Cruts, H. Backhovens, A. Wehnert, C. van Broeckhoven. (1992) Unique sequence homology in the pericentromeric regions of the long arms of chromosomes 13 and 21. Genomics 12, 158-160.

4. W. van Hul, G. van Camp, L. Stuyver, J. Delabar, M. McInnis, A. Warren, S. Antonarakis, C. van Broekchoven (1993) A contiguous physical map of the pericentromeric region of chromosome 21 between D21Z1 and D21S13E. Genomics 15, 626-630.

5. W. van Hul, C. van Broeckhoven (1993) A long-range restriction map from the APP gene to the centromere of chromosome 21. "Alzheimer's Disease: Advances in Clinical and Basic Research". Edited by B. Corain, K. Iqbal, M. Nicolini, B. Winblad, H. Wisniewski, P. Zatta. John Wiley & Sons Ltd.

6. M.L. Yaspo, N. Crete, Z. Chettouh, J.L. Blouin, Z. Rahmani, D. Stehelin, P.M. Sinet, N. Creau-Goldberg, J.M. Delabar (1992) New chromosome 21 DNA markers isolated by pulsed field gel electrophoresis from an ETS2 containing Down syndrome Chromosomal Region. Hum. Genet. 90, 427-434.

3. Yacs and cosmids cloning and mapping

1. N. Crete, P. Gosset, D. Theophile, M. Duterque-Coquillaud, J.L. Blouin, C. Vayssettes, P.M. Sinet, N. Creau-Goldberg (1993) Mapping the Down syndrome Chromosome Region: establishment of a YAC contig spanning 1.2 Megabases. Eur. J. Hum. Genet.1, 51-63.

2. M.C. Dufresne-Zacharia, N. Dahmane, D. Theophile, R. Orte, Z. Chettouh, P.M. Sinet, J.M. Delabar (1994) 3.6 Mb Genomic and Yac physical map of the Down syndrome chromosome region on chromosome 21. Genomics 14, 462-469

3. A. Dutriqux, J. Rossier, W. van Hul, D. Nizetic, D. Theophile, J.M. Delabar, C. van Broeckhoven, M.C. Potier. Cloning and characterization of a 135-500 kbp region of homology on the long arm of human chromosome 21. (submitted for publication).

4. J. Kumlien, T. Labella, G. Zehetner, R. Vatcheva, D. Nizetic, H. Lehrach. Efficient identification and regional positioning of YAC and cosmid clones to human chromosome 21 by radiation fusion hybrids. (submitted for publication).

5. D. Nizetic, L. Gellen, R. Hamvas, R. Mott, A. Grigoriev, R. Vatcheva, G. Zehetner, M.L. Yaspo, A. Dutriaux, C. Lopes, J.M. Delabar, C. van Broeckhoven, M.C. Potier, H. Lehrach. An integrated YAC overlap and "cosmid-pocket" map spanning > 90 % of the human chromosome 21. (submitted for publication).

6. M.C. Potier, W.L. Kuo, A. Dutriaux, J. Gray, M. Goedert (1992) Construction and characterization of a yeast artificial chromosome library containing 1.5 equivalent of human chromosome 21. Genomics 14 :481-483

7. M.T. Ross, D. Nizetic, C. Nguten, C. Knights, R. Vatcheda, N. Burden, C. Douglas, G. Zehetner, D.C. Ward, A. Baldini, H. Lehrach (1992) Selection of a human chromosome 21 enriched YAC sub-library using a chromosome-specific composite probe Nature Genetics 1, 284-290.

4. Mapping of diseases related to chromosome 21

1. S.E. Antonarakis, M.B. Petersen, M.G. McInnis, P.A. Adelsberger, A.A. Schinzel, F. Binkert, C. Pangalos, O. Raoul, S.A. Slaugenhaupt, M. Hafez, M.M. Cohen, D. Roulston, S. Schwartz, M. Millelsen, L. Tranebjaerg, F. Greenberg, D.I. Hoar, N.L. Rudd, A.C. Warren, C. Metaxotou, C. Bartsocas, A. Chakravarti. (1992) The meiotic stage of nondisjunction in trisomy 21: Determination by using DNA polymorphisms. Am J Hum Genet 50, 544-550.

2. O. Bartsch, U. Konig, M.B. Petersen, H. Poulsen, M. Mikkelsen, F. Palau, F. Prieto, E. Schwinger (1993) Cytogenetic, FISH and DNA studies in 11 individuals from a family with two siblings with dup (21q) Down syndrome. Hum Genet 92, 127-132.

3. O. Bartsch, M.B. Petersen, I. Stuhlmann, G. May, M. Frantzen, E. Schwinger, S.E. Antonarakis, M. Mikkelsen. "Compensatory" uniparental disomy of chromosome 21 in two cases. J Med Genet (submitted).

4. C. Brahe, F. Gurrieri, S. Zappata, M.G. Pompono, A. Mazzei, G. Neri. Further definition of the Wolf-Hirschhorn and Down syndrome critical regions through two sibs with partial deletion of chromosome 4p and duplication of 21q. Journal of Medical Genetics (submitted).

5. W. Courtens, M.B. Petersen, J.C. Noel, J. Flament-Durand, N. van Regemorter, D. Delneste, P. Cochaux, M.R. Verschraegen-Spae, N. van Roy, F. Speleman, U. Koenig, E. Vamos. Proximal deletion of chromosome 21 confirmed by in situ hybridization and molecular studies. Am J Med Genet (submitted).

6. G.E. Davies, C.M. Howard, M.J. Farrer, M.M. Coelman, L.M. Cullen, R. Williamson, R.K.H. Wyse, A.M. Kessling (1993). Unusual genotypes in the COL6A1 gene in parents of children with trisomy 21 and major congenital heart defects. Human Genetics (in press).

7. G.E. Davies, C.M. Howard, M.J. Farrer, M.M. Coleman, L.M. Cullen, R.K.H. Wyse, J. Burn, R. Williamson, A.M. Kessling. Molecular genetics of congenital heart defects in trisomy 21: outcome is influenced by parental genetic variation in the COL6A1 region. Am J Hum Genet (submitted).

8. G.E. Davies, C.M. Howard, L.M. Gorman, M.J. Farrer, A.J. Holland, R. Williamson, A.M. Kessling (1992) Polymorphisms and linkage disequilibrium in the COL6A1 and COL6A2 gene cluster: novel DNA polymorphisms in the region of a candidate gene for congenital heart defects in Down's syndrome. Hum. Genet. 90, 521-525.

9. J.M. Delabar, D. Theophile, Z. Rahmani, Z. Chettouh, J.L. Blouin, M. Prieur, B. Noel, P.M. Sinet. (1993) Molecular mapping of 24 features of Down Syndrome on chromosome 21. Eur. J. Hum. Genet. 1,114-124.

10. M.J. Mc Ginniss, H.H. Kazazian Jr, G. Stetten, M.B. Petersen, H. Boman, E. Engel, F. Greenberg, J.M. Hertz, A.A. Johnson, Z. Laca, M. Mikkelsen, S.R. Patil, A.A. Schinzel, L. Tranebjaerg, S.E. Antonarakis (1992) Mechanisms of ring chromosome formation in 11 cases of human ring chromosome 21. Am J Hum Genet, 50, 15-28.

11. M.J. Mc Ginnis, C. Rosenberg, G. Stetten, A.A. Schinzel, F. Binkert, M.B. Petersen, W.G. Kearns, H.H. Kazazian Jr, P.L. Pearson, S.E. Antonarakis (1993) Unbalanced translocation, t(18;21), detected by fluorescence in situ hybridization (FISH) in a child with 18q- syndrome and a ring chromosome 21. Am J Med Genet 46, 647-651

12. L. Hendriks, C.M. van Duijn, P. Cras, M. Cruts, W. van Hul, F. van Harskamp, A. Warren, M.J McInnis, S.E. Antonarakis, J.J. Martin, A. Hofman, C. van Broeckhoven (1992) Presenile dementia and cerebral haemorrhage linked to a mutation at codon 692 of the b-amyloid precursor protein gene. Nature Genetics 1, 218-221

13. B. Hertz, C.A. Brandt, M.B. Petersen, S. Pedersen, U. Konig, H. Stroemkjaer, P.K.A. Jensen (1993) Application of molecular and cytogenetic techniques to the detection of a de novo unbalanced t(11q;21q) in a patient previously diagnosed as having monosomy 21. Clin Genet 44, 89-94.

14. C.M. Howard, G.E. Davies, M.J. Farrer, L.M. Cullen, M.M. Coleman, R. Williamson, R.K.H. Wyse, F. Palmer, A.M. Kessling (1993) Meiotic crossing over in nondisjoined chromosomes of children with trisomy 21 and a congenital heart defect. Am. J. Hum. Genet. 53, 462-471.

15. C.G. Pangalos, C.C. Talbot Jr, J.G. Lewis, P.A. Adelsberger, M.B. Petersen, J.L. Serre, M.O. Rethore, M.C. de Blois, P. Parent, A.A. Schinzel, F. Binkert, J. Boue, E. Corbin, M.F. Croquette, S. Gilgenkrantz, J. de Grouchy, M.F. Bertheas, M. Prieur, O. Raoul, F. Serville, J.P. Siffroi, F. Thepot, J. Lejeune, S.E. Antonarakis (1992). DNA polymorphism analysis in families with recurrence of free trisomy 21. Am J Hum Genet 51, 1015-1027.

16. M.B. Petersen, S.E. Antonarakis, T.J. Hassold, S.B. Freeman, S.L. Sherman, D. Avramopoulos, M. Mikkelsen (1993). Paternal nondisjunction in trisomy 21: excess of male patients. Hum. Mol. Genet. 2, 1691-1695.

17. M.B. Petersen, O. Bartsch, P.A. Adelsberger, M. Mikkelsen, E. Schwinger, S.E. Antonarakis (1992). Uniparental isodisomy due to duplication of chromosome 21 occuring in somatic cells monosomic for chromosome 21. Genomics 13, 269-274.
18. M.B. Petersen. M. Frantzen, S.E. Antonarakis, A.C. Warren, C. van Broeckhoven, A. Chakravarti, T.K. COX, C. Lund, B. Olsen, H. Poulsen, A. Sand, N. Tommerup, M. Mikkelsen (1992). Comparative study of microsatellite and cytogenetic markers for detecting the origin of the nondisjoined chromosome 21 in Down syndrome. Am J Hum Genet 51, 516-525.
19. A.C. Warren, M.G. Mc Innis, J. Blaschak, M. Kaliatsidaki, M.B. Petersen, A. Chakravarti, S.E. Antonarakis (1992) Dinucleotide repeat (GT)n markers on chromosome 21. Genomics 14, 818-819.
20. M.L. Yaspo, D. Theophile, A. Aurias, N. Crete, N. Creau-Goldberg, C. Bastard, A.M. Suberville, F. Valensi, F. Viguier, R. Berger, P.M. Sinet, J.M. Delabar (1992). Molecular analysis of eleven patients with the (8;21) translocation and M2 acute myelogenous leukemia Genes, Chromosomes & Cancer 5, 166-177.

5. CDNA Identification and mapping

1. I. Khan, R.A. Ficher, K. Johnson, M. Bailey, M.J. Siciliano, A. Kessling, M. Farrer, B. Carrit, T. Kamalati, L. Buluwela. The SON gene encodes a conserved DNA binding protein mapping to human chromosome 21. Am Hum Genet (in press).
2. M.C. Potier, A. Dutriaux, B. Lambolez, P. Bochet, J. Rossier (1993). Assignment of the human glutamate receptor gene GluR5 to 21q22 by screening a chromosome 21 YAC library. Genomics 15, 696-697.
3. M.L. Yaspo, M.A. North, H. Lehrach (1993) Exon-enriched probe derived from a human chromosome 21 YAC by exon-amplification. Nucleic Acids Research 21, 2271-2272.
4. M.L. Yaspo, P. Sanseau, D. Nizetic, B. Korn, A. Poustak, H. Lehrach. Integrated transcriptional maps of large DNA regions: towards a transcriptional map of human chromosome 21. Plenum Press (in press).

6. Report of the Fourth International Workshop on Human Chromosome 21

1. J.M. Delabar, N. Creau, P.M. Sinet, O. Ritter, S.E. Antonarakis, M. Burmeister, A. Chakravarti, D. Nizetic, M. Ohki, D. Patterson, M.B. Petersen, R.H. Reeves, C. van Broeckhoven (1993). Report of the Fourth International Workshop on human chromosome 21. Genomics 18, 735-744.

Contract number: GENO-CT91-0024
Contractual period: 1992- 1993

Coordinator
Dr. J.M. Delabar
Laboratoire de Biochimie Génétique
CNRS 1335 - Clin. R. Debre
Hôpital Necker-Enfants Malades
149, rue de Sèvres
F - 75743 Paris Cedex 15
France
Tel: 33 1 44 49 47 56
Fax: 33 1 42 73 06 59

Participants
Dr. Nicole Creau (P1)
CNRS URA 1335 - Hôpital Necker
149, rue de Sèvres
75743 Paris Cedex 15
France
Tel: 33 1 43 06.92.64
Fax: 33 1 42.73.06 59
E-mail DELABAR@.CITI2.FR
E-mail CREAU@.CITI2.FR

Dr. Christina Brahe (P2)
Istituto di Genetica Umana
Universita Cattolica del Sacro Cuore
1 Largo Francesco Vito
I- 00168 Roma
Italy
Tel: 39 6 355 00 877
Fax: 39 6 305 00 31
E-mail SERRA @MVX36CSATA.IT

Dr. Elisabeth Fisher (P3)
Dpt of Biochemistry and Molecular Genetics
St. Mary's Hospital Medical School - Norfolk Place
London, W21 PG
United Kingdom
Tel: 44 71 723 1252 Ext 5468
Fax: 44 71 706 3272
E-mail e.fisher@sm.ic.as.uk

Dr. Anna Kessling
Dpt. of Biochemistry and Molecular Genetics
St. Mary's Hospital Medical School - Norfolk Place
London, W21 PG
United Kingdom
Tel: 44.71.723.1252 Ext 5479
Fax: 44.71.706.3272
E-mail a.kessling@uk.ac.ic.sm.dka

Dr. Marie-Claude Potier (P4)
Institut Alfred Fessard
Laboratoire de Physiologie Nerveuse
CNRS, Avenue de la Terrasse
F - 91198 Gif sur Yvette
France
Tel: 33 1 69/82 34 40
Fax: 33 1 69 82 43 43
E-mail Bobby@IAF.CNRS-GIF.FR

Dr. Dean Nizetic (P5)
Imperial Cancer Research Fund Laboratories
Dpt of Genome Analysis - Lincoln's Inn Fields
PO Box 123, London WC2A EPX
United Kingdom
Tel: 44.71.269.3080
Fax: 44.71.269.3068
E-mail D_NIZETIC@ICRF.AC.UK

Dr. Michael B. Petersen (P6)
The John F. Kennedy Institute
Department of Medical Genetics
7GL, Landevej
DK-2600 Glostrup
Denmark
Tel: 45 42 45 22 28
Fax: 45 43 43 11 30

Dr. Christine Van Broeckhoven (P7)
Neurogenetics Laboratory
Born Bunje Foundation
Department of Biochemistry
University of Antwerp (UIA)
Building T, Room 5.35
Universiteitsplein 1
B - 2610 Antwerpen
Belgium
Tel: 32 3 820 2601
Fax: 32 3 820 2541
E-mail cvbroeck@reks.ia.ac.be

Human Genome Analysis Programme
M. Hallen and A. Klepsch (Eds.)
IOS Press, 1995

NOVEL MOLECULAR APPROACHES TOWARDS A HIGH RESOLUTION GENETIC AND PHYSICAL MAP OF CHROMOSOME 11

M. Lathrop,
Centre d'Etude du Polymorphisme Humain (CEPH), Paris, France

1. Background information

High density genetic and physical maps of the genome are prerequisite for systematic identification of the genes involved in human disease. This is reflected in the initial goals of the genome program which consists of completing genetic maps of approximately 2 cM resolution, and a contig maps defined by STSs spaced approximately every 300kb throughout the genome. Recently, the program has also focused on the creation of a transcript map that provides the locations for expressed sequences.

Modern techniques of genetic mapping rely principally on PCR-based microsatellite markers to obtain primary assignments and high-resolution localisation of disease loci. The production of microsatellite markers by genome-wide strategies has proven to be effective in producing a high-density linkage map, but it may be necessary to adopt a targeted approach which focuses on under-represented regions to bring the map to completion. An integrated map which provides the relative positions of transcribed sequences and microsatellite markers would be a powerful tool for identifying genes responsible for a disease once its location is available. Although expressed sequences are being identified at an increasing rate, the mapping of these has lagged behind their identification. Ultimately, a complete integrated map will be facilitated by the construction of a robust, complete physical contig, using YACs or other sources. In the meantime, the arduousness of STS screening of YACs on a large-scale, and complications due to YAC chimaerisms and instability will slow down the fulfilment of this goal. Alternative strategies, such as radiation hybrid mapping, offer an intermediate solution to several of these mapping problems.

We undertook a pilot project to determine the feasibility of producing high resolution integrated maps on a chromosome specific basis using the example of chromosome 11. The approaches that we adopted consisted of targeted microsatellite marker development taking into account maps from Généthon and other groups, radiation hybrid mapping of microsatellites and expressed sequences, and the construction of contigs with YACs.

2. Objectives and primary approaches

The principal goal of the programme was to provide a high resolution genetic and physical map of human chromosome 11 containing over 150 polymorphic markers, integrated with RFLP probes, cloned genes and PCR loci generated by Alu-PCR or simple STSs using radiation hybrid mapping. In addition, cosmids and YACs were mapped by high resolution *in situ* hybridisation. Polymorphic microsatellite markers were to be developed on a focused approach using previously localised cosmids and YACs, and new technology developed for resolving microsatellite genotypes. YAC contigs were to be constructed for 11qcen-11q13 and 11q22-q23.

We subsequently modified the goals of the project to increase the density of the map to more than 500 markers. The development of new technology for resolving microsatellite genotypes was dropped in favour of techniques developed at Généthon, and the use of commercial technology available from Applied Biosystems.

3. Results and discussion

A high density radiation hybrid map was constructed consisting of 506 STS markers spanning human chromosome 11 (James et al. 1994). The map includes 143 unique map positions that could be ordered with respect to each other with odds greater than 1,000:1. Based on the estimated length of 144 Mb for the chromosome, this provides a framework map with a resolution of approximately 1 Mb. Overall, there are 299 unique map positions with an average resolution of 1 position for 480 kb. Although terminal map positions have not been defined by isolation of the telomeres, comparison of the genetic and physical maps with the estimated length of the chromosome, and *in situ* data generated in one of the collaborating laboratories, leads to the conclusion that most distal loci are close to the telomeres. The pericentric region is extremely well-defined in the radiation hybrid map.

The STSs included of 256 polymorphic microsatellite markers. The ordering of these loci in the radiation hybrid maps produces a high density set of markers for genetic studies of this chromosome. On average, the genetic markers have a spacing of 1.2-1.5 cM throughout the chromosome. Fifty-six new microsatellite are included in the map, and others from diverse sources are integrated into a single map for the first time. Genetic linkage data were available for 98 of the microsatellite markers which allowed us to make the first detailed comparison of physical and genetic maps across a whole chromosome.

We mapped 151 genes, including 26 ESTs, representing the vast majority of genes known to reside on chromosome 11. Since these are integrated with genetic markers, it is now possible to obtain candidate genes rapidly from a region of interest that has been defined by linkage studies. The chromosome 11 radiation hybrid map and DNA from the panel provides a resource for further studies, and it should be easy to integrated new candidate genes as these are identified. The results of this pilot study strongly supports the application of radiation hybrid mapping by whole-genome approaches as an integral part of the human genome project.

In addition to producing an integrated map of STSs, the radiation hybrid map provides a high resolution ordering of STSs that will have a significant impact on the construction of other physical maps. Initially, these will be STS-based maps using YAC contigs. As an illustration of this approach, we constructed a YAC contig spanning 2.8 Mb from the 11q12-q13 region (Stafford et al. 1994). This was chosen because of its biological interest, in that one of the collaborating groups had linkage data supporting the presence of a gene implicated in atopy in this region. The YAC contig contained 15 STSs which were ordered physically; the order of most of these could be confirmed in the radiation hybrid map. Seven genes were placed in the contig map, including the high affinity immunoglobulin E receptor which is now thought to harbour variants implicated in atopy. A second contig was constructed in the region of chromosome 11q22-23 which contains a gene responsible for ataxia-telangectasia (publication in preparation).

The success of these two projects led us to examine the possibility of identifying a complete set of YACs spanning the whole of chromosome 11 based on STS information from the radiation hybrid map. This work is presently in progress in one of the collaborating laboratories, and is expected to be finished early in 1995.

Fluorescence *in situ* hybridisation (FISH) has played an important role in the above studies. A substantial number of YACs have been mapped throughout chromosome 11, with particular attention to 11q22-q23. Using a series of YACs, it was shown that a constitutional familial chromosome deletion 11q23.3-qter was a true deletion and not a hidden translocation. Thus, this deletion can now be used for further mapping studies. The localisation of the chromosomal breakpoint of the constitutional translocation t (11;22) has been refined by finding with FISH YAC clones encompassing the breakpoint. YACs and other clones were also mapped to regions of interest on other chromosomes.

The ordering of cosmid probes on interphase nuclei was also investigated by FISH. The chromosome region selected for this purpose was the long arm of chromosome 11 around band 11q23. Our aim was to order cosmid probes which could not be ordered by other methods (no polymorphims for recombination studies, and co-localisation on the same chromosome band or subband.) To avoid some ambiguities, an interspecific somatic cell hybrid containing only one copy of chromosome 11 was used for FISH experiments. The results of these studies have led to a novel technique for ordering markers on interphase nuclei (Cherif et al., 1994). Additional work was undertaken on the identification of acquired translocation of leukaemia's involving band 11q23, and more precise determination of chromosome breakpoints. These studies led to the recognition of complex translocations, and to the demonstration that some putative deletions were actually translocations.

4. Major scientific breakthroughs and/or industrial applications

The principal result of this collaborative effort has been the production of the first high-resolution integrated map of a human chromosome. Novel technologies have been evaluated for physical mapping, and the necessary background information has been obtained for construction of a complete contig of chromosome 11. During the course of the program, contigs were already for regions of specific interest.

5. Major co-operative links

Important co-operative links were maintained between all the groups during this study. STSs were developed through co-ordinated sequencing efforts in Paris (M. Lathrop's group) and Oxford (J. Bell's group). These were mapped on radiation hybrids in Paris (M. Lathrop's group), and YAC or other clones were transferred from M. Lathrop's group to the laboratory of R. Berger (Paris) for FISH analysis. Dr. Cookson's group (Oxford), who have collaborated very closely with the Dr. Lathrop's group on the study of the 11q12-13 region in atopy were able to exploit radiation hybrid data for confirmation of the order of STSs in their YAC contig of this region. The links were maintained by many exchanges of personnel between the laboratories during this period.

Joint/individual publications and patents:

- Cherif D. et al. Chromosome painting in acute monocytic leukemia. Genes Chrom Cancer, 107-112, 1993.
- Cherif D. et al. Ordering markers in the region of the ataxia-telangiectasia gene (11q22-q23) by fluroescence in situ hybridization (FISH) to interphase nuclei. Hum Genet 93: 1-6, 1994.
- Cherif D. et al. Hunting 11q23 deletions with fluorescence in situ hybridization. Leukemia 8: 578-586,

1994.
- Fatakkag D.M. et al. Molecular cloning and assignment to chromosome 5q31.2 of a novel human HSP cDNA. J Immunol, in press, 1994.
- Le Coniat M. et al. A novel translocation t(9;11)(q33;q23) involving the IIRX gene in an acute monocytic leukemia. CR Acad Sci Paris, Sc de la Vie 316: 692-697, 1193.
- James M. et al. A radiation hybrid map of 506 STS markers spanning human chromsome 11. Nature Genetics, in press, 1994.
- Richard I. et al. Mapping of the formin gene and exclusion as a candidate gene for the autosomal recessiver form of limb-girdle muscular dystrophy. Hum Mol Genet 1: 621-624, 1992.
- Romana S.P. et al. t(12;21) a new recurrent translocation in acute lymphoblastic leukemia. Genes Chrom Cancer 9: 186-191, 1994.
- Stafford A. et al. A 2.8 Mb YAC contig in 11q12-q13 localizes candidate genes for atopy: FcεR1B and CD20. Hum Mol Genet 3: 779-785, 1994.

Contract number: Geno-CT-91 0025 (SSMA)
Contractual period: 1 February 1992 to 31 January 1994

Coordinator
Professor G.M. Lathrop
Inserm U.358
16, rue de la Grange aux Belles
F - 75010 Paris
France
Tel: 33 1 44 52 75 45
Fax: 33 1 42 40 10 16

Participants
Dr. R. Berger
INSERM U301
27 rue Juliette Dodu
F - 75010 Paris
France
Tel: 33 1 42 49 9277
Fax: 33 142 06 9531

Dr. J. Bell
Institute of Molecular Medicine
John Radcliffe Hospital
University of Oxford
Oxford
United Kingdom
Tel: 44 865 221 339
Fax: 44 865 222 502

Dr. B. Cookson
Nuffield Department of Medicine
John Radcliffe Hospital
University of Oxford
Oxford
United Kingdom
Tel: 44 865 221 335
Fax: 44 865 750 506

Human Genome Analysis Programme
M. Hallen and A. Klepsch (Eds.)
IOS Press, 1995

TWO-DIMENSIONAL DNA TYPING OF HUMAN INDIVIDUALS
FOR MAPPING GENETIC TRAITS

A.G. Uitterlinden and E. Mullaart
INGENY B.V., Leiden, The Netherlands

1. Background information

A major goal of the human genome project is to provide investigators an optimal infrastructure for finding and characterizing new genes (for a review, see Olson, 1993). The availability of genetic and physical maps of the human genome will greatly accelerate the identification of human genes, including disease genes, and to subsequently characterize those genes. Such gene discovery programs will lead to new insight into the organization and functioning of the human genome and its role in the etiology of disease. In view of the growing recognition of a genetic basis for most human health problems, this could greatly benefit cost-effective healthcare through the availability of new highly accurate diagnostic and prognostic tests. Ultimately, the availability of fully characterized genes encoding a variety of functions could provide the raw material for various new rational forms of therapy, including gene therapy (for the impact of the Human Genome Project on medicine, see Hoffman, 1994).

A rational starting point for the identification and (positional) cloning of disease genes has proven to be its genetic/physical location in the genome. Such information can be obtained through genetic mapping studies on families with multiple affected members. By following the co-inheritance of the disease with genetically mapped DNA markers the position of the gene in the genome can be determined. Once this has been accomplished, the disease gene can be found and cloned by searching the genomic region, to which it was mapped, for expressed sequences and, finally, for the mutant gene of the trait one was looking for.

In the generation of genetic linkage maps much progress has been made since Southern's technique made it possible to measure RFLPs (Southern, 1975). In 1987, the first global human genetic map, based on RFLPs was published (Donis-Keller et al., 1987) and since then many chromosome-specific maps have followed (e.g. Keith et al., 1990). More recently, Weissenbach et al. (1992) published more than 800 sequences for CA-repeat PCR primer pairs distributed throughout the genome. These markers are microsatellites and belong to the VNTR (variable number of tandem repeat) type of polymorphism. Most of these markers have heterozygosities of >70% and an average spacing of about 5 cM. This major accomplishment makes genetic mapping of monogenic diseases relatively easy.

However, the common diseases of the aged (e.g. heart disease, adult-onset cancers, diabetes, rheumatoid arthritis) are mostly multifactorial. Such diseases can be approached either by a variant of the linkage approach, termed sib-pair analysis or through association studies (Clerget-Darpoux and Bonaïti-Pellié 1992). The latter is based on linkage disequilibrium and involves measuring differences in allele frequencies (of the markers) between patients and the control population. This situation requires an extreme map density in order to have a reasonable chance of detecting linkage disequilibrium. At a map density of 1-2 cM, IBD (Identity by Descent) methods can be employed through the identification of conserved haplotypes for gene localisation in multifactorial systems (Lander and Schork, 1994).

Both linkage and association approaches when applied on a total genome scale rely on cheap, fast and efficient methods for genotyping large numbers of individuals for many markers (thousands) simultaneously. In spite of the virtual completion of a 2-5 cM genetic map and an upcoming STS-based physical map it is still an open questions as to how useful and accessible these maps will be for large-scale gene identification. Indeed, for genetic mapping projects involving hundreds to thousands of individuals it would be necessary to use methods of scale to serially analyze a thousand and more individual microsatellite loci. The required investments in robotics (e.g. sample preparation, pipetting, PCR) and consumables (oligonucleotide primers, Taq polymerase) may be quite formidable and therefore gene discovery programs might be restricted to only a few, factory-based, genome analysis centers. While such a development might be desirable, it would also be reasonable to ask the question of whether disease gene mapping and analysis can possibly be carried out in a decentralized way, be made more cost-effective and be more widely accessible. In addition, the present genetic maps are still incomplete with several areas with thinly spread markers.

Therefore, to optimally benefit from the accomplishments of human genome analysis there is a need for efficient techniques to compare individual genomes, in a comprehensive way, for sequence variations. Thusfar, the serial approach has been predominant. That is, the analysis of DNA fragments one by one using either electrophoretic or hybridization techniques. Alternative approaches are under development, most notably the DNA chip approach in which multiple oligonucleotides are screened by the target nucleic acid of interest by hybridization (Fodor et al., 1993). In this way a pattern of hybridization is obtained that potentially reveals sequence variation down to the basepair level. Ultimately, this system should allow sequencing by hybridization (Drmanac et al., 1993). However, although great progress has recently been made in turning this concept into a reality, as yet the methodology is still considered as immature.

Thusfar, several total genome approaches have been proposed, of which Genomic Mismatch Scanning (GMS; Nelson et al., 1993), which is designed to identify DNA sequences two genomes have in common, and Representational Difference Analysis (RDA; Lisitsyn et al., 1993), which seeks to identify the differences between two genomes, have emerged as most promising. However, while RDA offers no real advantages in the speed with which genetic markers can be analyzed, GMS can not be easily applied to the complex human genome.

An alternative more classical approach involves two-dimensional separation of DNA fragments to increase the efficiency of gene and genome analysis. Analogous to proteins, DNA fragments can be separated in two dimensions using size separation and separation in denaturing gradients as the two independent criteria. This system was pioneered by Fischer and Lerman, who showed that it was possible to two-dimensionally resolve the entire E. coli genome and detect differences (Fischer and Lerman, 1979). Subsequently it was shown that in analyzing higher genomes it is possible to combine 2-D separation according to Fischer and Lerman with hybridization analysis to reveal multiple fragments homologous to the probe used. When using micro- or minisatellite core elements as probe hundreds of spot-giving alleles, many representing polymorphic loci, can be screened simultaneously (Uitterlinden et al. 1989). Subsequent rounds of hybridization with micro- and minisatellite core probes allows the rapid screening of thousands of such spots in a short period of time.

It was demonstrated that excellent separation patterns could be obtained when using G+C-rich core probes, allowing the target sequence to act as a stable GC-clamp (Uitterlinden and Vijg 1991). From simulation and empirical data the practical informativity of 2-D DNA typing for positional cloning studies has been elucidated (te Meerman et al., 1993). One data set related to the CEPH panel and another data set to the problem of finding linkage with a monogenic trait in cattle. The results indicated that in spite of a reduction in informativity, 2-D DNA typing is already a cost-effective system for rapidly mapping genetic traits. However, its informativity could be increased in a relatively simple manner through the identification of spots as alleles from specific loci, which is the purpose of the present study.

Finally, although the initial step in disease gene identification can be cumbersome the second (finding candidate genes) and third (finding disease-causing mutations) steps may be even more problematic. Indeed, once a trait has been assigned a particular chromosomal region, it will be necessary to scrutinize that region in order to find candidate genes. Analogous to studying genomic variation in 2 dimensions, entire reverse transcribed cell messages, i.e. total cDNA, can be resolved in the 2-D format and hybridized to specific probes, e.g. cosmid contigs, YACs, motif sequences, to reveal the transcripts of interest and sequence variations therein. Finally, taking the 2-D approach single genes can be analyzed in one single test for the presence of all possible mutations, based on the virtually 100% accuracy of the denaturing gradient principle to detect such sequence differences (Vijg et al., 1994; Wu et al., 1994).

Therefore, 2-D DNA electrophoresis allows complete coverage of the entire cycle from mapping a gene corresponding to a given trait to its comprehensive analysis for all possible mutations, including trinucleotide expansions. This is schematically depicted in Figure 1 (see also Uitterlinden and Vijg, 1994).

References

- Alderton, R.P., Kitau, J., Beck, S. Automated DNA hybridization. Anal Biochem 1994, 218, 98-102.
- Botstein, D., White, R., Skolnick, M., Davis, R. Construction of a genetic linkage map in man using restriction fragment length polymorphisms. Am J Hum Genet 1980, 32, 314-331.
- Brown, D.L., Gorin, M.B., Weeks, D.E. Efficient strategies for genomic search using the affected-pedigree-member method of linkage analysis. Am J Hum Genet 1994, 54, 544-552.
- Clerget-Darpoux, F., Bonaïti-Pellié, C. Strategies based on marker information for the study of human diseases. Ann Hum Genet 1992, 56, 145-153.
- Collins, F., Galas, D. A new five-year plan for the U.S. human genome project. Science 1993, 262, 43-46.
- Donis-Keller, H., Green, P., Helms, C., et al. A genetic linkage map of the human genome. Cell 1987, 51, 319-337.
- Drmanac, R., et al. Science 1993, 260, 1649-1652.
- Fischer, S.G., Lerman, L.S. Length-independent separation of DNA restriction fragments in two-dimensional gel electrophoresis. Cell 1979, 16, 191-200.
- Fodor, S.P.A., Rava, R.P., Huang, X.C., Pease, A.C., Holmes, C.P., Adams, C.L. Nature 1993, 364, 555-556.
- Hoffman, E.P. The evolving genome project: current and future impact. Am. J. Hum. Genet. 1994, 54, 129-136.
- Hoheisel, J.D. and Lehrach, H. Use of reference libraries and hybridization finger-printing for relational genome analysis. FEBS Lett, 1993, 325, 118-122.
- Keith, T.P., Green, P., Reeders, S.T., Brown, V.A., Phipps, P., Bricker, A., Falls, K., Rediker, K.S., Powers, J.A., Hogan, C., Nelson, C., Knowlton, R., Donis-Keller, H. Genetic linkage map of 46 DNA markers on human chromosome 16. Proc Natl Acad Sci USA 1990, 87, 5754-5758.
- Lander, E.S. and Schork, N.J. Genetic dissection of complex traits. Science, 1994, 265, 2037-2048.

- Lathrop, G.M., Lalouel, J.M. Easy calculations of lodscores and genetic risks on small computers. Am J Hum Genet 1984, 36, 460-465.
- Lisitsyn, N., Lisitsyn, N., Wigler, M. Cloning the differences between two complex genomes. Science 1993, 259, 946-951.
- Mullaart, E., de Vos, G.J., te Meerman, G.J., Uitterlinden, A.G., Vijg, J. Parallel genome analysis by two-dimensional DNA typing. Nature 1993, 365, 469-471.
- Nelson, S.F., McCusker, J.H., Sander, M.A., Kee, Y., Modrich, P., Brown, P.O. Genomic mismatch scanning: a new approach to genetic linkage mapping. Nature Genet 1993, 4, 11-18.
- NIH/CEPH collaborative mapping group A comprehensive genetic linkage map of the human genome. Science 1992, 258, 67-86.
- Olson, M.V. The human genome project. Prod Natl Acad Sci USA 1993, 90,4338-4344.
- Ott, J. (1992) Analysis of Human Genetic Linkage. The John Hopkins University Press, Baltimore.
- Risch, N. Linkage Strategies for genetically complex traits. II. The power of affected relative pairs. Am J Hum Genet 1990, 46, 229-241.
- Risch, N. A note on multiple testing procedures in linkage analysis. Am J Hum Genet 1991, 48, 1058-1064.
- Southern, E.M. Detection of specific sequences among DNA fragments separated by gel electrophoresis. J Mol Biol 1975, 98, 503-517.
- Te Meerman, G.J., Mullaart, E., van der Meulen, M.A., den Daas, J.M.G., Uitterlinden, A.G., Vijg, J. Linkage analysis by two-dimensional DNA typing. Am J Hum Genet 1993, 53, 1289-1297.
- Uitterlinden, A.G., Slagboom, P., Knook, D.L., Vijg, J. Two-dimensional DNA fingerprinting of human individuals. Proc Natl Acad Sci USA 1989, 86, 2742-2746.
- Uitterlinden, A.G., Vijg, J. Locus-specific electrophoretic migration patterns of minisatellite alleles in denaturing gradient gels. Electrophoresis 1991, 12, 12-16.
- Uitterlinden, A.G., Vijg J. (1994) Two-dimensional DNA typing: A Parallel Approach to Genome Analysis. Ellis Horwood PTR Prentice Hall Biotechnology Series, Chichester, Englewood Cliffs.
- Vijg, J., Wu, Y., Uitterlinden, A.G., Mullaart, E. Two-dimensional DNA electrophoresis in mutation detection. Mutation Res 1994, 308, 205-214.
- Weeks, D.E., Lange, K. A multilocus extension of the efedted-pedigree-member method of linkage analysis. Am J Hum Genet 1992, 50, 859-868.
- Weissenbach, J., Gyapay, G., Dib, C., Vignal, A., Morisette, J., Millasseau, Vaysseix, G., Lathrop, M. A second-generation linkage map of the human genome. Nature 1992, 359, 794-801.
- Wu, Y., Dijkstra, D-J., Scheffer, H., Uitterlinden, A.G., Mullaart, E., Buys, C.H.C.M., Vijg, J. Comprehensive and accurate mutation scanning of the CFTR-gene by two-dimensional DNA electrophoresis. 1994, submitted.

2. Objectives and primary approaches

To optimally profit from the reaps of the human genome project efficient methods are needed to comparatively analyze individual genomes for sequence variation. One way to achieve this is by high-resolution 2-dimensional analysis of DNA fragments, employing both size and sequence separation. By sequential re-hybridization analysis with multiple micro- and minisatellite core probes thousands of spots representing alleles of polymorphic loci can be addressed in a short time. This method, which has recently been automated, is cost-effective, but less informative than single-locus DNA typing where both alleles can be recognized and the locus is known. Here we propose to turn 2-D genome typing into a universally applicable human genotyping system by mapping individual spots to specific chromosomal positions and determine allelic and haplotype relationships, through co-segregation analysis of the CEPH panel of reference pedigrees and by direct isolation of the spot-forming alleles. As we see it, 2-D genome typing could be especially useful to rapidly assign traits to specific genetic regions through linkage and association analysis (based on e.g., conserved haplotypes); further, more refined mapping activities in that region can then occur with hyper-polymorphic microsatellites. Additionally, this project would help to fill up the holes in the present genetic maps.

The short-term objectives of the project were:

1. To characterize a limited set of micro- and minisatellite core probes as to their suitability for detecting informative VNTR loci in the human genome.
2. To develop procedures for direct isolation and cloning of spot-giving alleles from 2-D gels.
3. To genetically map a limited set of 2-D spot markers by co-segregation analysis of CEPH pedigrees.
4. To develop procedures for direct hybridization of short sequences to human genomic YAC and cosmid libraries.
5. To develop procedures for in situ mapping of isolated spot-giving alleles using primed in situ labelling (PRINS).

The long-term objectives of the project are the following:

1. To generate a 1-2 cM 2-D spot genetic map through co-segregation analysis of at least 4000 spot variants with the complete 60-pedigree CEPH marker panel.
2. To establish allelic relationships and informational haplotypes.
3. To isolate the micro- or minisatellite fragments corresponding to the variant spots and physically map the corresponding sequences.

The major experimental lines were the following:

2.1 Central aim

The central aim of mapping spots in 2-D genome typing patterns onto the human genome is to obtain a universally applicable cost-effective gene mapping system. As such it should allow a more optimal use of the, soon to be available, complete genetic and physical maps. The project therefore should result in a system for the rapid and economical assignment to chromosomal regions of genetic traits, especially the more complex ones. Once that is accomplished hyper-polymorphic microsatellite markers from that region can take over for more refined mapping if necessary. For genetic regions less dense with markers, the 2-D approach would offer the possibility to obtain such markers through the isolated and cloned spot-markers themselves and through its link-up to the physical map.

2.2 Mapping spots through linkage analysis

To obtain a 2-D genetic map we will work out segregation patterns of core-probe-detected spots in the CEPH panel and run the results against the CEPH marker database. For a standard CEPH pedigree with 12 children and four grandparents, the expected lodscore and variance (obtained in simulation studies) gives an indication of the possibility of genetic mapping of 2-D spots. For 40 CEPH pedigrees of the type of pedigree 1322, with 11 children and 4 grandparents, the expected lodscore is 27.2, with a standard deviation of 6.8, assuming 0.5 as frequency of the spot-giving allele against 0.2 as frequency of a 5-allele CEPH marker to do 2-point lodscore analysis with. This shows that most spots can be linked to at least one marker in the CEPH panel. Looking at informative meioses, there will in the worst case (lodscore two standard deviations below the expected value) about 45 informative meioses, enough for generating a rough genetic map.

2.3 Spot isolation and development of locus-specific probes

To develop suitable protocols for the isolation of the spot-giving alleles 3 experimental steps were considered crucial and therefore the subject of exhaustive testing. First, the elution of DNA underneath the spot of interest. Second, the amplification of these fragment in order to obtain a sufficiently high amount of starting material for the specific isolation. Third, the selective isolation of the core-probe specific fragment present in the mixture.

2.4 Hybridization of genomic libraries

Two sublines of research are distinguished:

1. To test a battery of short oligonucleotide probes by direct hybridisation to human genomic cosmid libraries for the purpose of obtaining fingerprints of the cosmid clones. This would, at the same time provide information for the other participants (Uitterlinden lab) as to which short (in particular tandemly repeated sequences) might serve as useful probes in 2-D DNA typing.
2. To develop simple ways of mapping the short genomic sequences to a specific chromosomal regions, and to provide access to larger clones from that region using a variety of cloning systems. This would enable the other participants (Uitterlinden and Kruse labs) to rapidly map sequences flanking 2-D variant loci, isolated by the "spot isolation procedure" (see co-ordinator's report), to the physical genomic map. This would give access to sets of overlapping genomic clones (contigs) defining the entire area-map around a 2-D variant locus.

2.5 In situ mapping

To establish suitable protocols for in situ mapping of the isolated spot-giving alleles by primed in situ labelling (PRINS), first one of the core probes (CAC) itself will be tested. Then, by the subsequent extension of this probe by adding specific sequences, locus-specificity should be obtained.

3. Results and Discussion

3.1 General configuration and reproducibility of 2-D DNA typing
(Uitterlinden/Mullaart)

Two-dimensional DNA typing was carried out using instruments that were modified after the one described by Fischer and Lerman (1979). We were able to develop a routinely applicable protocol for these instruments, which are used in combination with highly efficient electroblotting equipment with ceramic-coated electrodes (for the most recent protocols, see Uitterlinden and Vijg, 1994).

3.1.1 Experimental error (Uitterlinden/Mullaart, Kruse)

By repeated analyses of the same DNA sample the reproducibility in spot position was estimated. Table 1 gives the deviations observed in the position of a number of phage lambda fragments used as markers. The somewhat higher experimental error after hybridization analysis as compared to ethidium bromide staining is due to slight stretching of the gel during blotting.

Using the same series of gels the experimental error in the position of spots in the patterns obtained with minisatellite core probe 33.15 was assessed. Not surprisingly, the results in Table 1 indicate errors in spot position virtually identical to the errors found with the marker spots. Also results from the Kruse lab fall in the same range. The inter-lab reproducibility is currently being assessed as merged data from CEPH pedigree analysis from the two labs are being used in linkage analysis (see item 3. Mapping spots through linkage analysis).

Another source of error has been the absence of a spot known to be present in a given DNA sample and the occurrence of spots that should not be present but are due to dirt or other forms of contamination. The former occasionally occurred (Verwest et al., 1994). As yet, however, the reproducibility in spot-occurrence is virtually 100% provided the hybridization conditions are strictly controlled (de Leeuw et al., in preparation). In fact, an intensity difference of 50% (homozygous vs heterozygous) can still be detected although as yet we prefer to rely on genetic data to confirm this (see below).

These results indicate that theoretically at least 1600 spots can be independently displayed in a gel of 16 x 16-cm. However, due to unequal spot distribution, in practice with the probes used only about 500 spots can still be optimally evaluated by eye or by image analysis. Micro and minisatellite core probes seldom give more than 500 spots.

3.1.2 Marker-assisted calibration (Uitterlinden/Mullaart)

The use of marker DNA fragments facilitates 2-D gel comparisons and allows to correct for the inter-gel differences given in Table 1. The marker points serve to adjust for gel distortions and differences between electrophoretic runs. We routinely mix the DNA digests to be analyzed with sets of restriction fragments of lambda DNA. After co-electrophoresis, these markers can be visualized by ethidium bromide staining and by hybridization with labelled lambda DNA after or before the 2-D separation patterns have been probed with the core sequences. The resulting calibrated patterns are then subjected to the spot-scoring routines of the IngenyVision image analysis system (see also Mullaart et al., 1993 and Experimental Design Section of this proposal).

3.1.3 Automation (Uitterlinden/Mullaart)

Finally, by the recent development of automated instrumentation multiple gels can now be run simultaneously without manual interference (Mullaart et al., 1993). That is, it is no longer necessary to cut out the first-dimension lane and load it onto the second dimension gel. When many samples have to be run, as is the case in the present study, such a system is very useful. It may also increase the reproducibility of the system even further. The complete procedure that was developed on the basis of this instrument is schematically depicted in Figure 2.

3.2 Characteristics of the probes used (Uitterlinden/Mullaart, Kruse, Lehrach)

Much of our experimental work has focused on testing micro- and minisatellite core probes useful for 2-D DNA typing. Three characteristics are of major importance. First, the total number of spots detected. This should be at least several hundred to give 2-D DNA typing its major advantage over serial analysis by using locus-specific probes. Second, a major fraction of the spots should represent polymorphic loci. Third, the different probes used should be non-overlapping, that is, they should each detect different loci in the genome.

At least 12 of these probes were identified. Table 2 lists the numbers of spots, percentages of variant spots (on the basis of 10 unrelated individuals) and spot overlap for several core probes tested. The overlap in spot positions among these core probes was found to be low, on average. (It should be noted that there are minisatellite core probes that greatly overlap, like HBV-1 with 33.6.) In view of the high resolving power of the gel system it is unlikely that the low overlap is due to co-migration of fragments. Rather, cross-hybridization of one micro- or minisatellite to two or more core probes will occur. (Occasionally, co-migration of unrelated fragments was observed, which became apparent from segregation studies.)

From Table 2 it can be derived that about 80% of all spots detected by a given probe correspond to polymorphic loci. This figure may increase even more individuals are analyzed. The average heterozygosity level of the loci the alleles of which are detected as spots can be estimated to be about 50% (depending on the probe). On average spots may correspond to 3-allele systems, which is much lower than the highly polymorphic micro- and minisatellite loci which can easily have as many as 20 alleles per locus. Indeed, it would be impossible to accommodate such high numbers of different alleles on a 2-D gel. However, the system is polymorphic enough to be informative as became apparent from our segregation analysis.

With a limited number of spots obtained with probes 33.6 (214 spots) and CAC (213 spots) segregation analysis was performed on 2 CEPH pedigrees (Example in Fig. 3A and B). Figure 4 shows the transmission of the spots, which follow a basically Mendelian pattern. Comparison with the CEPH database of known markers allowed to tentatively map a number of spots to chromosomal positions. No evidence for extensive clustering of 33.6 or CAC loci in the genome was obtained. Table 3 provides the number of informative spots in these 2 pedigrees.

3.3 Mapping of spots through linkage analysis (Uitterlinden/Mullaart, Kruse)

To demonstrate the feasibilty to generate a 2-D genetic map, three large CEPH pedigrees have been analysed. These are pedigree nr 1362 (17 individuals), pedigree nr 1377 (11 individuals) and pedigree nr 1413 (19 individuals). Typings have been obtained with the microsatellite core probe $(CAC)_n$ and the minisatellite core probe 33.6. Linkage analysis was performed using all CEPH markers.

Results from the Kruse lab, where 9 CAC spots were analyzed in pedigree 1413, showed that 8 of these spots could be assigned to a particular chromosome on the basis of linkage with the CEPH markers (Børglum et al., Submitted). Furthermore, by segregation and linkage analysis, evidence was obtained for possible allelic relationships of two pairs of $(CAC)_n$ spots. Recently, an additional 15 $(CAC)_n$ and also 15 33.6 spots could be genetically mapped.

Results from the Uitterlinden/Mullaart lab showed a chromosomal assignment of 29 33.6 spots, out of the 214 spots followed in pedigree 1362 and 1377. Fig. 5 is a synthetic spot pattern obtained with probe 33.6 indicating the 29 spots mapped with a lod score higher than 3 (Table 4). Also here some evidence was obtained for allelic behaviour of certain spot pairs. Only 4 spot pairs (out of the 214 spots analysed) showed evidence for coupling; the other spots segregate as independent alleles.

These results obtained with only 1 (15 meioses) or 2 pedigrees (18 meioses) showed that in total already 68 spots could be mapped, which indicate the feasibility of the present project. We expect being able to generate a rough genetic map involving about 90% of all variant spots, detected by the core probes listed in Table 1, by using between 10 and 20 of the best typed families.

The typing of the CEPH pedigrees was somewhat delayed due to the fact that several of the CEPH DNA samples suffer from a rather high degree of single-strand breaks (as measured on an alkaline gel), which results in bad 2-D spot patterns. Attempts (by the Kruse Lab) to repair the breaks by ligation were only successful when extremely high amounts of ligase were used. Therefore, in some cases new DNA was isolated from cell lines obtained from Coriell Cell Respositories, Cambden, New Jersey, USA.

3.4 Spot isolation from 2-D gels and development into locus-probes
(Uitterlinden/Mullaart, Kruse, Bolund, Lehrach)

Recently we developed protocols for the isolation of the spot-giving alleles from the gel. The basic procedure followed is illustrated in Fig. 6. It is based on the elution of the genomic DNA fragments from a duplicate gel, corresponding to spots of interest indicated on the master gel hybridization patterns. Exact positions can be determined on the basis of the lambda marker fragments. The next step originally involved ligation in a plasmid, allowing to amplify the flanking regions of the repeats by using 2 different primers on the plasmid as well as the repeat core itself as the second primer. This should allow to specifically amplify the flanking regions of the repeat-containing genomic DNA fragments. Although we succeeded to directly isolate spot-giving alleles in this way, it turned out that the efficiency of this process is too low; hence, for many spots this procedure didn't work well enough to rapidly generate locus-specific markers.

A second protocol that we developed is simpler and appeared to be superior. This protocol, which is based on ligation of the eluted DNA fragments to small adaptors rather than large plasmids, is more efficient. After PCR with adapter primers, PCR products are cloned in plasmid vectors. Plasmid inserts are screened for micro- or minisatellite containing sequences using the core probes.

We are now isolating a number of spots for core probe 33.6 order to confirm the genetic mapping of these spots by hybridization (with the isolated spots as probe) of chromosome-specific blots (BIOS).

3.5 Testing of short oligonucleotide probes (Lehrach)

We tested 39 different mono- di- tri- and tetra-nucleotide simple tandem repeat sequence (microsatellite) probes in the form of 12 bases long oligonucleotides to a collection of 1536 random cosmids from the human X chromosome. Hybridisation was performed as described under near-zero-mismatch conditions (Nizetic et al., 1991) and each probe was washed at 3-4 different temperature points, to determine the optimal washing conditions. In parallel to cosmid colony filters, we hybridised filters bearing dot-blots of serial dilution's of human and E.Coli genomic DNAs. The ratio of the signals between the two series of dots was used to estimate the density of finds of each oligonucleotide sequence in the two genomes. Eight probes were found to have a high frequency in the E.Coli genome resulting in a high background on cosmid colony filters, which made the human insert-derived signals invisible. Three tandemly repeated sequences (CA, GA and AAAC) were found to have frequencies higher than 10% among cosmids. Seventeen sequences gave good signals, but were relatively low frequency (<3%). Eleven sequences gave frequencies high enough for potential use in 2-D mapping (see co-ordinator's report) i.e. between 3-10% of cosmids (D. Nizetic et al. unpublished). Several of these sequences have been successfully used by the Uitterlinden lab to detect 2-D DNA typing variations (see co-ordinator's report).

These short oligonucleotide sequences are a powerful addition to other mapping techniques such as the use of YAC, P1 and cosmids as probes in hybridisations to high density arrays of genomic cosmid libraries. The pattern of probe hybridisation generates a fingerprint of each cosmid, allowing overlaps to be deduced and eventually resulting in continuous sets of overlapping clones spanning entire chromosomes (Hoheisel et al., 1993). A battery of 30 short tandemly repeated and similar sequences have been hybridised to a 15 genome equivalent cosmid library of human chromosome 21. The expected hybridisation frequencies were found. These data are being analyzed using image analysis and contig construction software under development in the Lehrach Laboratory, and will eventually be integrated with hybridisation data from YACs used as probes against the chromosome 21 cosmid library. A cosmid and YAC contig of human chromosome 21 is at an advanced stage of construction (D. Nizetic; unpublished).

3.6 Resource development for mapping 2-D variants (Lehrach)

This participant has developed a set of techniques (Lehrach et al., 1990) which can enable rapid mapping of a large number of short flanking sequences form 2-D variant loci. The sequences obtained by spot isolation procedures (see co-ordinator's report) can be hybridised to human genomic YAC libraries.

The Lehrach laboratory has four YAC libraries stored in microtitre plates. These are the ICRF YAC library, two CEPH YAC libraries and the ICI YAC library with respective average insert sizes of 630, 450, >1000 and 350 kilobases. Providing a 15 fold human genome coverage.

In addition to expanding the YAC library collection, progress has been made in handling the libraries. Firstly, a faster robot for arraying YAC clones at high density on nylon membranes has been constructed. This robot spots clones from microtitre plates, and can produce 12 membranes (22x22 cm) carrying 20,000 clones in less that 2h. Secondly, upgrading the density of storage by commissioning manufacture of quadruple density microtitre plates. These plates hold 384 clones (wells) in the same space as a conventional microtitre plate. This storage format has also increased the speed of high density membrane generation and reduces handling time (plate replication). Thirdly, optimisation of the preparation procedures for the high density membranes of YAC colonies to be used as hybridisation targets. Fourthly, a PCR robot has been constructed allowing library scale PCR (40,000 clone capacity) to be carried out in customised 384 well microtitre plates (Meier-Ewert et al., 1991). Procedures have been optimised to allow DNA preparation from individual yeast clones in microtitre wells and inoculation of PCR reactions from these plates for successful inter-Alu PCR. Spotting protocols have been developed allowing PCR products to be arrayed at high density on membranes for hybridisation (as for YAC colonies). These membranes are being used in contiging strategies. They could also be of use for identification of YACs corresponding to 2-D variant flanking sequences if these contain Alu sequences. The advantage of these DNA arrays in the very high level of sensitivity they offer. At a later stage in the 2-D typing project inter-Alu products may provide polymorphic markers.

These YAC resources are being used in several genome wide mapping projects in the Lehrach laboratory. These libraries (in the form of hybridisation membranes) are also distributed to laboratories world wide as a reference library system, allowing additional probe hybridisation data to be stored in the database. These experiments are resulting in the generation of contigs.

Once a YAC is identified it can be mapped to a particular cytogenetic region of a particular human chromosome by means of fluorescence in situ hybridisation (FISH) to human metaphase chromosome spreads. To facilitate and speed up this process, the Lehrach laboratory in collaboration with other groups at ICRF, developed protocols that enable the direct use of YAC colony material as the template for the inter-repeat PCR, generating products which have successfully been used in FISH-mapping (Baldini et al., 1992). This acceleration of the mapping procedure (from YACs to a chromosomal location) will be important for the mapping of the large number of 2-D spot-variant loci likely to be generated.

Once the chromosomal location of a YAC bearing a 2-D spot variant locus is known, it can be used as a probe (Ross et al., 1992) against one of the human chromosome cosmid sub libraries constructed in the Lehrach Lab (Nizetic et al., 1991). To date eleven chromosome cosmid sub libraries have been constructed for chromosomes 1,5,6,7,11,13,17,18,21,22 and X. Further libraries are under construction. If a chromosome cosmid library does not exist for a particular YAC then a high density gridded human genomic phage P1 library (average insert size of 85 kbp), constructed in the Lehrach Laboratory will be used instead.

3.7 In situ mapping (Bolund)

The mapping in situ of the clones obtained were technologically the more demanding part of the project. In brief the status is now that though no sequence has as yet been mapped, significant progress has been made.

As a starting point the CAC repeat itself was used to induce PRimed IN Situ labelling (PRINS). As expected all chromosomes were strongly stained with the signal appearing as a diffuse banding pattern. Thus, the CAC repeat was shown to be an efficient primer for PRINS.

We then proceeded to test the next hypothesis, namely that modification of the 3'-end of the primer could be used to change and direct the specificity of the primer. In order to do so the sequence CTNAG was added to the end of the primer. This should lower the number of binding sites about 200-fold, and lead to a selective staining of a selected subset of the CAC repeats, namely those flanked by the sequence CTNAG. The results were in agreement with this assumption: The overall staining was much reduced with a few regions stronger labelled than the remaining genome.

The next step was then to increase the size of the addition to the 3'-end to make the primer locus specific. To ensure that the sequence chosen was really locus specific it was chosen from one of the clones obtained in the project. With this primer the diffuse chromosome staining was completely eliminated, indicating that the primer actually do not label other sites that the one of interest. Unfortunately, the week specific signals possibly appearing were to weak for positive identification. A fact that a number of technical modifications were unable to change. Thus, obtaining stronger signals seems to be the main problem left. Knowing ahead that sensitivity could become a critical parameter, a parallel study was undertaken to improve the sensitivity of the PRINS by doing the reaction repeatedly in a PCR like manner. Results on locus specific tandem repeat sequences have been promising with a 15-fold increase in signal intensity (manuscript submitted). In the continuation we will try to apply this approach also to the type of repeat dealt with in this project.

Apart from the intensity of the signals, the detection of the signals may also be a problem. In the near future we will get access to a cooled CCD camera which will enable us to detect weaker signal, possibly solving the sensitivity problem.

3.8 Joint/individual manuscripts

- Børglum, A.D., Mullaart, E., Kvistgaard, A.B., Uitterlinden, A.G., Vijg, J. and Kruse, T.A. Two-dimensional DNA typing as a genetic marker system. Submitted.
- Mullaart, E., Verwest, A.M., Børglum, A.D., Uitterlinden, A.G., te Meerman, G.J.,Kruse, T.A. and Vijg, J. Two-dimensional DNA typing of human pedigrees. Spot pattern characterization and segregation. Submitted.
- De Leeuw, W.J.F. Verwest, A.M., Feenstra, M.F., Sugiyama, A., Mullaart, E., Uitterlinden, A.G. and Vijg, J. Cloning of micro-and minisatellite containing sequences from two-dimensional DNA typing gels. Isolation of polymorphic DNA markers. In preparation.

References

- Baldini, A., Ross, M., Nizetic, D., Vatcheva, R., Lindsay, E.A., Lehrach, H. and Siniscalco, M. Chromosomal assignment of human YAC clones by fluorescence in situ hybridization. Use of single-yeast-colony-PCR and multiple labelling. Genomics, 14, 181-184, 1992.
- Baxendale, S., Bates, G., MacDonald, M., Gusella, J. and Lehrach, H. The direct screening of cosmid libraries with YAC clones. Nucleic Acids Res., 19, 6651, 1991.
- Fischer, S.G., Lerman, L.S. Length-independent separation of DNA restriction fragments in two-dimensional gel electrophoresis. Cell 1979;16:191-200.
- Hoheisel, J.D., Maier, E., Mott, R., McCarthy, L., Grigoriev, A.V., Schalkwyk, L.C., Nizetic. D., Francis, F. and Lehrach, H. High resolution cosmid and P1 maps spanning the 14 Mbp genome of the fission yeast S.Pombe. Cell, 73, 109-120, 1993.
- Lehrach, H., Drmanac, R., Hoheisel, J.D., Larin, Z., Lennon, G., Monaco, A.P., Nizetic, D.., Zehetner, G. and Poustka, A. Hybridization fingerprinting in genome mapping and sequencing. In: Genome Analysis, Eds. K.E. Davies and S. Tilghman. Cold Spring Harbor Lab. Press, Cold Spring Harbor (NY), pp 39-81, 1990.
- Meier-Ewert, S. Maier, E., Ahmadi, A., Curtis, J. and Lehrach, H. An automated approach to generating expressed sequence catalogues. Nature, 361, 375-376, 1991.
- Mullaart, E., de Vos, G.J., te Meerman, G.J., Uitterlinden, A.G., Vijg, J. (1993) Parallel genome analysis by two-dimensional DNA typing. Nature, 365, 469-471.
- Nizetic, D., Zehetner, G., Monaco, A.P., Gellen, L., Young, B.D. and Lehrach, H. Construction, arraying and high density screening of large insert libraries of the human chromosomes X and 21: their potential use as reference libraries. Proc. Natl. Acad. Sci. USA, 88, 3233-3237, 1991.
- Nizetic, D. Drmanac, R. and lehrach, H. An improved colony lysis procedure enables direct DNA hybridization using short (10,11 bases) oligonucleotides to cosmids. Nucleic Acids Res., 19, 182, 1991.
- Ross, M.T., Hoheisel, J.D., Monaco, A.P., Larin, Z., Zehetner, G. and Lehrach., H. High density gridded YAC filters: their potential as genome mapping tools. In: Techniques for the analysis of complex genomes, Eds. R. Anand, Academic Press, New York, pp 137-154, 1992.
- Uitterlinden, A.G., Vijg J. (1994) Two-dimensional DNA typing: A Parallel Approach to Genome Analysis. Ellis Horwood PTR Prentice Hall Biotechnology Series, Chichester, Englewood Cliffs.
- Verwest, A.M., de Leeuw, W.J.F., Molijn, A.C., Andersen, T.I., Börresen, A.-L., Mullaart, E., Uitterlinden, A.G. and Vijg, J. (1994) Genome scanning of breast cancers by two-dimensional DNA typing. Br. J. Cancer, 69, 84-92.

4. Major scientific breakthroughs and/or industrial applications

This project has led to at least one scientific breakthrough: for the first time it has been shown feasible to analyse the genome at a large number of loci simultaneously without loss of informativity. Hence, genome scanning for individual differences that could be associated with human disease has now become reality. Industrial applications include the development of automated instrumentation and cumputer programs to facilitate large-scale application and rapid implementation of the system worldwide. This task has already been undertaken by one of the participants in the project: Ingeny B.V. (Leiden, NL).

5. Major cooperative links

The project has led directly to the establishment of a reference network for 2-D DNA typing, first for validating the automatic instrument and software, and then to generate human genetic information to be stored in a centrally maintained database system. All participants of the network will meet at least once a year in Europe. This meeting cycle will be sponsored by Ingeny B.V.

Contract number: GENO-CT91-0021
Contractual period: 1 February 1992 to 1 February 1994

Coordinator
Dr. A.G. Uitterlinden
and Dr. E. Mullaart
INGENY B.V.
Einsteinweg 5
NL-2300 AR Leiden
The Netherlands
Tel: 31 71 21 4575
Fax: 31 71 21 0236

Participants
Dr. Torben Kruse
and Dr. Lars Bolund
Institute of Human Genetics
The Bartholin Building
DK - 8000 Aarhus C
Denmark
Tel: 45 86 139 711
Fax: 45 86 191 277

Dr. Hans Lehrach
Imperial Cancer Research Funds
Genome Analysis Laboratory
44 Lincoln's Inn Fields
UK - London WC2A 3PX
United Kingdom
Tel: 44 71 269 3308
Fax: 44 71 405 4303

No. of joint/individual publications + patents: 3.

Table I   Reproducibility of the 2-D DNA typing method

Variation in position of lambda marker spots detected after ethidium bromide staining (n = 7)

	x-coordinate (mm)	y-coordinate (mm)
Between samples on the same gel	1.2	0.92
Between samples on different gels	2.36	3.86

Variation in position of lambda marker spots detected after hybridization with lambda (n = 7)

	x-coordinate (mm)	y-coordinate (mm)
Between samples on the same gel	2.14	1.62
Between samples on different gels	3.18	5.32

Variation in position of 33.15 spots detected after hybridization[a] (n = 7)

	x-coordinate (mm)	y-coordinate (mm)
Between samples on the same gel	1.94	2.58
Between samples on different gels	2.64	4.76
Between samples run in different laboratories	2.4	3.6

[a] About 30 spots were selected for measurements of their position on the different gels.

Table II   **Probe characteristics**

Probe	Nr of spots and spot variants			Informative spots		
	Ind.[1]	Pedigree[2]	Total[3]	Ind.[1] (%)	Pedigree[2] (%)	Total[3] (%)
33.6	356	437	508	82 (23)	164 (38)	371 (73)
33.15	382	466	nd	84 (22)	168 (36)	nd
HBV-2	196	237	nd	41 (21)	82 (35)	nd
HBV-5	351	425	nd	73 (21)	146 (34)	nd
INS	159	193	nd	34 (22)	68 (35)	nd
16C6	125	151	nd	26 (21)	52 (34)	nd
Enhance	75	92	nd	17 (22)	34 (36)	nd
TELO	63	73	114	10 (16)	20 (27)	78 (75)
(CAC)$_n$	470	583	689	113 (24)	226 (36)	510 (74)
(TCC)$_n$	460	608	nd	138 (30)	276 (45)	nd
(AGC)$_n$	209	263	nd	56 (28)	112 (43)	nd
(GAC)$_n$	202	284	nd	82 (40)	164 (58)	nd
Total		3812	±4500[4]		1512	±3200[4]

[1] Number of spots and spot variants present in one individual (when compared to an other individual).
[2] Number of spots and spot variants present in total in the two parents of a given pedigree.
[3] Total number of spots and spot variants found in 8 unrelated individuals.
[4] Estimated on basis of data obtained with 33.6, (CAC) and TELO.
Overlap between the probes is less than 5%.

Table III   Informativity of 2-D DNA typing patterns

	Spots	Informative spots[1]		Heterozygous spots[2]	Genetically informative spots[3]
		Total	homozygous		
Probe 33.6					
Pedigree # 1362	184	66 (36%)	5	29 (16%)	80 (43%)
Pedigree # 1377	187	79 (42%)	9	23 (12%)	93 (50%)
1362/1377[4]	214	116 (54%)	14	46 (21%)	134 (63%)
Probe (CAC)$_n$					
Pedigree # 1362	191	82 (42%)	1	43 (23%)	120 (63%)
Pedigree # 1377	177	53 (30%)	1	23 (13%)	75 (43%)
1362/1377[4]	213	110 (51%)	2	58 (27%)	147 (68%)

[1] Present in only one parent
[2] Present as a single copy in both parents since not all children receive this spot.
[3] The total number of spots containing genetic information is the number of informative spots minus the homozygous ones, plus the heterozygous spots.
[4] Spots present in at least one of the pedigrees

Table IV Genetic mapping of 2-D DNA spot variants in human

Chromosome nr	2-D spot nr
1	1-29; (1-123)
2	3-5; 3-9
3	1-49
4	1-47; (1-194)
5	1-115
6	1-91
7	1-10; 1-79; 1-190
8	1-169; 3-6; 3-7; (1-132)
9	1-64; 1-139
10	1-52; 1-257
11	3-8; (1-132)
12	-
13	1-128; 1-254
14	-
15	-
16	1-50
17	1-156; (1-194)
18	-
19	1-147
20	1-80; (1-123)
21	3-4
22	1-145; 1-148; 3-1; 3-2

Based on the analysis of two CEPH pedigrees #1377 and 1362 for 33.6 and one pedigree #1413 for CAC.
The spot numbers between parentages are mapped to two chromosomes

1-* : 33.6 spots
3-* : CAC spots

In total **29** spots mapped to one chromosome and 3 to two chromosomes.

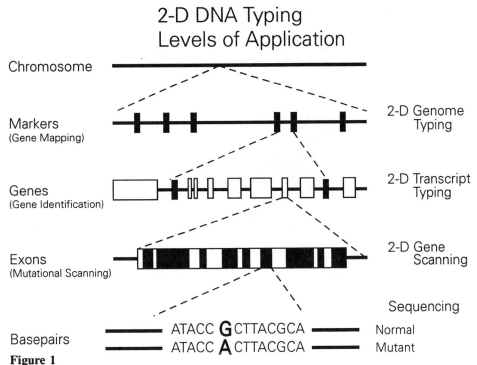

Figure 1
Schematic depiction of the use of 2-Delectrophoresis in the entire cycle from genome mapping to mutational analysis of a gene.

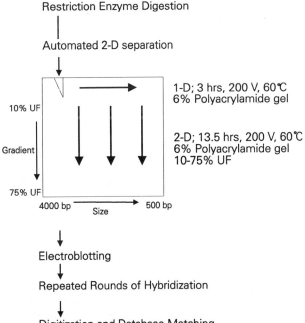

Figure 2
Experimental set-up of semi-automated 2-D DNA typing

CEPH Pedigree 1377

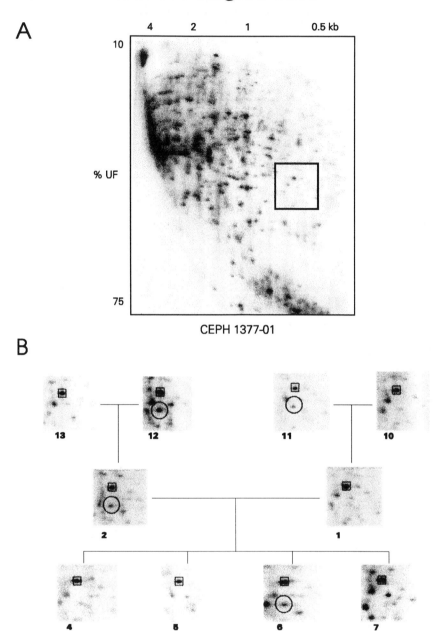

Figure 3
(A) Two-dimensional genome typing patterns of human genomic DNA hybridized 33.6. (B) Examples of the transmission of spots and spot variants detected with probe 33.6. Each square indicate a constant spot and each circle indicates the presence of a spot variant. Pedigree numbers are as follows: 1 and 2 = parents, 3-12 and 17 = children and 13-16 = grandparents.

Transmission of spot variants

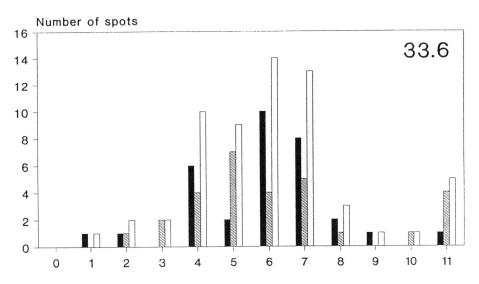

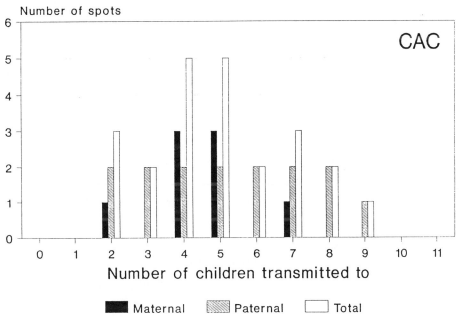

Figure 4
The percentage of paternal and maternal spot variants detected by probe 33.6 (A)
and $(CAC)_n$ (B) transmitted to the children of pedigree 1362.

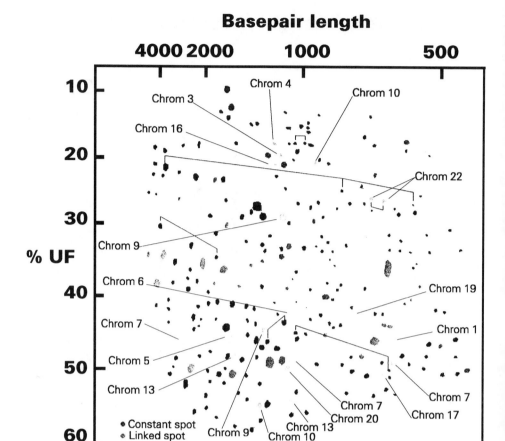

Basepair length

Probe 33.6

Figure 5
Two-dimensional DNA spot map of probe 33.6 Constant spots are indicated as well as linked or allelic spots. Furthermore, the spots coupled to each other and allelic spot pairs are indicated. The spot pattern of individual 1362-01 (father) is used as master and the other spots (not present in 1362-01) are positioned in this pattern on basis of their position relative to the constant spots.

Isolation of spots from 2-D DNA gels

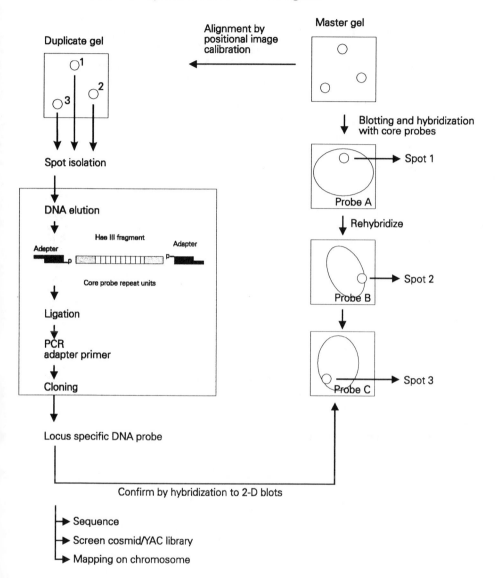

Figure 6
Basic procedure for the isolation of spots from 2-D gels.

Human Genome Analysis Programme
M. Hallen and A. Klepsch (Eds.)
IOS Press, 1995

APPROACH TO THE PHYSICAL AND FUNCTIONAL MAPPING OF HUMAN GENOME IN METAPHASE AND INTERPHASE CHROMOSOMES BY *IN SITU* HYBRIDIZATION AND 3-DIMENSIONAL CONFOCAL LASER SCAN MICROSCOPE IMAGING

M. Robert-Nicoud
Université Joseph Fourier, Grenoble, France

1. Background information

The aim of this project was *to develop approaches for the physical mapping of DNA sequences on metaphase and interphase chromosomes*. To reach this goal the development of fluorescent procedures for *the detection of in situ hybridization (ISH) DNA probes* was combined with the development of *systems for 2D and 3D digital imaging of the fluorescence signals*. These systems were optimized for *maximal spatial resolution, sensitivity and optimal discrimination of multiple fluorescent probes*.

This project was carried out jointly by *two research laboratories* and *two industrial companies*. The two laboratories are experts in the fields of *cytogenetics*, and *cell biology* and with methodologies and technologies used of *in situ analysis* of the structural and functional organization of cells and tissues. The two industrial companies are specialized in the fields of *microscopy* and *image analysis* respectively.

Key words: Genome physical and functional mapping; Interphase cytogenetics; Fluorescence *in situ* hybridization; Confocal microscopy; 2D and 3D image analysis.

2. Objectives and primary approaches

The research activity carried out by the four contractors did converge towards: (i) the development of a *routine fluorescent multicolor reproducible ISH approach* to locate probes on chromosomes and in cell nuclei, and (ii) the development of a *specific high resolution digital imaging system* for the detection of fluorescent ISH signals, by improving the confocal laser scan microscope and interfacing the microscope with the *image processing and analysis dedicated workstations*.

The work carried out has been divided into 4 complementary workpackages:
- *Workpackage PM*: Physical mapping of DNA sequences on metaphase and interphase chromosomes by means of fluorescent ISH-probes (Robert-Nicoud and Cremer);
- *Workpackage CL*: Confocal laser scan microscopy improvement for fluorescent ISH-probes imaging (Robert-Nicoud and Faltermeier);
- *Workpackage IP*: Image pre-processing for detection of fluorescent ISH probes (Robert-Nicoud and Adelh);
- *Workpackage MA*: ISH-map construction tools (Robert-Nicoud, Cremer and Adelh).

3. Results and Discussion

3.1 Workpackage PM: Physical mapping of DNA sequences on metaphase and interphase chromosomes by means of fluorescent ISH-probes (Robert-Nicoud and Cremer)

A sex chromosome and 2 autosomes were selected as models for testing various techniques of fluorescent *in situ* hybridization and for checking the general usability of the tools developed.

Subpackage PM/MET/X: Mapping X-specific YAC contigs on metaphase chromosomes (Cremer)

39 YAC clones were mapped by FISH to bands on the long and short arms of human X chromosome. For this purpose, Alu-PCR amplification products of these clones were generated, using a protocol developed by Dr. Cremer. With these probes, two-color "bar codes" (CBCS) were generated. In contrast to conventional G- or R-bands, the chromosomal position, extent, individual color and relative signal intensity of each "bar" could be modified, depending on probe selection and labeling procedures. Probes from up to twenty YAC clones were used simultaneously to produce CBCS on selected human chromosomes. Evaluation using a cooled CCD camera and digital image analysis confirmed the high reproducibility of the bars from one metaphase to another. Combinatorial FISH with mixtures of whole chromosome paint probes can be used along with a set of YAC clones which map to these chromosomes. Using this approach analytical chromosomal bar codes were constructed and adapted to particular needs of cytogenetic investigations and automated image analysis. Multicolor FISH with cosmid and YAC clones was used e.g. for the simultaneous visualization of deletion prone regions in the dystrophin gene.

Subpackage PM/INT/X: Mapping X-specific YAC contigs in interphase chromosomes (Cremer)

The resolution limit of gene mapping by FISH using metaphase or prometaphase chromosomes is in order of several Mb. Using interphase nuclei, DNA targets which are some hundred Kb apart can be readily resolved. Dr. Cremer has demonstrated the usefulness of histone depleted Halo-DNA preparations for high resolution mapping with FISH. This new approach was applied to map overlapping clones from a cosmid contig from the X-specific human dystrophin gene using multicolor FISH.

Subpackage PM/MET/A: Mapping cosmid probes on autosomes (Robert-Nicoud)

Mapping chromosomes 11q13 specific cosmid probes was realized by Professor Robert-Nicoud in collaboration with the group of P. Gaudray in Nice. Using FISH techniques it was possible to confirm the scattering of breakpoints from the MTC to CCND1 in centrocytic lymphomas, as was previously reported in experiments based on molecular biology approaches. The arrangement of this new set of cosmid probes was particularly suitable for studies in the frame of this project, since this contig covers distances suitable for interphase mapping.

Subpackage PM/INT/A: Mapping cosmid probes on interphase chromosomes (Robert-Nicoud)

Pairs of cosmid probes spanning the regions 9q13 and 11q13 were used for *in situ* hybridization on interphase nuclei in order to measure distances between sequences with known positions on the physical map of loci.

9q13 contig: Series of distance measurements were carried out using various pairs of probes from a contig spanning a region of 450kb in 9q13 (YAC 700F 10). This contig is constituted of 13 probes. Combinations of probes were chosen with distances ranging from 90 to 715kb. *In situ* hybridization was carried out on interphase lymphocyte nuclei fixed with acetic acid/methanol (2D analyses) or with paraformaldehyde (3D analyses). For 2D analyses, images were acquired using a fluorescence microscope equipped with a cooled CCD camera (Hamamatsu Photonics) and processed in different ways for distance measurement. Software packages from Dr. Adelh were used for this purpose.

A method for measuring distances between the ISH spots even in the case where the two signals overlap was developed. Measurements were carried out on raw images and on images processed by using deconvolution algorithms (see Workpackage MA). The results of the measurements performed before and after deconvolution of the images demonstrate the improvement obtained after deconvolution. The distances measured varied between 0.45μm (probes distant by 100 kb and $0,75\mu$m (probes distant by 700 kb).

11q13 contig: In order to measure distances between sequences separated by less than 100kb, probes from a contig spanning a region of 250kb in 11q13 were chosen. This contig is constituted of a set of probes for sequences separated by 25kb for the two closest ones, and by 215kb for the two most distant ones. 5 pairs of probes were used for *in situ* hybridization on interphase lymphocyte nuclei fixed with acetic-acid/methanol (2D-analyses) or paraformaldehyde (3D-analyses). Images were acquired with a conventional fluorescence microscope equipped with a cooled CCD camera (Hamamatsu Photonics) and processed in different ways for distance measurements. Software packages from Dr. Adelh were used for these measurement. Measurements were carried out on raw images and on images processed by using deconvolution algorithms (see Workpackage MA). The distances measured vary between 0.24μm (probes distant by 50kb) and 0.45μm (probes distant by 160kb).

3D analyses were performed on lymphocyte and fibroblast nuclei by confocal laser scanning microscopy. Various types of fixation were tested in order to define the conditions for best preservation of the 3D structure of the nuclei. 3D analyses were performed on paraformaldehyde fixed nuclei using the new confocal laser scanning microscope LSM4 provided by Dr. Faltermeier. This instrument gives a higher flexibility to exchange filters and beamsplitters, has a better collection efficiency and more detector channels than the LSM3. Various types of objective lenses were used for these measurements, among them a new designed water immersion lens newly designed by Dr. Faltermeier.

3.2 Workpackage CL: Confocal laser scan microscopy improvement for fluorescent ISH-probes imaging (Faltermeier)

It was the task of Dr. Faltermeier to support the project by developments on the microscope technology and to provide the Contractors with information and hardware necessary to reach the sensitivity and the resolution of the confocal microscope which is necessary to do the biological research work.

Subpackage CL/RWL: Registration between ISH fluorescent spots of various wavelength (Faltermeier)

The originally planned development of special filters for different dyes was stopped. Early investigations indicated difficulties in optimizing the fluorescence filters in the Confocal Laser Scanning Microscope of Professor Robert-Nicoud. A decision was made to replace the instrument LSM3 by a new type of instrument LSM4. This instrument gives very high flexibility to exchange all filters and beamsplitters.

Subpackage CL: HRI/High resolution of ISH fluorescent probes (Faltermeier)

Objective lenses for microscopes are designed for a variety of applications. For particular applications like in this project, special consideration had to be taken into account concerning the use of lenses. The Zeiss lenses used in the project are PlanNeofluar 40/1.3; PlanNeofluar 100/1.3 and PlanApo 63/1.4 For these 3 lenses computer modelling was made under the special circumstances of those application. The refractive index of the embedding medium, which is actually used in the experiment, was measured. Because of a difference in index from the index of the immersion oil for thick samples image degradation appears if the lens is focused deep into the sample.

A new method for simulation of the imaging of the confocal microscope was developed. This method describes the imaging of the confocal microscope along the full imaging path. The imaging path includes illumination beam path and emission beam path of the microscope. The model covers different cases including geometrical and diffraction optical properties of the system. A series of calculations was made for different depth of penetration into the sample. Using the measured refractive index of the embedding media, which is fairly closed to the index of standard immersion oil, the lens could be used up to a penetration depth of about 30 μm. Up to this depth the imaging of the lenses is fairly good. The drop in energy detected through the pinhole is about 30% of the energy measured directly below the coverglass.

If the refractive index of the immersion oil (1.52) and the embedding media are very different (for example water 1,33) the image quality gets poor at a depth of a few microns in the sample. In that case the intensity of the confocal signal drops down to 50% within a depth of 5μm. Therefore thick water samples cannot be imaged with an oil immersion lens. A water immersion lens was developed (C. Apochromat 40X) which fits to the need of water samples and confocal microscopy. The lens is a 40X lens with a numerical aperture of 1.2 and is optimized for a spectral range from 400 to 700 nm. This lens was optically completely new designed and requires the use of well calibrated cover glasses and has correction for refractive index differences. It was made available to Professor Robert-Nicoud and used in his laboratory for comparative 3D-analyses on *in situ* hybridization preparations.

3.3 Workpackage IP: Image pre-processing for detection of fluorescent ISH probes (Robert-Nicoud and Adelh)

Connection between a Confocal Laser Scanning Microscope and a Workstation:
File server programmes were written by contractor 01 for exchanging image files through GPIB communication between the LSM410 (keithley-board) and a Silicon Graphics Indigo workstation (NS-GPIB/SCSI).

- On the LSM side: a windows 3.1 application working in the background (ICON only) and checking every half-second if there is an incoming request on the GPIB port. If there is no request then the programme returns to a sleep state. If there is request the scanning frequency of the port is increased and the programme comes to active mode. Incoming commands are dealt with until a sleep request is received.
- On the SGI side: the programme uses a window-menu-dialog interface. The programme makes the LSM disk visible as if it was a volume mounted on the SGI workstation. The programme also treats a series of LSM.TIFF images as if it was only file stating at *000.tiff. The series is transferred and converted to the 3D compressed file format compatible with our applications. Files can also be imported one by one with no conversion.

Subpackage SRI: Storage, Retrieval and Interface (Adelh)

The main achievements of this part of the work were:
- Development of image data base facilities;
- Investigation of different media for image archiving;
- Specifications of the image preprocessing and processing methods.

Image data base: The storage of all the necessary information describing the image, the nature of the observed object and the conditions of its acquisition in a sufficiently flexible but simple way, requires to use a data base able to handle multimedia information. As the objective of the project is to provide an environment for fluorescence image quantification at an affordable price the target system which has been choosen is a PC-AT compatible. In this environment a wide variety of products commercially available exist concerning data base management systems. These products are not all able to handle image information even if their editors claim they are. Besides the conventional data base management systems, document oriented management systems have appeared. These software packages have integrated the management of images and offer specific processing capabilities able to optimize the management of the very large amount of data that images represent. Among these dedicated services are:
- the display of images in various formats,
- the possibility to select images from their contents by offering multiple images display on a single screen in a so called gallery mode,
- the ability to compress image information in order to reduce the volume needed to store them.

Product comparison: A study was made in order to compare the pros and cons of different products for data base management systems in order to select the most adapted one for purpose of the project. Two products have been selected for this comparison:
- one is relational data base provided by MICROSOFT in the Windows environment: ACCESS,
- the second one is a document oriented data management system provided by DCI: TAURUS.
The conclusions of this study are:
Although ACCESS reveals to be easier to use concerning non image data handling, particularly concerning the availability to exploit existing tables issued from other software packages such as Btrieve, dBase, Paradox, etc, it is too poor concerning

specific functionalities for image handling. The limitations concerning the compression mechanisms which are not adapted to quantitative fluorescence applications can be overcome through an adaptation consisting of rewriting some of the modules, especially those in charge of accessing the images in order to allow other compression techniques to be accessible. As a conclusion TAURUS is better compromise than ACESS regarding the specific constraints of the application. The necessary adaptations do not prevent to use the product now but will improve the ergonomy and the user friendliness of the software.

Physical support for image archiving: The requirements of the application concerning data storage are such that the amount of available memory in the system must be sufficient in order to allow for the storing of a large number of images corresponding to the experiences to be conducted. It can be envisaged that several thousands of images will have to be stored in order to document all the combinations between probes, dyes, acquisition conditions, etc.

The size of an image may vary between 0.25 Mbyte for a monochrome 512x512 image to 3 Mbytes for a 3 wavelengths 1024x1024 image. The total storage capacity is thus certainly higher than the typical capacity of a hard disk using magnetic technology. Moreover, the images have to be archived in order to allow a safe storage and the necessary back up of the hard disk to prevent data loss in case of disk failure. Several technologies have been envisaged: magnetic tape back up, optical disk (WORM), magneto optical disk.

Techniques comparison: The various technologies have specific benefits and constraints. Magnetic tapes such as streamers offer with the DAT technology a high capacity. They are particularly adapted to back up applications since they provide a sequential access allowing to store in one run a very high amount of data. They are also providing a high speed transfer that is interesting for images. The draw back is that the limitations due to the sequential access which do not permit to rewrite selective parts of the tape but only to rewrite the tape entirely or to add at the end. The previously written data remaining unchanged.

Optical disks using Write Once Read Many (WORM) technology, are providing a direct access to data at the difference of the streamers. They allow a quick access to a specific image on a disk. The data storage is permanent: an image can not be overwritten and the life time is very long over 10 years and certainly more. The main draw back is that data cannot be overwritten and so the storage can only be applied to data that are definitive and will not be modified: archiving activities are the main applications.

Magneto Optical Disks are comparable to optical disks with a large difference concerning the data modification since data may be rewritten at any time.

The conclusions of this study are:

The Magneto Optical Disks provide the best compromise for image storage. They provide the following advantages which are:

- *Flexibility*: since the access to data is direct, data may be rewritten and the disk cartridge is removable thus offering,
- *Access*: time which is higher than a magnetic disk but much shorter than a streamer,
- *Performance to cost ratio*: price is in the range of 5 000 ECUs for the drive and 200 ECUs for each disk cartridge,
- *Data life time* providing both storage and archiving on a single support and in a single operation.

User environment: The user environment is made of several functions providing the following services: acquisition, image storage and retrieval, image display, image preprocessing, measurement. These functions will be described in the next paragraphs.

Acquisition: This function is implemented through the standard package delivered with the confocal microscope by Carl Zeiss. The result is made of TIFF images which can be read by the other software packages.

Image storage and Retrieval - Data base principles: Storage and retrieval are built using the tools provided by the data base management system. The basic concept supporting information management and organisation is the "card". A card is made of two parts: one is *descriptive* and provides the information attached to the image(s), the other is made of the documents which are constituting the *pictorial* information of the card.

The main achievements concerned the development of the image preprocessing and processing software environment called *EXPLORER*. Taking into account the requirements and the investigations performed by the different laboratory partners, this environment was designed having in mind to provide an open environment able to be applied to a variety of processing tasks in the field of fluorescence.

The next chapter describes the main functions of the environment and the rationale of the choices made during the development to decide between the different possible options.

Subpackage PRE: Image pre-processing for colour registration and improved spatial resolution - EXPLORER basic concepts (Adelh)

Protocols: The EXPLORER software has been designed to provide a user friendly environment due to the diversity of applications which can be addressed with this software package, there is a large number of parameters which allow to set up correctly the program to take into account application specificity. These parameters define the way to acquire the images, to display them or to register them. It defines the number of wavelengths and other characteristics which are application dependent but more rarely sample dependent.

To overcome the corresponding confusion and workload induced to the user when setting up the program for a given application, the concept of *protocol* has been introduced. A protocol allows to group under a unique name of values (or a range of values) for the set of parameters defining the program behaviour. Selecting a given protocol automatically configures the program for the associated application.

In order to provide enough flexibility, it is possible after having selected a given protocol for a sample, to modify it in order to take into account sample specificity. This protocol is only valid for this sample and does not interfere with the default protocol which is left unchanged and thus can be used for other samples.

References Images: Two types of reference images have been introduced. The first one is for background subtraction corresponding to black currents and the second one is for shading correction. In the case of CLSM images as there is a single detector, the P.M. tube, the black current images is not very important since it is uniform over the entire image frame. However the shading correction is still of interest since the shading may be due to the optics. These two images have been introduced because images coming from other sources than the CLSM may be used:

for example cooled CCD cameras are more and more present in the genetic laboratory and have to be accepted as input devices.

Analysis: In order to facilitate the task in managing and organizing the information, the data exploited by *EXPLORER* are grouped into *Analysis*. An analysis is a composite set of data of various kinds: images, protocol, measurements, comments. These data are associated to a sample and may correspond to several images of the same sample corresponding to different organizations of the acquisition. They may correspond to a stack of images of the same field acquired at different heights and/or to different fields of the sample. This data structure allows to easily store all the required information and provide a fast access to image data while facilitating the tracking of the conditions of the various acquisition, display, preprocessing and processing phases.

Measuring with EXPLORER: A set of the most useful tools for measuring has been developed to be offered to the user. These tools are of three categories: densitometric, dimensional, profiles. The dimensional tools allow to measure distances between objects such as probes. They are two ways to compute distances: using the conventional Euclidean, using the distance along the chromosome axis.

Chromosome axis extraction: As described in the above paragraph, in case of bent chromosomes, it may be necessary to measure distances between probes along the axis of the chromosome instead of measuring the Euclidean inter probes distances. This operation implies that the axis has been already extracted and, it is available as a succession of segment extremities forming a polygonal line. There are two possibilities to compute the chromosome axis which are: to manually draw the polygonal line forming the axis, to automatically extract the axis through computer extraction. The manual mode will not be described here since it is just based on the standard interactive tools for drawing of the basic *SAMBA* image processing library.

Image registration: When acquired at different wavelengths, images do not match exactly a point of the image emitting light at two wave lengths will not contribute to the same pixels in the image. Making these two images matching is called registration.

Two different approaches were envisaged to solve this problem: (i) modeling the transfer function of the system depending on the wavelength. Then registration problem becomes a general problem of finding a solution by interverting the model, (ii) experimentally record the matching error and correct the image by applying the inverse of the error. It was decided to focus on the second approach for the following reasons: (i) it applies for any type of instruments and thus this approach is more general than the model based approach,(ii) it is more robust because no assumption is made on the shape of the distortion except that is supposed to be continuous which is the case.

Measuring the registration error: After having investigated the different practical means for measuring the registration error, it was decided to compute the registration automatically using a grid. The registration is made in the following manner: Providing that the miss match between the two images is not too large, localize automatically the crossing points on the grid image. It is supposed that the grid is first aligned in order that the centre of the grid is put in coincidence with the centre of the optical path.

The result is an "image" of the error of registration. For a pair of wavelengths, this image contains for the second wavelength the offset in X and Y which should be added to the coordinated of the pixel to make it matching with the corresponding pixel in the first wavelength image. This image can be seen as a spatial offset look up table in 2 dimensions. This look up table does not apply to the gray level but the position of each pixel that is coordinates in the image.

The correction of the registration error is performed in two phases:

1. the offset image is computed using a special sample displaying a grid of points,
2. the offset image is applied to the image of the second wavelength image for any pair of acquired images.

The offset image remains valid as long as any new setting of the instruments are not performed.

In conclusion, the design of this calibration method has allowed to:

- provide an automatic way to register the images. The automation induces less user errors and facilitates the handling of the system as compared to a tedious manual registration,
- the performances of the method are rather good and allow a precise spatial registration,
- an other advantage is also to provide a straightforward way to perform a spatial calibration in order to measure the distances accurately. Knowing the step of the grid, the pixel size can be derived locally to have a precise quantification of the distances.

Image filtering: The image filtering is set up to increase the perception and the detection of the probes on one side and the chromosome banding on the other side. The main difficulty in detecting these objects is resulting from the presence of noise in the images. Thus the problem is to identify signal in presence of noise. The basic assumption is that the spatial frequency of the noise is higher than the spatial frequency of the signal. The first operation is to remove or at least to reduce the noise present in the images. This operation is then followed by an operation for detecting the probes or the band.

Noise reduction: Depending on the nature of the noise, different approaches have to be applied: Impulse noise can only be reduced efficiently using non linear filtering such as the median filter. Additive zero mean Gaussian noise is easily reduced with a linear filtering knowing the spatial noise frequency.

Combination of noise reduction and probes detection: The problem of noise reduction can be envisaged alone or in conjunction with the problem of probe detection. In that case it can be formulated as the design of an optimal reverse filter to detect and localize the probes in a noisy image. The detection is made by the derivation of the smoothing filter response function. The probes correspond to the order 1 discontinuities.

Probes detection: We have already seen the use of optimal detection. However in practice, the parameters necessary to the application of these techniques are unknown. The only valid approach is thus to separately apply the noise reduction and the probe detection.

The probes detection is basically an impulse detection problem. Knowing the approximate probe diameter, probes can be easily detected using a non linear filtering and thresholding techniques as the Top Hat transform. The main

advantages of the Top Hat transform are:
- insensitivity to low frequency background variations often encountered in fluorescence imaging,
- ability to ignore regions larger than the diameter specified. This is particularly useful for probe detection where diameter can be easily determined.

In conclusion, the developments undertaken have permitted:
- to design methods robust enough to allow image registration,
- to automate the process of registration through the implementation of automatic grid template analysis,
- to perform a spatial calibration in the same process than spatial registration,
- to develop specific methods for computing distances along chromosome axis to correct for chromosome bending,
- to develop a method for computing profiles for precise location of probes on the banding structure of the chromosome and/or relatively to other probes along the chromosome axis,
- to specify linear and non linear filtering for improving the signal to noise ratio of probes and bands,
- to set up robust and sensitive methods for probes detection and segmentation.

These developments have been first prototyped using the development environment of *SAMBA* under the form of a set of macros which have been progressively enhanced and tuned.

The most significative results have been embedded in an open environment for fluorescent image quantification called *EXPLORER*. This environment may be used as a software running on the CLSM for confocal image analysis, or on a separate imaging workstation for processing of other fluorescent image types such one coming from cooled CCD.

3.4 Workpackage MA: ISH-map construction tools (Robert-Nicoud, Cremer and Adelh)

Given the biological specimens prepared according to Workpackage PM, this part of the proposal concerns the development of the dedicated software to analyze the fluorescent images of the *in situ* hybridization experiments and to derive maps which will contribute to detect, locate and order DNA sequences at the chromatid level.

Subpackage MA/QUI/2D: Two dimensional quantitative ISH probe imaging (Robert-Nicoud and Cremer)

Model experiments were designed to test the accuracy of fluorescence ratio measurements on single chromosomes. DNAs from up to five human chromosome specific plasmid libraries were labeled with biotin and digoxigenin in different hapten proportions. Probe mixtures were used for CISS-hybridization to normal human metaphase spreads and detected with FITC and TRITC. An epifluorescence microscope equipped with a cooled CCD-camera was used for image acquisition. Procedures for fluorescence ratio measurements were developed on the basis of commercial image analysis software. For hapten ratios 1/1, 1/2 and 1/4, fluorescence ratio values measured for individual chromosomes could be used as a single, reliable parameter for chromosome identification. Our findings indicate (i) a tight correlation of fluorescence ratio values with hapten ratios and (ii) the potential of fluorescence ratio measurements for multiple color chromosome painting. Three different ranges of fluorescence ratio could be distinguished without overlap for three hapten ratios. This result suggests that four spectrally separable fluorochromes in various proportions may be sufficient to distinguish all chromosomes of the human chromosome complement by fluorescent ratio measurements.

Based on these results a new possibility to search genomes for imbalanced genetic materials, termed comparative genomic *in situ* hybridization (CGH), was implemented. For CGH, labeled genomic test DNA, prepared from clinical or tumor specimens, was mixed with differently labeled control DNA, prepared from cells with normal chromosome complement. The mixed probe was used for chromosomal *in situ* suppression (CISS-) hybridization to normal metaphase spreads (46,XX or 46, XY). Hybridized test and control DNA sequences were detected via different fluorochromes, e.g. FITC and TRITC. The ratios of FITC/TRITC fluorescence intensities measured for each chromosome and chromosome segment, respectively, in the normal metaphase spread should then reflect the relative copy number in the test genome as compared to the control genome, e.g. 0.5 for monosomies, 1 for disomies, 1.5 for trisomies, etc. The feasibility of this approach was demonstrated in a series of examples, including genomic test DNAs, prepared from a patient with Down syndrome, from blood of a patient with T-cell prolymphocytic leukemia, from cultured and uncultured cell materials of a variety of solid tumors, including renal cell carcinomas, a bladder cancer, uveal melanomas and glioblastomas and astrocytomas. Tumor specific gains and losses as well as gene amplifications in these tumors genomes could be readily mapped on the normal metaphase chromosomes due to significant differences of fluorescence ratios as described above. The smallest chromosome segments for which a gain or loss could be identified so far were in the order of 30Mbp. In case of gene amplifications the smallest amplification unit which was mapped so far on normal human complements was 90 kbp present in 16-24 copies. It can be expected, however, that amplicons present in lower copy numbers or smaller amplicons will be detectable by this new approach.

Most recently, Cremer has extended this technique to the analysis of archival tumor specimens. Prior to CGH, the DNA from paraffin embedded tumor cells was amplified via PCR using a degenerated oligonucleotide as a primer (DOP-PCR) and labeled via nick-translation. The feasibility of this protocol to detect genetic imbalances in formalin-fixed tissue sections could be demonstrated. This allows for a comprehensive genotype/phenotype comparison of archival tumor materials.

Subpackages MA/QUI/LOC/2D: Two dimensional quantitative ISH probe imaging and 2D mapping tools (Robert-Nicoud)

Development of an editing and measurement tool for multichannel FISH: FISH generates many fluorescent images. These correspond to the imaging of the same specimen at different excitation and emission wavelengths. In order to handle and combine these images Robert-Nicoud developed a software (cytoFISH) on the Silicon Graphics workstation.

This programme handles three images (512x512 pixels with a dynamic range of 16 bits) corresponding to different channels. In order to make the programme compatible with a great number of sources we implemented the possibility of reading various images formats such as: grey-level TIFF, colour TIFF, raw binary format 8 bits and 16 bits, and Hamamatsu cooled CCD proprietary image format. Each image can be individually processed and edited.

The different processings available are:
- Noise filtering (apply to 8 and 16 bit images);
- Dynamic compression (apply to 16 bit images);
- Deblurring, resolution enhancement (apply to 8 and 16 bit images);

- Background equalization (apply to 8 and 16 bit images);
- Dynamic correction (apply to 8 bit images);
- Editing tool (apply to 8 bit images);
- Merge tool (apply to 8 bit images);
- Measurement tool (apply to 24 bit colour images).

Development of tools for increasing the resolution of 2D fluorescence imaging: By nature fluorescence images are blurred by glare and stray light. This makes it difficult to accurately measure distances between close fluorescent probes such as cosmid probes. To facilitate distance measurements it was necessary to develop a computational method that improve the resolution of the fluorescence images recorded with a cooled CCD camera. Professor Robert-Nicoud developed deconvolution routines based on iterative constrained algorithms such as the Jansson-van Citter, the Meinel and the Richardson-Lucy methods. These were implemented in the cytoFISH programme developed on a Silicon Graphics workstation. The algorithms were optimized in order to obtain computation times compatible with routine analysis.

The deconvolution based on a simplified PSF was used to enhance (i) the resolution of cosmid probes in interphase nuclei, and (ii) the resolution of G-banding of DAPI stained metaphase chromosome. In practice, the deconvolution of an image took between 20 and 30s, that is, durations of the same order as the integration time of the fluorescence image on the cooled CCD camera.

Subpackages MA/QUI/3D and MA/LOC/3D: Development of three-dimensional imaging tools (Robert-Nicoud)

Professor Robert-Nicoud developed a programme on the Silicon Graphics workstation for the edition of series of confocal sections (C language). It includes functions for the compression and storage of large three-dimensional data sets. A series of tools is available that allows to investigate the three-dimensional data set, interpole data, improve the fluorescence dynamics of the series of sections, filter out noise, reject out of focus glare to virtually improve the axial resolution of the microscope. These tools are:
- a 3D-browser tool;
- a fluorescence intensity compensation tool;
- a 3D median filter;
- a 3D morphological opening filter;
- a 3D sharpening filter;
- a 3D nearest neighbour deconvolution;
- a 3D reconstruction tool based on surface rendering;
- a 3D reconstruction tool based on ray-tracing.

Development of three dimensional image analysis tools: In parallel to the development of the 3D editing programme we have developed a library of functions dedicated to 3D image analysis. These functions are:
- Segmentation tools: two methods of segmentation were developed. The first method is based on a simple grey level thresholding algorithm. The second method is based on a more sophisticated approach, and is more convenient for the segmentation of signals with fuzzy borders such as chromosomes or chromosome domains in interphase nuclei;
- Labelling tool: we developed a specialized automatic 3D labelling tool that is based on a 3D "seed-fill" algorithm. This makes it possible to identify and give a unique label to every segmented object in the 3D volume;

- Distance transform tool: this tool is used to characterize the topology of a 3D volume. The principle is to generate isosurfaces in the object such that all voxels belonging to one isosurface are located at the same distance from the border of the object. This way a distance map of all voxels is constructed. For example, the distance transform may be applied to a segmented nucleus in order to locate structures in it as a function of the distance from the border of the nucleus;
- Topographic analysis tool: these statistical tools are used to translate the spatial distribution of signal in a nucleus. They combine the masks of segmentation of the signals with the topographical map of the nucleus given by the distance transform tool.

Morphological algorithms based on Voronoï and Delaunay graphs: For 3D image analysis an algorithm adapted form computational geometry was developed. The basic idea of this algorithm is to tesselate the image into convex polyeder ("Voronoï polyeder") according to a set of given points ("seeds") in the image space. A Voronoï polyeder is associated with one seed in the following sense: each point belonging to a polyeder is closer to its seed than to anay other seed in the image space. The resulting tesselation is called the three-dimensional Voronoï diagram. Simultaneously a second structure called the Delaunay graph is built which represents the neighborhood of polyeder in the Voronoï diagram the following sense: two seeds are connected in the Delaunay graph if and only if their respective polyeder have one face in common.

Segmentation of chromosome territories performed independently by another investigator in a subset of 30 nuclei yielded very similar results. Despite of a pronounced variation in individual chromosome territory sections, the total size calculated for all exterior and interior areas of the chromosome territory sections was roughly similar (53% exterior versus 47% interior). Accordingly, the observed distribution of the dystrophin gene signals is significantly different from the distribution expected in case of their random placement within the interior or exterior part. Notably, dystrophin signals located outside of the exterior boundary of the segmented X-chromosome territories were not observed in this experiment and only rarely (<3%) in several cell types including genes located on different chromosomes. These results indicate that individual DNA-loops carrying such genes which would extend far away from the periphery of a chromosome territory into the nuclear space are rare events, if they occur at all in intact nuclei. The observation of such events in hypotonically treated nuclei fixed with acetic acid/methanol may reflect artefacts. Such treatments, while useful for interphase gene mapping are less favorable for the preservation of the three-dimensional nuclear and chromosome territory structure. The dystrophin gene is known to be actively transcribed in myotubes, but also shows low level transciption in other cell types. The level of transcription in HeLa cells is presently under investigation. A preferential distribution in the chromosome territory periphery has also been obtained for two other genes known to be active and inactive, respectively, in various cell types.

Application of morphological algorithms for studying the size and shape of X-chromosome territories: For a long time experimental investigations of the threedimensional topology of chromosomes in cell nuclei have not been possible. Only recently with the event of fluorescence *in situ* hybridisation (FISH) and new microscopic techniques as confocal laser scanning fluorescence microscopes (CLSM) it became possible to prove the hypothesis already proposed by Rabl and Boveri at the beginning of this century that chromosomes occupy distinct territories in cell nuclei. Since then intensive studies were made to investigate a correlation between genetic activity and the threedimensional organisation and compaction of chromosome territories.

In this context investigations have been concentrated on the threedimensional structure of active and inactive X-chromosome territories in female, mammalian cell nuclei. During early development in each female somatic cell one of the two X-chromosomes becomes genetically largely inactivated (Xi), while the other remains genetically active (Xa). Xi can be identified in the cell nucleus as a compact structure called the Barr body. A widely held view assumes that Xa is largely decondensed as compared to the strongly condensed Xi and, consequently, that genes contained in the heterochromatic chromatin territory may become inaccessible for factors involved in the expression of their homologs in the active chromosome.

This predicted large difference in volume, however, could not be confirmed experimentally but these investigations are still limitated in their quantitative results. The interactive image analysis using two dimensional segmentation algorithms as simple thresholding and interpolation aberrations between subsequent image slices could result in a strong influence on the results obtained. Using a wide range of possible thresholds for segmentation of chromosome territories resulted in an equivalent range of possible results. Consequently, until now it has not been possible to differentiate uniquely between active and inactive X-chromosome in female cell nuclei using the size of volume or twodimensional extension of X-territories only.

To study this problem, the X-chromosome territories and territories of chromosome 7 in human amniotic fluid cell cultures were painted entirely with the fluorochrome FITC. Additionally the pericentrometric region of chromosome 7 (p7c1) was painted by fluorescence *in situ* hybridization (FISH) with Cy5 to differ between the territories of chromosome 7 and the X-chromosomes. The Barr body was identified in DAPI stained nuclei and images recorded with a CCD camera. After chromosome painting and FISH the nuclei were counterstained with propidium iodide. With a confocal laser scanning microscope (CLSM) series of 12 to 35 optical sections were obtained at intervals of 250 nm or 300 nm in the FITC, Cy5 and propidium iodide channels from each of 54 nuclei with well separated, painted territories.

For image analysis 3D-data-volumes of nuclei, chromosome territories and centrometric regions of chromosome 7 were tesselated by Voronoï polyhedra structured in a graph environment. Using this graph structure a 3D-segmentation was performed and morphological parameters such as volume, surface and roundness factor (shape) of each chromosome territory were computed.

In most (51 out of total 54) nuclei it was possible to differentiate between active and inactive X-territories with regard to their shape and surface. Such a differentiation was not possible considering only the volume. In contrast, the territories of chromosome 7 show a highly significant ($p > 0.99$) smaller difference in surface and in shape as compared to the X-territories. No significant difference ($p < 0.95$) was observed regarding the difference in volumes of the X-territories and the territories of chromosome 7 respectively. These results strongly support a model which proposes that the genetic activity of chromosome territories in the cell nucleus is correlated with their threedimensional shape and surface.

Distribution of the dystrophin gene in X-chromosome territories: Little is known about the spatial organization of coding and non-coding sequences within the chromosome territories. As an approach to study the localization of the dystrophin gene in X-chromosome territories, HeLa cells were fixed with buffered paraformaledhyde and subjected to two color CISS-hybridization using a digoxigenin-labelled X-chromosome specific DNA-library in combination with a pool of five biotinylated genomic cosmid clones which extend from exon 47 to 51 of the dystrophin gene. While volume measurements of active and inactive X-chromosomes were performed in hybridized nuclei subjected to pepsin digestion, this step was avoided in the following experiments. Permeabilization was achieved with 0.5% Triton X-100 and 0.5% Saponin. Digitized optical sections of the chromosome territory (TRITC-signal) and the gene (FITC-signal) were obtained with a Zeiss LSM 10 confocal laser scanning microscope. To avoid any prejudice with regard to the localization of the FITC-signal, a threshold yielding a reasonable segmentation of chromosome territory boundaries was first applied to the TRITC-mages. After overlay of the TRITC and FITC images the localization of the dystrophin gene signal within an interior or exterior part of the territory section was determined. Analysis of 250 chromosome territories revealed that 208 (83%) of the gene signals were located in the exterior part, 37 (15%) of the signals were located within the interior part, while for 5 signals (2%) such a decision was not possible.

4. Major scientific breakthroughs and/or industrial applications

New methodologies and technologies:

1. Development of a new approach for the construction of *analytical chromosomal bar codes* adaptable to the particular needs of cytogenetic investigations and automated image analysis.
2. Development of a new approach for the rapid *detection of amplifications and losses of genetic material in tumor cells*, based on the simultaneous hybridization of tumoral and normal DNA to metaphase chromosomes, and on the measurement of fluorescence intensities ratios.
3. Development of a new method for simulation of the *imaging pathway in the confocal laser scanning microscope*. A *water immersion lens* was newly designed (C Apochromat 40x1.2W Korr) which fits to the need of water samples and confocal microscopy. This lens is optimized for a spectral range from 400 to 700 nm and has correction for refractive index differences. During the project the lens was computed, designed and produced in a series of 4 prototypes.
4. Development of a special *software version for the new laser scanning microscope LSM4*, dedicated to the *measurement of distances in space*. This functionality gives the possibility to measure distances between different ISH fluorescent spots in interphase nuclei.
5. Development of a *software package (cytoFISH)* on a Silicon Graphics workstation for *2D quantitative ISH probe imaging and 2D mapping*. This package offers the following image processing facilities: noise filtering, dynamic compression, debluring, resolution enhancement, background equalization, dynamic correction, editing, merging and measurement tools.
6. Development of an *image preprocessing and processing software environment* called *EXPLORER*. EXPLORER was designed with the aim of providing an open environment able to be applied to a variety of processing tasks in the field of fluorescence imaging. This environment may be used as a software running on the CLSM for confocal image analysis, or on a separate imaging workstation for processing of other fluorescent images types such as those coming from a cooled CCD camera.

7. Development of *3D quantitative ISH probe imaging and mapping*. Morphological algorithms based on Voronoï and Delaunay graphs were developed. The basic idea of this algorithm is to tesselate the image into convex polyeder ("Voronoï polyeder") according to a set of given points ("seeds") in the image space. It consists of two steps, initialization and propagation, and is followed by an extraction and parametrization step.

This morphological algorithm was applied for studying the *size and shape of chromosome territories in the cell nucleus*. The results obtained strongly support a model which proposes that the genetic activity of chromosome territories in the cell nucleus is correlated with their three-dimensional shape and surface, but not with their volume.

5. Major cooperative links

Meetings between members of the two laboratories (Contractors 01 and 02) and of the two industrial companies took place at a frequency of:

one per month (Contractors 01-03)
one per trimester (Contractors 01-02, 01-04)
one per semester (Contractors 03-04, 02-03, 02-04).

In addition, the partners had the chance to meet at the occasion of several international meetings.

Two members of the laboratory of Contractor 01 went to Heidelberg for short stays (1-2 weeks) in the laboratory of Contractor 02.

One member of the laboratory of Contractor 02 went to Grenoble for a stay of 3 weeks in the laboratory of Contractor 01.

Two *general meetings* with all the Contractors and several members of their laboratories were organized:

one on May 20, 1992 in Nijmegen (NL),
the other one on February 26, 1993 in Basel (CH).

Bibliography

- Bertin E., Parazza F., Chassery J.M., (1993). Segmentation and measurement based on 3D Voronoï diagram: application to confocal microscopy. Computerized Medical Imaging and Graphics, Vol. 17, 175-182.
- Bischoff A., Schmidt J., Kharboush I., Stelzer E., Cremer T., Cremer C. (1993). Differences of size and shape of active and inactive X-chromosome domains in human amniotic fluid cell nuclei. Microscopy Research and Technique, 25: 68-77.
- Cremer C., Cremer T., Lichter P. The interchromosome domain compartment: a model for the structural and functional compartmentalization of the cell nucleus. Manuscript in preparation.
- Cremer T., Kurz A., Zirbel R., Dietzel S., Rinke B., Schröck E., Speicher M.R., Mathieu U., Jauch A., Emmerich P., Scherthan H., Ried T., Cremer C., Lichter P. (1993). The role of the chromosome territories in the functional compartmentalization of the cell nucleus. Cold Spring Harbor Symp Quant Biol. 58, DNA and chromosome, in press.
- Du Manoir S., Speicher M.R., Joos S., Schröck E., Popp S., Döhner H., Kovacs G., Robert-Nicoud M., Lichter P., Cremer T. (1993). Detection of complete and partial chromosome gains and losses by comparative genomic *in situ* hybridization. Human. Genet., 90: 560-610.
- Eils R., Bertin E., Saracoglu K., Schröck E., Dietzel S., Usson Y., Robert-Nicoud M., Stelzer E.H.K, Cremer T., Cremer C. Morphology of territories of chromosome X and 7 in human amniotic fluid cell nuclei determined by laser confocal sectioning and 3D-Voronoi diagrams. Manuscript in preparation.
- Eils R., Dietzel S., Schröck E., Bertin E., Usson Y., Robert-Nicoud M., Cremer C., Cremer T. Shape and surface of active and inactive X-chromosome territories studied in human amniotic fluid cell nuclei. Manuscript in preparation.

- Joos S., Scherthan H., Speicher M.R., Schlegel J., Cremer T., Lichter P. (1993). Detection of amplified DNA sequences by reverse chromosome painting using genomic tumor DNA as probe. Hum. Genet. 90: 584-589.
- Jouk P.S., Usson Y, Michalowicz G., Parazza F. Methods for the mapping of the orientation of myocardial cells by means of polarized light. Microscopial Research & Technics, in press.
- Leger I. Measuring fluorescent nuclei acid probes. In: Cell & Tissue Culture: Laboratory Procedures. J.R. Griffiths, A. Doyle & D.G. Newell (eds), John Wiley & Sons, Ltd, Chichester, 1993, 10B, 8.1-8.14.
- Leger I., Robert-Nicoud M., Brugal G. (1994) Combination of DNA *in situ* Hybridization and Immunocytochemical Detection of Nucleolar Proteins - A contribution to the Functional Mapping of the Human Genome by Fluorescence Microscopy. Journal of Histochemistry & Cytochemistry, 42: 149-154.
- Leger I., Thomas M., Ronot X., Brugal G. (1993) Detection of chromosome 1 aberrations by fluorescent *in situ* hybridization (FISH) in the human breast cancer cell line. Anal. Cell Pathol., 5: 299-309.
- Lengauer C., Speicher M.R., Popp S., Jauch A., Taniwaki M., Nagaraja R., Riethman H.C., Donis-Keller H., D'Urso M., Schlessinger D., Cremer T., (1993). Chromosomal bar codes produced by multicolor fluorescence *in situ* hybridization with multiple YAC clones and whole chromosome painting probes. Hum. Mol. Genet., 2: 505-512.
- Leroux D., Seite P., Hillion J., Le Marc'Hadour F., Pegourie-Bandelier B., Jacob J.C., Sotto J.J. (1993). t(11;18)(q21;q21): A karyotypic anomaly characterizing lymphocytic lymphoma with extranodal site? Genes Chrom. Cancer: 7: 54-56.
- Marcelpoil R. Normalization of the minimum spanning tree (1993). Anal. Cell. Pathol., 5:177-186.
- Monier K., Usson Y, Mongelard F, Gaudray P, Robert-Nicoud M, Vourc'h C. Metaphase and interphase mapping by fluorescent *in situ* hybridization: amelioration of chromosome banding and signal resolution by means of iterative deconvolution. Cytogenetics and Cell Genetics, (submitted)
- Parazza F., Humbert C., Usson Y. (1993) Method for 3D volumetric analysis of intranuclear fluorescence distribution in confocal microscopy. Computerized Medical Imaging and Graphics, 17: 189-200.
- Popp S., Jauch A., Schindler D., Speicher M.R., Lengauer C., Donis-Keller H., Riethman H.C., Cremer T. (1993). Identification of a small, unbalanced translocation by multiple fluorescence *in situ* hybridization with chromosome specific DNA libraries and YAC clones. Hum. Genet., 92 : 527-532.
- Raynaud S.D., Bekrl S., Leroux D., Grosgeorges J., Klein B., Bastard C., Gaudray P., Simon M.P. (1993). Expanded range of 11q13 breakpoints with differing patterns of Cyclin D1 expression in B-cell malignancies. Genes Chrom. Cancer: 8: 80-87.
- Rinke B., Bischoff A., Schröck E., Scharschmidt R., Hausmann M., Stelzer E.H.K., Cremer T., Cremer C. (1994). Volume ratios of chromosome territories determined for chromosome 5, 7 and X homologs in human cell nuclei. Manuscript in preparation.
- Tocharoentanaphol C., Cremer M., Schröck E., Kilian K., Cremer T., Ried T. (1994). Multicolor fluorescence *in situ* hybridization on metaphase chromosomes and interphase Halo-preparations using cosmid and YAC clones for the simultaneous high resolution mapping od deletions in the dystrophin gene. Hum. Genet. 93, 229-235.
- Usson Y., Humbert C. (1992) Methods for topographical analysis of intranuclear Brd-Urd-tagged fluorescence. Cytometry, 13: 595-602.
- Usson Y., Parazza F., Jouk P.S., Michalowicz G. (1994) Method for the study of the three-dimensional orientation of the nuclei of myocardial cells in fetal human heart by means of confocal scanning laser microscopy. J. Microscopy, 174: 101-110.
- Volm T., Scherthan H., Fischer C., Speicher M.R., Cremer T. (1994). Size correlated differences of chromosome distribution in cultured amniotic fluid cell nuclei. Manuscript in preparation.
- Vourc'h C., Taruscio D., Boyle A., Ward D.C. (1993) Cell cycle dependent distribution of telomeres, centromeres and chromosome specific subsatellite domains in the interphase nucleus of mouse lymphocytes. Exp. Cell Res., 205: 142-151.

Contract number: GENO-CT91-0029
Contractual period: 1 February 1992 to 31 January 1994

Coordinator
Professor M. Robert-Nicoud (01)
Université Joseph Fourier
Grenoble 1
Faculté de Médecine
Domaine de la Merci
F-38706 La Tronche Cedex
France
Tel: 33 76 54 94 61
Fax: 33 76 54 94 14

Participants
Dr. Th. Cremer (02)
Laboratory of Molecular Cytogenetics
Institute of Human Genetics and Anthropology
Ruprecht-Karls-Universität
Im Neuenheimer Feld 328
D-6900 Heidelberg
Germany
Tel: 49 6221 563 896
Fax: 49 6221 565 332

Dr. D. Adelh (03)
Alcatel TITN Answare
"L'Epilobe"
35 Chemin du Vieux Chêne
F-38240 Meylan
France
Tel: 33 76 41 71 72
Fax: 33 76 41 06 31

Dr. B. Faltermeier (04)
Carl ZEISS
Postfach 1369
F-7082 Oberkochen
Germany
Tel: 49 7364 202 969
Fax: 49 7364 204 258

No. of joint/individual publications: 20 (3 joint and 17 indiv. publications)

Human Genome Analysis Programme
M. Hallen and A. Klepsch (Eds.)
IOS Press, 1995

DEVELOPMENT OF HIGH-SPEED DNA-SEQUENCING TECHNOLOGY FOR SEQUENCING AND STS MAPPING OF HUMAN cDNAs AND MICROSATELLITE DNA

W. Ansorge
European Molecular Biology Laboratory, Heidelberg, Germany

1. Background information

The analysis of human genome, as well as of genomes of other organisms, will require development of advanced technologies, with the aim to increase the sequencing throughput, accuracy and reliability of the data and to lower the cost per base.

The EMBL group works on the automation of the DNA sequencing process. This includes development of automated DNA sequencing devices, procedures and automation of optimized DNA template preparations and DNA sequencing reactions. An automated DNA sequencing system using fluorescent DNA labelling techniques was developed and has been commercially distributed to several hundred sites all over the world.

The increasing number of genome analysis projects requires sequencing systems with an increased throughput compared to the commercially available standard devices. This increased throughput can be achieved by increasing the (i) sequencing speed (high speed sequencing system) or (ii) number of clones sequenced simultaneously (two dye sequencing system).

The Aarhus laboratory works on analysis of expressed genes in human keratinocytes. In the course of this grant efforts were continued to identify proteins in the comprehensive 2-D gel database of human keratinocytes. So far, about 900 proteins have been identified using a combination of procedures that include (i) comigration with purified proteins (ii) 2-D gel immunoblotting, (iii) microsequencing followed by database searches, (iv) microsequencing in combination with mass spectrometry and (v) expression of cDNAs in the vaccinia virus system. To date, about 450 proteins recorded in the database have been microsequenced, and about 100 annotation entries ranging from protein identity to chromosomal mapping have been established.

An increasing number of inherited deseases is described and the responsible genes are identified and mapped to their chromosomal location. Gene loci of several inherited deseases are located on human chromosome 21. For further detailed analysis these genes are sequenced and characterised. To accomplish this task a fine map of chromosome 21 needs to be established. Highly polymorphic CA-repeats are valuable tools for the generation of a high resolution map, since they are evenly distributed across the genome. The Barcelona group works on the fine mapping of human chromosome 21 using polymorphic microsatellite markers to accomplish this task.

2. Objectives and primary approaches

The objective of the project was to develop new advanced sequencing technology and methodology in functional prototypes and demonstrate their function and applicability to the analysis of the human genome.

Part of this objective was the construction of a DNA sequencing system with a sequence output of 30-50 kilobases/device/day. During the course of this project a number of human cDNAs as well as polymorphic microsatellite DNAs were to be sequenced and analyzed in parallel, contributing to the analysis of the human genome.

2.1 Development and construction of a high speed DNA sequencer, increasing 10 times the sequencing output compared to standard state of the art technology

The methodology is based on the principles of the automated fluorescent DNA sequencing device developed at EMBL previously:
- Detector system generating time and position resolved gel data. Detector with a detection limit of less than 10^6 fluorescent DNA fragments, imaging 10 to 20 clones from the gel onto 256 independent channels. The expected sequence throughput of 500 bases/hour/clone requires sampling rates of 5 Hz or more.
- Development of analog to digital converter electronics for fast data acquisition with 256 channels, a dynamic range of 16 bits and sampling rates of 50 Hz/channel. Interfacing this AD electronics to a computer system for data storage and process control.
- Development of data acquisition software. Implementation of real time data acquisition program for the control of sequencing device, read out of the AD electronics, graphical display and storage of data on disk.

2.2 Two-dye sequencing system

Construction of a two-dye system to further increase the throughput by a factor of two. Projection of two laser beams with distinct wavelengths across the gel to enable detection of two independent sets of sequencing reactions labelled with two different fluorescent dyes in the same lanes on the gel.

Analysis and feasibility tests are carried out to evaluate the resolution when double amount of DNA is loaded on the gel, as well as bleaching effects on the dyes which could lead to lower sensitivity with one of the two dyes.

2.3 Development of an automated gel casting system for ultrathin gels

Modification of the existing gel moulds for the thin gel technology.
Re-loading and use of gels for several runs as well as testing of new gel matrices.

2.4 Development of solid support techniques for DNA sample preparation and its adaptation to the existing robotic workstations

Testing of various approaches to automate DNA template preparations including glass fiber filters, already used for automated preparation of single stranded DNA, with the aim to avoid centrifugation steps.

2.5 Identification of the human cDNA clones

Identification and cloning of the cDNAs based on the established comprehensive cell type specific 2D protein gel data base.

2.6   Sequencing the human cDNAs

In the test sequencing phase, the methodology is based on the existing automated DNA sequencing devices. After 12 months testing of newly developed high speed sequencing system in the analysis of cDNA clones.

2.7   The cDNA sequence data is used to generate genomic sequence tagged sites (STS) by PCR which are mapped to the genome

Determination of STS sequences derived from the cDNAs and their mapping to the chromosomes.

2.8   Identification of human polymorphic microsatellite DNAs

Identification of new polymorphic microsatellite probes from human chromosomes 21 by using oligonucleotide probes recognizing simple repeat sequences (e.g. CA-GT, TA-AT and GATC) in hybridization experiments with human chromosome 21 specific genomic libraries. Development of probes by PCR cloning.

2.9   Sequencing the identified polymorphic DNAs

Parallel sequencing of large numbers of microsatellite DNAs. In the test sequencing phase, the methodology consists of the use of existing automated DNA sequencing devices. After 12 months testing of newly developed system in the analysis of the microsatellite DNA clones.

3. Results and discussion

3.1   DNA Sequencer

Basic physical parameters for the high speed DNA sequencer have been identified. Due to electrophoretic variations in the gel, caused among others by the high electric fields, DNA bands do not migrate as straight as in the standard system with low electrical fields. A new detector system was needed which compensates shifts of the tracks on the horizontal axis.

We have developed a continuous detector array for simultaneous DNA sequencing of 20 clones on the standard gel format (Fig. 1). The detector contains 180 photosensitive elements, covering a width of 305 mm, and spherical lenses in the optics. Spacing of the sample wells was reduced to 3.4 mm, each sample track covered by two detector elements. Ultra thin slab gels have been successfully tested in combination with this new detector system. Since the DNA bands do not migrate ideally straight on gels thinner than about 0.3 mm, standard commercial sequencing devices with only one photodiode per track are not efficient with ultrathin gels. In order to reduce the Joule's heating, usually high in the standard gels, the thickness of the gel was reduced down to 100 μm. Using low concentration gels, sequencing runs were performed at speeds of up to 500 bases per hour.

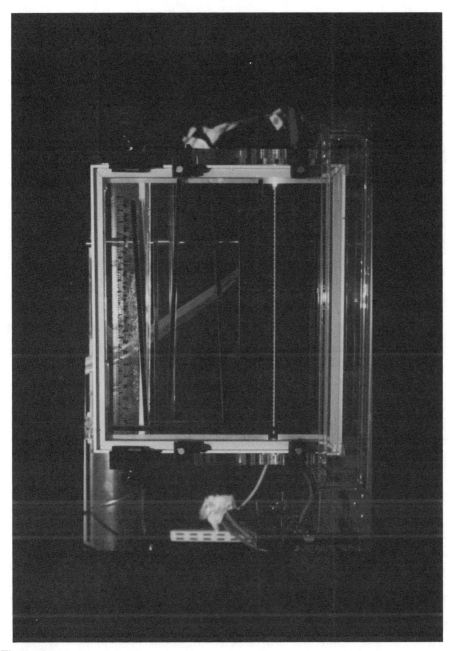

Figure 1
Device for the simultaneous on-line detection of 20 clones loaded on one gel,
fluorescein label, Argon laser, $\lambda_{emission} = 488$ nm.

3.2   Two-dye sequencing system

The development of the two-dye sequencing system has been completed based on the
previous EMBL technique (Fig. 2). Based on this sequencer a novel strategy has been

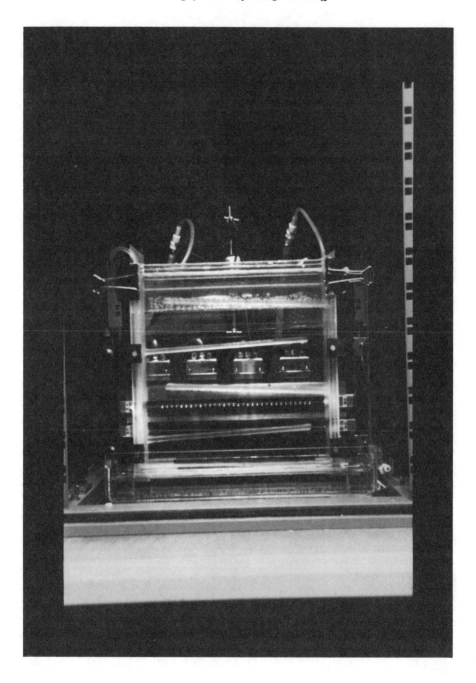

Figure 2
Image of the two dye sequencing system (8 clones per fluorophore). Laser beams Argon
(Ar) laser ($\lambda_{emission}$ 488 nm, P= 3 mW) and Helium-Neon (HeNe) laser ($\lambda_{emission}$ 543
nm, P= 2 mW) are coupled into the gel with help of two light coupling plate placed
between spacers on either side of the gel.

developed allowing to sequence on both strands of a double stranded template simultaneously in the same sequencing reaction, and to detect both sequences on-line (Fig. 3, 4; Wiemann *et al.*, 1994 in press).

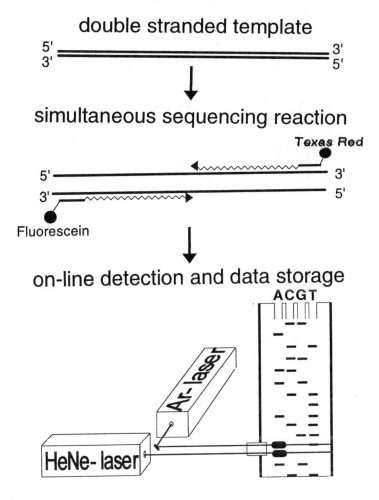

Figure 3
Schematic diagram of the sequencing reaction and gel electrophoresis for simultaneous sequencing on both strands of a double stranded template. After denaturation and neutralization the two differently labeled primers have annealed to the complementary strands of the template. Sequencing reactions are performed in the same tubes and the products are loaded in the same lanes of the sequencing gel (A,C,G and T). Sequencing products carrying a Texas red label are symbolized by red bands, products carrying a Fluorescein label by green bands. Bands where both a Texas red and a Fluorescein labeled sequencing product co-migrate are drawn in black. The gel is traversed from either side by two laser beams, generated with Ar and HeNe lasers. The Texas red label is excited only by the HeNe laser and Fluorescein label solely by the Ar laser while respectively labeled sequencing products pass the beams. Data are monitored with two sets of detectors, one for each laser, placed behind the notched glass plate and stored on-line in a computer ready for automated base calling.

Figure 4
Double stranded plasmid DNA containing a CA/GT microsatellite was sequenced simultaneously with a Fluorescein labeled reverse primer (A) and a Texas Red labeled universal primer (B). Fragments were separated on a sequencing gel and detected on-line and independently with the Ar and HeNe laser/detector systems of the newly developed DNA sequencer.

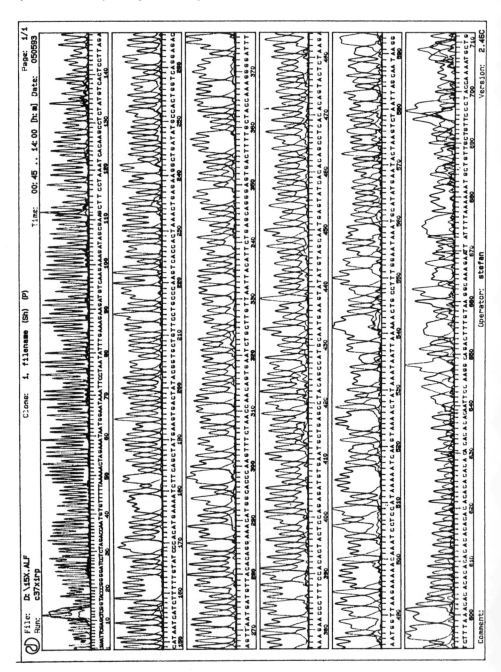

Figure 4A

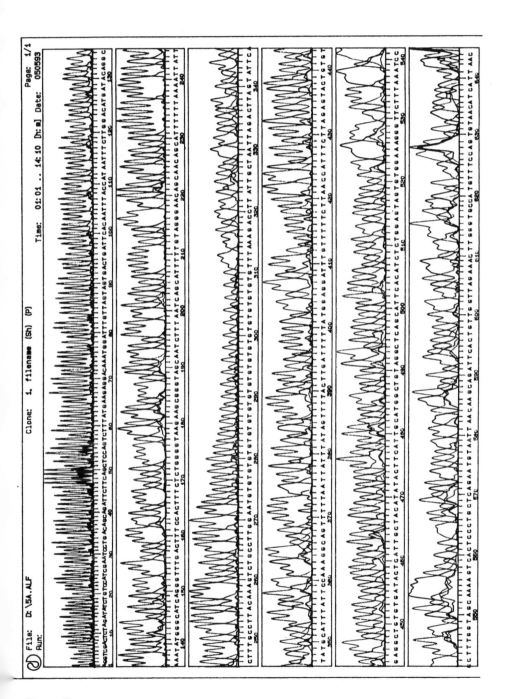

Figure 4B

New detectors have been designed for the collection of the fluorescent light emitted by the DNA samples labelled with two different fluorophores, allowing 8 samples per each fluorophore.

To avoid cross excitation of the two different dyes with the not-corresponding laser beam and cross detection of the emission from the not-corresponding dye, excitation and detection of the two different dyes was arranged geometrically separated. Different laser/fluorophor systems have been tested. For the first dye the standard system, argon laser 488 nm / fluorescein, is used. For the second dye a helium/neon laser is used for excitation, with fluorophores texas red and tetramethylrhodamine.

3.3   Development of an automated gel casting system for ultrathin gels

A technique with vibrating elements shows the greatest promise for automated casting. Its testing and extension to formats larger than 30x30 cm is under way.

3.4   Development of solid support techniques for DNA sample preparation and its adaptation to the existing robotic workstations

Existing methodology developed for the preparation of M13 single stranded DNA was modified and tested for its applicability for the purification of double stranded DNA. Different membrane materials were tested with respect to their DNA binding ability and capacity, e.g. glassfiber and silica membranes.

For efficient automation of DNA preparations centrifugation steps should be omitted if possible. Filtration steps were tested for their ability to replace centrifugations, performed in part with use of gradient filters. One centrifugation step for the final precipitation of DNA turned out to be essential even with the modified protocols. The developed procedures work well, but the final recovery of DNA (about 1 mg) needs to be increased for routine sequencing with T7 DNA polymerase. Work is continued to increase the amount of DNA obtained in the preparations.

3.5   Identification of the human cDNA clones, using probes derived from cell type specific 2D protein gels

About 600 randomly picked cDNA clones from a normal keratinocyte cDNA library have been picked and sequenced from the ends. About 15% of the clones coded for unknown proteins and another 15% were full length clones coding for known proteins that had not previously been mapped in the keratinocyte protein 2-D gel database. We have so far recombined 24 of the full length clones into the vaccinia virus system and expressed the proteins in human AMA cells. This allowed the mapping of these proteins to spots in the 2-D gel database.

3.6   Sequencing human cDNAs

The total output was 42 kilo bases of sequence data. More than 10 full length unknown cDNA clones have been completely sequenced, additional 20 cDNA clones have been partially sequenced. Some of the cDNA clones coded for interesting proteins that are unknown in human but known in other species, including a cDNA that is homologous to a Drosophila tumor suppressor gene. We have used these partial cDNAs as probes for screening cDNA libraries, and have isolated the corresponding full length clones. These will be sequenced and recombined into vaccinia virus.

The clones were first sequenced simultaneously with universal and reverse primers on the two dye sequencing system. The sequencing was completed using the walking primer strategy, and labelled dNTPs. Our work clarified an additional rule for the design of sequencing primers with internal labelling: Within three bases following the primer a labeled dNTP has to be incorporated in order to ensure efficient labelling of the DNA strands. Primers designed according to this rule resulted in strong signals allowing reliable and accurate sequence determination. Primers not meeting this rule did not result in usable results (Wiemann *et al.*, submitted).

3.7 Sequencing human polymorphic microsatellite probes

A total of 190.000 bases of sequence have been collected. In the course of the project 154 human polymorphic microsatellite clones have been analyzed. The clones were first sequenced simultaneously with universal and reverse primers on the two dye sequencing system. The inserts of several clones were discovered to be short enough to finish the sequence on both strands already in the simultaneous sequencing reaction with standard primers. The final sequence of longer inserts was completed using the walking primer strategy. The identified CA repeats are analyzed for their degree of polymorphism and interesting repeats are mapped to human chromosome 21. Reference CEPH families are analyzed: About 20 CA repeats have been completed so far.

4. Major specific breakthroughs and industrial applications

A high speed two dye sequencing system has been developed in the course of this project allowing the detection of two independent sets of sequencing reactions labelled with two different dyes, in the same lanes on the gel. Both the high speed sequencing and throughput, as well as its proven performance, will serve as the basis for the next gerneration of high speed automated DNA sequencers, and be attractive for the industry.

A particularly interesting application of the two dye system is the high accuracy sequencing of templates (e.g. of PCR products) in double stranded form which can now be accomplished in only one sequencing reaction, thereby reducing by 50% the effort and costs for preparation of DNA templates, sequencing reactions and casting of gels.

5. Major cooperative links

The human cDNAs / polymorphic microsatellites were cloned in Aarhus / Barcelona. Sequence analysis was performed at Heidelberg using the newly developed equipment, hardware and software. Final analysis of clones has been carried out in Aarhus and Barcelona. The groups maintained frequent collaborative contacts meeting about 5 times a year in their laboratories or at conferences.

6. List of joint/individual publications

- Wiemann S., Stegemann J., Grothues D., Bosch A., Estivill X., Schwager C., Zimmermann J., Voss H., and Ansorge W. (1994) Simultaneous on-line DNA sequencing on both strands with two fluorescent dyes. *Anal. Biochem.* in press
- Wiemann S., Rupp T., Zimmermann J., Voss H., Schwager C., and Ansorge W. Primer design for automated DNA sequencing utilizing fluorescein 15-dATP as internal label; Submitted for publication
- Wiemann S., Voss H., Schwager C., Rupp T., Stegemann J., Zimmermann J., Grothues D., Sensen C., Erfle H., Hewitt N., Banrevi A., and Ansorge W. (1993) Sequencing and analysis of 51.6 kilobases on

the left arm of chromosome XI from *S. cerevisiae* reveals 23 open reading frames including the FAS1 gene. Yeast **9**, 1343-1348

- Wiemann S., Stegemann J., Voss H., Schwager C., Rupp T., Zimmermann J., and Ansorge W. (1993) Simultaneous DNA sequencing on both strands with two dyes: Application to human polymorphic microsatellites and cDNA clones. Meeting: Genome Mapping and Sequencing Cold Spring Harbor, NY., 271

- Stegemann J., Schwager C., Erfle H., Hewitt N., Voss H., Zimmermann J., and Ansorge W. (1991) High speed DNA sequencing on a commercial automated sequencer using 0.3 mm thin gels. Meth. Mol. Cell. Biol. **2**, 292-293

- Stegemann J., Schwager C., Erfle H., Hewitt N., Voss H., Zimmermann J., and Ansorge W. (1991) Automated DNA sequencing on ultrathin slab gels. Meth. Mol. Cell. Biol. **2**, 182-184

- Stegemann J., Schwager C., Erfle H., Hewitt N., Voss H., Zimmermann J., and Ansorge W. (1991) High speed on-line DNA sequencing on ultrathin slab gels. Nucleic Acids Res. **19**, 675-676

- Banchs I., Bosch A., Guimera J., Lazaro C., Puig A., and Estivill X. New alleles at microsatellite loci in CEPH families mainly arise from somatic mutations in the lymphoblastoid cell lines. Human Mutation, in press.

- Bosch A., Nunes V., Patterson D., and Estivill X (1993). Isolation and Characterization of 14 CA-repeat microsatellites from Human Chromosome 21. Genomics **18**: 151-155

- Bosch A., Wiemann S., Guimera J., Ansorge W., Patterson D., and Estivill X (1993). Two dinucleotide repeat polymorphisms at 21q22.3 (D21S416 and D21S1235) Hum. Mol. Genet. **2**: 1744

- Bosch A., Wiemann S., Ansorge W., Patterson D., and Estivill X (1994). Three CA/GT repeat polymorphisms from loci D21S414 and D21S1234 on Human Chromosome 21. Hum. Genet. **93**: 359-360

- Bosch A., Guimera J., Beckmann J., and Estivill X. EUROGEM human chromosome 21 genetic map, submitted for publication.

- Chumakov I., Rigault P., Bosch A., Estivill X., *et al.* (1992). Continuum of overlapping clones spanning the entire human chromosome 21q. Nature **359**, 380-386

- Celis J.E., Rasmussen H.H., Olsen E., Madsen P., Leffers H., Honore B., Dejgaard K., Gromov P., Hoffman H.J., Nielsen M., Vassilev A., Vintermeyr O., Hao J. Celis A., Basse B., Lauridsen J.B., Ratz G.P., Andersen A.H., Walbum E., Kjaergaard I., Puype M., Van Danme J., and Vandekerckhove J. (1993) The human keratinocyte two-dimensional gel protein database: Update 1993. Electrophoresis **14**, 1091-1198

- Leffers H., Madsen P., Rasmussen H.H., Honore B., Andersen A.H., Walbum E., Vandekerckhove J., and Celis J.E. (1993) Molecular cloning and expression of the transforation sensitive epithelial marker stratifin. J. Mol. Biol., **231** 982-998

- Dejgaard K., Leffers, H., Rasmussen H.H., Madsen P., Kruse T.A., Gesser B., Nielsen H., and Celis J.E. (1994) Identification, molecular cloning, expression and chromosome mapping of a family of transformation upregulated hnRNP-K proteins derived by alternate splicing. J. Mol. Biol. **236**, 33-48

- Celis J.E., and Olsen E. (1994) A qualitative and quantitative protein database approach identifies individual and groups of functionally related proteins that are differentially regulated in simiam virus 40 (SV40) transformed human kertinocytes. Electrophoresis **15**, 309-344

Contract number: GENO-CT91-0015
Contractual period: 1 April 1992 to 31 March 1994

Coordinator
Prof. W. Ansorge
European Molecular Biology Laboratory
Meyerhofstr. 1
D-69117 Heidelberg
Germany
Tel: 49 6221 387 355
Fax: 49 6221 387 306

Participants
Prof. J. Celis
Institute of Medical Biochemistry
Aarhus University
Ole Worms Alle
building 70
DK-8000 Aarhus
Denmark
Tel: 45 894 228 66
Fax: 45 861 311 60

Prof. X. Estivill
Institut de Recerca Oncologica
Hospital Duran i Reynals
Autovia de Castelldefels km. 2,7
L'Hospitalet de Llobregat
E-08907 Barcelona
Spain
Tel: 34 3 263 0039
Fax: 34 3 263 2251

Human Genome Analysis Programme
M. Hallen and A. Klepsch (Eds.)
IOS Press, 1995

MASS SPECTROMETRY OF POLYNUCLEOTIDES BY
MATRIX-ASSISTED LASER DESORPTION/IONIZATION (MALDI-MS)

F. Hillenkamp
Institute for Medical Physics and Biophysics, Münster University, Germany

1. Background information

Since its introduction in 1988 by Karas and Hillenkamp[1], MALDI-MS has become an established method for desorbing ions of proteins with molecular weights up to 500 kDa[1-6]. The determination of molecular masses with an accuracy of up to 0.01% is possible. Typical sample amounts required are 1 pmol, but a sensitivity in the low femtomol range can be achieved[7,8]. The key idea of this technique is to embed the macromolecules (the analyte) in a suitable matrix of molecules having a strong absorption at the laser wavelength and present in high molar excess over the analyte. This induces an efficient transfer of the laser-pulse energy to the analyte and results in a "soft" desorption process. It is suggested that the matrix molecules also play a role in the ionization of the analyte molecules.[9] Different lasers and wavelengths in the UV (mainly 266 nm, 337 nm and 355 nm) and IR (mainly 2.94 μm, 2.79 μm and 10.6μm) have been used for this technique. Complex mixtures of proteins and peptides are routinely mass analysed. Carbohydrates[10], glycoproteins, lipoproteins and lipids, as well as many other synthetic and natural polymers[11], are also amenable to MALDI-MS. In all of these cases the key to successful analysis of a new class of analyte molecules has been to find a specifically suited combination of matrix and laser wavelength.

Provided that the right conditions for desorption of nucleic acids of > 100 nucleotides could be found, rapid DNA sequencing could be possible by direct mass spectrometric analysis of the Sanger reaction products[12], replacing the time consuming gel electrophoretic procedure. In many other fields of nucleic acid research such as the chemical synthesis of modified oligonucleotides for e.g. antisense DNA applications a quick and precise mass determination of oligonucleotides of 10 to 30 bases, would also be of high interest. Typical modifications such as labelling with a fluorescence marker, the addition of a hydrophobic group to the 5'- or 3'-end, for an increased cell-uptake, or the introduction of thiophosphate groups, etc. could easily be verified by a determination of the accurate molecular mass. Further examples for potential and promising applications are the mass spectrometric characterisation of UV-light-demaged DNA or RNA, of photo-cross-linking products in the study of protein-nucleic acid interaction, and of the interaction products of cytostatics, as e.g. cis-platinum, routinely applied in cancer treatment, and model- as well as native DNA and RNA.

Keywords: Mass Spectrometry; MALDI-MS; Polynucleotides; DNA; Sequencing.

2. Objectives and primary approaches

The overall objective of this one-year pilot project was to explore the potential and the limits of matrix-assisted laser desorption/ionization mass spectrometry (MALDI-MS) in nucleic acids analyses. A routine MALDI-MS technique would be valuable in the whole field of molecular biology; e.g. for the verification of the synthesis of modified oligonucleotides, for the identification of naturally modified nucleic acids and the development of alternative DNA sequencing procedures.

At the beginning of the project, all experiments on nucleic acids had been performed with matrix/laser combinations which had proven successful for the analysis of peptides or proteins. However, extensive fragmentation of the analyte molecule was observed, setting an upper limit of approx. 15 nucleotides above which the molecular ion could not be identified. Thus, a search for improved combinations of matrices and laser wavelengths was the most important initial goal. A range of lasers emitting in the infrared and ultraviolet were investigated in combination with many new potential matrices, mainly small organic compounds.

Another important goal was to develop a sample preparation procedure that would ensure preparation of a homogeneous sample. Due to the strong acidic (highly negatively-charged) phosphodiester backbone, nucleic acids have a strong tendency to form multiple salts with different and differing numbers of cations in MALDI, thus generating nominally identical analyte molecules with a broad mass distribution. This significantly reduces both the mass resolution and the ion yield. Based on experiments with electrospray-ionization MS on oligonucleotides[13], introduction of ammonium as the counter ion for the phosphodiester groups appeared promising. Upon desorption in electrospray-ionization MS, the ammonium salts dissociate into ammonia and the free acid of the oligonucleotide giving rise to a homogeneous analyte- molecule-ion mass. Keeping in mind that the sample procedure should be fast and simple, different procedures with ammonium salt incubations and precipitation as well as ion exchange materials were evaluated.

We also wanted to determine the upper mass limit of oligonucleotides amenable to MALDI-MS analysis under improved experimental conditions. To address this problem, synthetic oligodeoxyribonucleotides, oligoribonucleotides as well as RNA transcripts prepared in vitro were used because these types of analytes can easily be made in large quantities. In-vitro transcripts were employed to explore the upper mass limit for RNA samples because the chemical synthesis of RNA is more difficult and less established than that of DNA.

Finally, analyses of mixtures containing nested series of oligonucleotides, in which each species differs from the previous by one nucleotide, were planed. The aim was to evaluate the potential of the method for the analysis of oligonucleotide ladders, as e.g. generated in the "Sanger"-sequencing reaction. Here, both mixtures of synthetic oligodeoxynucleotides and chemically degraded polynucleotides were investigated.

3. Results and discussion

Significant progress in all addressed fields has been achieved and has led to four publications[14-17]. For details of the results, the reader is referred to these publications; they are not repeated in detail here.

Among the tested matrices and laser wavelengths for desorption (266 nm, 337 nm and 355 nm in the ultraviolet region; 2.79 μm, 2.94 μm and 10.6 μm in the infrared region), the best results have been obtained with the combinations: succinic acid as matrix and a laser wavelength of 2.94 μm and with 3-hydroxypicolinic acid as matrix and 337 or 355 nm laser wavelength. The first combination was discovered in the Münster group 1992, the latter was reported by Wu et al. in spring 1993 as a new promising combination for the MALDI analysis of oligodeoxynucleotides[18]. A high accuracy of 0.01-0.02% for molecular mass determination and a sensitivity in the low picomolar range have been achieved with both desorption schemes. The problem with heterogeneous counterions on the phosphate groups of the nucleic acids has been solved (see Fig. 1). Besides a simple purification of the matrix solutions with a ion-exchange-column, an in situ exchange, of alkali cations with ammonium ions, is performed in the sample droplet just prior to the introduction into the mass spectrometer. This leads to oligonucleotides almost exclusively associated with ammonium counterions. During desorption/ ionization, NH_3 is lost and the sample ions become fully protonated resulting in a single ion mass. The in situ ion exchange is very simple, cheap and fast. A detailed description of this technique can be found in the enclosed papers.

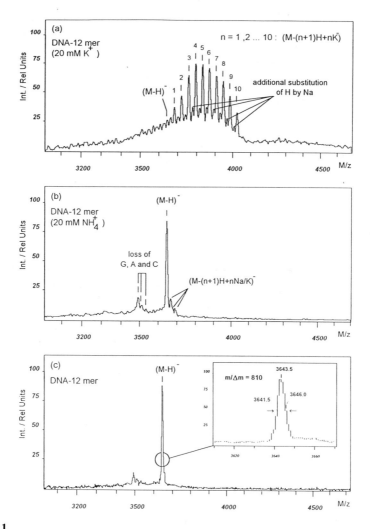

Figure 1

IR-MALDI mass spectra of the oligodeoxynucleotide 12-mer 5'-CCT TTT GAA AAG-3' under three different conditions: in the presence of (a) 20 mM potassium bromide or (b) 20 mM ammonium acetate in the analyte solution; (c) 15-20 cation exchange polymer beads loaded with ultra pure ammonium acetate, but without the addition of salt. 5 pmoles oligodeoxynucleotide were loaded for each measurement. All spectra are the sums of 10 single-shot spectra.

In the high mass range, results differ for DNA and RNA samples. DNA oligo-nucleotides give well resolved signals up to the 30 mer level. Above this size metastable molecule-ion fragmentation, dominated by single and multiple base losses, degrades the quality of the spectra. For DNA UV-MALDI with the 3-hydroxypicolinic acid matrix is superior to the IR-desorption scheme in terms of accessible mass range (Fig. 2). The latter one causes a stronger fragmentation with increasing mass of the analyte molecules and yields additionally to some extent prompt fragment ions, resulting from backbone cleavages, which offer valuable structure (sequence) information ("sequence ions")[16].

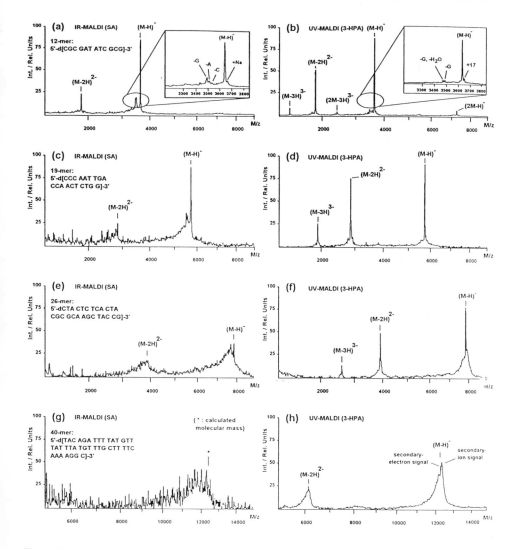

Figure 2

Comparison of negative-ion RTOF-mass spectra of oligodeoxynucleotides with increasing sequence length (12 to 40 deoxynucleotides) obtained with IR-MALDI at 2.94 μm laser wavelength and succinic acid as matrix (**a, c, e, and g**) and with UV-MALDI at 355 nm laser wavelength and 3-hydroxypicolinic acid as matrix (**b, d, f, and h**). Total oligodeoxynucleotide load for each measurement: 5 pmol. All spectra are the sums of ten single-shot spectra.

The frequency of loss of G, A and C is observed in that sequence. No loss of T has been found. Mass differences observed for the loss of a single base correspond to the molecular mass of the free nucleobases (111 Da : C, 135 Da : A, and 151 Da for G). A intramolecular proton-catalyzed 1,2-trans-elimination has been proposed as the corresponding fragmentation reaction[16]. The higher susceptibility of the purine bases for their elimination agrees with the higher stability of the N-glycosidic bond of purine bases compared to the one of pyridine bases. The stability of T can be rationalized by the fact that the base in this nucleotide has no basic function, thus, protonation is rather unlikely, increasing the polarization of the N-glycosidic bond.

For RNA, much larger molecules like in vitro transcribed RNA's of 67 and 104 nucleotides and in addition tRNA from brewers yeast and E. coli (MW app. 24,900 Da and 23,800 Da, respectively), multimers of the tRNAs (up to over 100,000 Daltons), 5S rRNA from E. coli (MW app. 38,500 Da) have been successfully desorbed and mass analysed (Fig. 3). The differences in the results obtained with IR- and UV-MALDI and the above mentioned matrices are much less pronounced here. The main reason for the different results for DNA and RNA is related to the higher stability of the N-glycosidic bond of the nucleobases in RNA. This increased stability is a well know phenomenon and can be ascribed to the 2'-hydroxyl group in the ribose ring of RNA. The fact that RNA can easily be analysed at high masses by MALDI-MS is of interest for further applications (e.g. sequencing of DNA using RNA-transcript-sequencing ladders (e.g. employing RNA polymerase and 3'-deoxynucleosidetriphosphates as terminators[19]) and for the characterization of modified mRNAs, tRNAs and rRNAs).

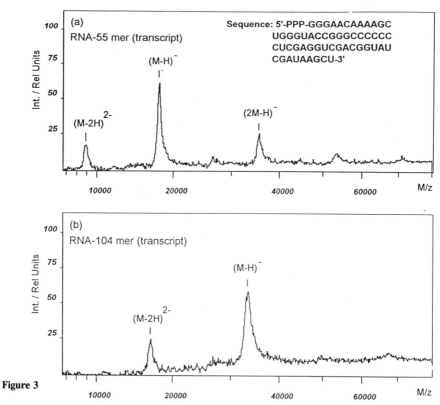

Figure 3

IR-MALDI mass spectra of RNA transcripts of (a) 55 nucleotides, and (b) 104 nucleotides. Total RNA load: 5 pmoles for each measurement. Both spectra are the sums of 10 single-shot spectra.

For the analysis of mixtures of oligodeoxynucleotides, very promising results have been obtained for a mixture of oligothymidylic acids[14] and of chemically degraded polyuridylic acids[15] (Fig. 4). Because the different oligonucleotides in a mixture have more uniform physicochemical properties (they are all water soluble and easy to charge) than different peptides, mass analysis of mixtures of the former turned out to be easier than for peptides and proteins. This result is of high relevance for sequencing applications based on the MALDI analysis of oligonucleotide ladders.

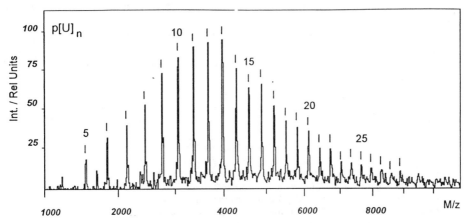

Figure 4

IR-MALDI mass spectrum of a mixture of oligouridylic acids generated by limited hydrolysis of Poly-U. Ca. 7 pmoles oligoribonucleotide were loaded. The spectrum is the sum of ten single-shot spectra.

Substitution of up to 30% of the matrix by urea, a common reagent used to denature double stranded DNA into single stranded DNA, can be tolerated for both matrices. Also in negative-ion mode, addition of peptides or proteins like cytochrome C, bovine insulin or human angiotensin I, in concentrations comparable to those of the oligonucleotides, does not disturb the analysis. Protein and peptide signals are suppressed in the presence of nucleic acids because of a higher ionization efficiency for negative ions of the latter. These results are also of interest for the future use of matrix-assisted laser desorption/ionization mass spectrometry for DNA sequencing because (a) denaturation of DNA is an essential step in sequencing and (b) proteins like the sequencing enzyme DNA-polymerase need not necessarily be removed prior to the analysis.

Excellent results have been obtained for the analysis of modified DNA samples of up to 25 nucleotides in length in cooperation with the group of Prof. Engels of the university of Frankfurt, FRG (antisense oligodeoxynucleotides) and Prof. Cech, university of Berlin, FRG (PEG linked DNA). A joint publication of these results is in preparation.

4. Major scientific breakthroughs and/or industrial applications

The development of a fast and efficient method for preparing homogeneous analyte solutions combined with a precise mass determination of pmol-amounts of analyte in both IR- and UV-MALDI-MS has received a great deal of attention among scientists in nucleic acid research. It is normally very laborious to verify the introduction of modifications in oligonucleotides but an accurate mass determination by MALDI-MS can be done in less than 30 minutes. As a result, the groups both in Münster and Odense have performed analyses for several outside research groups. Partly, the results of these cooperations are presented in the included publications.

5. Major cooperative links

- Prof. Dr. J. Engels, Institute of Organic Chemistry, Johann Wolfgang Goethe-Universität, 60439 Frankfurt am Main, Germany.
- Prof. Dr. C. Cech, Institute ofr Bioorganic Chemistry, Humboldt-Universität, 10115 Berlin, Germany.
- Prof. Dr. V. Erdmann, Institute of Biochemistry, Freie Universität Berlin, 14195 Berlin, Germany.

References

[1] Karas M. and Hillenkamp F. (1988) *Anal. Chem.*, **60**, 2299.
[2] Karas M., Bahr U. and Hillenkamp F. (1989) *Int. J. Mass Spectrom. Ion Proc.*, **92**, 231.
[3] Hillenkamp F. and Karas M. (1990) *Methods Enzymol.*, **193**, 280.
[4] Beavis R.C. and Chait B.T. (1989) *Rapid Commun. Mass Spectrom.*, **3**, 233.
[5] Beavis R.C. and Chait B.T. (1989) *Rapid Commun. Mass Spectrom.*, **3**, 432.
[6] Beavis R.C. and Chait B.T. (1989) *Rapid Commun. Mass Spectrom.*, **3**, 436.
[7] Strupat K., Karas M. and Hillenkamp F. (1991) *Int. J. Mass Spectrom. Ion Proc.*, **111**, 89.
[8] Karas M., Bahr U., Ingendoh A., Nordhoff E., Stahl B., Strupat K. and Hillenkamp F. (1990) *Anal. Chim. Acta*, **241**, 175.
[9] Ehring H., Karas M. and Hillenkamp F. (1992) *Organic Mass Spectrom.*, **27**, 472.
[10] Stahl B., Steup M., Karas M. and Hillenkamp F. (1991) *Anal. Chem.*, **63**, 1463.
[11] Deppe A., Bahr U., Karas M. and Hillenkamp F. (1992) *Anal. Chem.*, **64**, 2866.
[12] Sanger F., Nicklen S. and Coulson A.R. (1977) *Proc. Natl. Acad. Sci. USA*, **74**, 5463.
[13] Stults J.T. and Marsters J.C. (1991) *Rapid Commun. Mass Spectrom.*, **5**, 359.
[14] Nordhoff E., Ingendoh A., Cramer R., Overberg A., Stahl B., Karas M., Hillenkamp F., and Crain P.F. (1992) *Rapid Commun. Mass Spectrom.*, **6**, 771.
[15] Nordhoff E., Cramer R., Karas M., Hillenkamp,F., Kirpekar F., Kristiansen,K., and Roepstorff,P. (1993) *Nucleic Acids. Res.*, **21**, 3347.
[16] Nordhoff E., Karas M., Hillenkamp F., Kirpekar F., Kristiansen K., and Roepstorff P. (1993) *Proceedings of the 41th ASMS Conference on Mass Spectrometry and Allied Topics*, pp 246a-b.
[17] Svendsen M.L., Wengel J., Dahl O., Kirpekar F. and Roepstorff P. (1993) *Tetrahedron Lett.*, **49**, 11341.
[18] Wu K.J., Stedding A. and Becker C.H. (1993) *Rapid Commun. Mass Spectrom.*, **7**, 142.
[19] Axelrod V.D. and Kramer F.R. (1985) *Biochemistry*, **24**, 5716.

List of joint/individual publications:

1. Nordhoff E., Ingendoh A., Cramer R., Overberg A., Stahl B., Karas M., Hillenkamp F., and Crain P.F. (1992) *Rapid Commun. Mass Spectrom.*, **6**, 771.
2. Nordhoff E., Cramer R., Karas M., Hillenkamp F., Kirpekar,F., Kristiansen K., and Roepstorff P. (1993) *Nucleic Acids. Res.*, **21**, 3347.
3. Nordhoff E., Karas M., Hillenkamp F., Kirpekar F., Kristiansen K., and Roepstorff P. (1993) *Proceedings of the 41th ASMS Conference on Mass Spectrometry and Allied Topics*, pp 246a-b.
4. Svendsen M.L., Wengel J., Dahl O., Kirpekar F. and Roepstorff P. (1993) *Tetrahedron Lett.*, **49**, 11341.

Contract number: GENO-CT93-0022
Contractual period: 1 January 1993 to 30 June 1993

Coordinator
Prof. F. Hillenkamp
Institute of Medical Physics and Biophysics
Münster University
D-48149 Münster
Germany
Tel: 49 251 835 103 (835104)
Fax: 49 251 835 121

Participants
Prof. P. Roepstorff
Department of Molecular Biology
Odense University
DK-5230 Odense
Denmark
Tel: 45 66 158 600
Fax: 45 65 932 781

No. of joint/individual publications + patents: 4

Human Genome Analysis Programme
M. Hallen and A. Klepsch (Eds.)
IOS Press, 1995

MAPPING THE HUMAN X CHROMOSOME
BY TELOMERE INDUCED BREAKAGE

H. Cooke
MRC Human Genetics Unit, Edinburgh, United Kingdom

1. Background Information

A minimalist view of a chromosome is of a DNA molecule with replication and segregation functions; linearity imposes the further requirement of specific structures which result in non-recombinogenic ends and permit the complete replication of the molecule. In the fission yeast S. cerevisiae this simple view of a chromosome has been proven correct by the use of cloned centromeres, origins of replication and telomeres to create artificial chromosomes (YACs).

These three elements result in a DNA molecule which is maintained as a stable, linear entity in the cell. Of these three essential chromosomal components only telomeres have been molecularly characterized in humans to date. All vertebrate telomeres consist of the simple sequence (T2AG3) arranged as tandem repeats. The ability to define telomeres in vertebrates is a direct consequence of the apparent conservation of the basic strategy used by many organisms to replicate the end of a DNA molecule. All known DNA polymerases replicate DNA in a 5' to 3' direction from a primer. At the end of a molecule there is no DNA to which the primer can anneal and hence the 3' end of the molecule can not be replicated. Organisms with linear chromosomes therefore require a specialised replication mechanism. In the absence of such a mechanism a gradual loss of DNA will occur which will eventually result in loss of an essential gene. A more immediate and catastrophic consequence of telomere loss is probably chromosome instability caused by the fusion of non telomeric DNA ends and thus the setting up of breakage-fusion-bridge cycles caused by the resulting dicentric chromosomes.

Terminal arrays of repeated sequences were first studied in detail in ciliates, such as tetrahymena, which have a large number of small chromosomes in their macronuclei. A consensus sequence of known repeats can be derived but the key feature seems to be strand assymetry in base composition. In theory this has the consequence that the G rich strand can form a variety of non Watson Crick structures but these have not been shown to have any functional significance in vivo. These repeated sequences are synthesised by an RNA dependent DNA polymerase, telomerase, as first shown in tetrahymena. This enzyme is a ribonuclear protein and the RNA contains one and a half copies of the terminal repeat sequence which is used as a template on which the enzyme extends one strand of the chromosome end. Although the enzyme has not been fully purified from any source similar activities have been detected in a number of other organisms including humans.

The number of terminal repeats present at a telomere is variable. However, in yeast the average number is constant suggesting a regulated process. Indeed, mutations in a number of loci in yeast affect telomere length suggesting that many factors may be involved in telomere maintenance. A mutation in one of these loci, est1 (Ever Shorter Telomeres), causes the gradual loss of telomeric repeats, aneuploidy and senescence. Similar phenotypes have been generated by altering the sequence in tetrahymena telomerase RNA and hence the sequence incorporated into the tetrahymena telomeres themselves. Loss of telomerase activity would seem likely to result in these phenotypes.

We had previously shown that introduction of DNA constructs containing telomeres into immortal Chinese hamster cells carrying a human X chromosome resulted in terminalistion of the construct in the chromosome implying that telomerase was sufficiently active in these cells to allow the introduced telomeric sequences to seed terminal repeat addition. A possible mechanism by which this might have been happening was chromosome breakage by the integration of the exogenous telomeres followed by telomerase mediated stabilisation of the chromosome. If this was the case we would be producing terminally deleted X chromosomes which, by analogy with classical end labelling and partial digest mapping, are good substrates for long range restriction digest mapping. Indeed this has been demonstrated for the only chromosomal end which could previously be analysed in this way, the pseudoautosomal telomere.

Keywords: Chromosome Telomere Breakage X.

2. Objectives and primary approaches

The aim of this program was to show if telomeres added to cells resulted in chromosome breakage and if we could make terminally deleted X chromosomes for use in probe/STS derivation, long range restriction mapping and YAC isolation.

The primary approach we have taken is outlined in figure 1. By electroporating telomeric constructs into a hybrid line carrying a human X chromosome and applying appropriate selections we were able to isolate a number of cell lines which on the basis of their phenotype were candidates for lines which carried terminally deleted X chromosomes. These lines were analysed further. Chromosome analysis by metaphase in situ hybridisation was used to screen for the absence of gross chromosomal abnormalities (Edinburgh). Marker loss was assayed in Cambridge using a panel of established STS,s. In combination these approaches established that these cell lines, some fifty in total, represented un rearranged terminal deletions of the X chromosome. Cell lines were transferred to Paris for terminal restriction mapping and in Edinburgh and Cambridge the process of cloning terminal restriction fragments was started.

This proved to be possible only for a subset of cell lines which gave rise to terminal genomic fragments which were not too large to give problems in cloning.

A number of such clones were isolated and sequence data derived from them. The clones or the STS primer pairs derived from their sequences were mapped back on the panel of hybrid lines. This revealed an un-expected result - the terminal genomic sequences from 80% of the end clones mapped more proximally than the deletion point determined by marker loss in the cell line from which they were derived and in these cell lines Southern Blot analysis revealed that the original genomic restriction fragment was retained in addition to the fragment derived from it by addition of a telomere. Taken together these results imply an inverted terminal duplication of the chromosome.

McKlintock's original observations on breakage fusion bridge cycles in cells may provide the clues for understanding the processes involved in creating these inverted duplications. One such scheme is outlined in figure 2. Although it provides a mechanism for creating duplications it does not explain why duplicated fragments are more abundant than non duplicated since healing of the breakage product of a dicentric should give duplicated and non duplicated chromosomes with equal probability.

These aspects of the work have been reported (Farr et al. 1992). Subsequently we have taken a number of approaches to develop our understanding of the biology, to exploit the resources we have developed and to extend them.

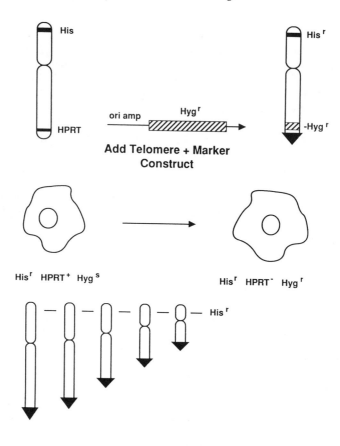

Figure 1
X Chromosome fragmentation

We have investigated the duplicated lines by in situ hybridisation (Edinburgh) and banding techniques on extended chromosomes and PFG electrophoresis (Paris). These approaches have shown that in the majority of the duplicated lines the duplications can not be less than about 2 mbp since single PFG fragments which hybridise to terminal genomic fragments are not found. The majority of duplications can not be larger than about 5 mbp since in situ hybridisation with terminal genomic fragments does not reveal resolvable double dots. The duplications clearly make these cell lines unsuitable for deriving terminal restriction maps to build up an overall X chromosome map.

We have used cell lines derived in these experiments to ask questions about the effect on the positioning of centromeric and telomeric parts of a chromosome of moving a telomere from its normal position on the chromosome to a previously internal position (Edinburgh). There is no significant effect on the position of the chromosome in the interphase nucleus. We have asked about the effects of partial deletion of X chromosome alphoid DNA (the current best candidate for human centromere DNA) caused in some of our lines by deletion of essentially all the long arm of the X (Edinburgh and Cambridge) and find no measurable effect on the fidelity of chromosome segregation with an alphoid block reduced by about 30%.

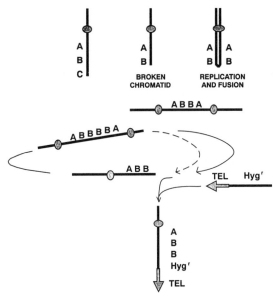

Figure 2

To extend the panel of hybrids for mapping purposes and to demonstrate the methods ability to manipulate chromosomes in the living cell we have (Cambridge) attempted to take the most deleted X chromosome from these experiments and repeat the approach on the short arm to create a second panel of deletions which would include a defined mini-chromosome consisting essentially only of telomeres, selectable markers and minimal centromere.

To start to use the information derived from the panel of X chromosome long arm deletions STS's have been developed (Pavia). STSs were mapped on the breakpoint panel. Mapping on the panel demonstrated that the end clones were not telomeric: they were all contained in telomere hybrids with more proximal breakpoints as mentioned above.

STS from HyTM157	was positive up to 23
STS from 20	was positive up to 42
STS from 16	was positive up to 58 and 26
STS from 84	was positive up to 80, 47, 45 and 9

The STSs were used to identify YAC clones from the ICI total human YAC library. YACs were also isolated using STS derived from known markers which were mapped on the telomere hybrid panel (Farr et al). A panel of 10 YAC clones was ordered along Xq, from Xq11 to Xq24 which could be used to map breakpoints in Xq.

We used them to map breakpoints in X autosome balanced translocations in Xq associated with gonadal dysgenesis. YACs were used as probes in in situ hybridisations on metaphases of six different translocations and demonstrated two regions in Xq21 were the breakpoints were clustered. A YAC contig of about 2 Mb was obtained, spanning all the breakpoints, and work is in progress to clone the breakpoints and establish if and how many genes are involved in this form of gonadal dysgenesis, which is frequently associated with rearrangements in Xq.

3. Major Scientific Breakthroughs

Previously we had reported probable breakage of chromosomes by telomere containing constructs. In the course of this program we have proven this and used the method in a number of ways. This work is internationally recognised as innovative and setting a precedent for chromosome engineering, for example in a review by Carol Greider in Current Opinion 4 it is cited as a paper "of outstanding interest".

4. Major co-operative links

There has been a full exchange of materials, both of DNA constructs cell lines and primer pairs between all program members. Regular meetings between members and the use of Internet links has facilitated the exchange of information. In situ hybridisation technology has been transfered to Pavia by the visit of one person to Edinburgh for three weeks.

Joint Publications

- Farr C.J., Stevanovic M., Thomson E.J., Goodfellow P.N. and Cook H.J., Telomere-associated chromosome fragmentation: applications in genome manipulation and analysis. Nature Genetics 2, 275-282, 1992.
- Bayne R.A.L., Broccoli D., Taggart M.H., Thomson E.J., Farr C.J. and Cooke H.J., Sandwiching of a gene between a functional telomere and centromere does not result in silencing. Hum Molec Genet (in press)
- Bayne, R., Taggart, M. T., Farr, C., Petit, C., Guilford, P., Toniolo, D., Sala, C., and Cooke H.J. Cytogenetics and Cell genetics 64 175 1993

Individual publications

- Broccoli D. and Cooke H., Aging, healing, and the metabolism of telomeres. Am J Hum Genet 52, 657-660, 1993.
- Broccoli D. and Cooke H.J., Effect of telomeres on the interphase location of adjacent regions of the human X chromosome. Exp Cell Res (in press)
- McKay S., Thomson E. and Cooke H., Sequence homologies and linkage group conservation of the human and mouse CENP-C genes. Genomics (in press)

Contract number: GENO-CT91 0014
Contractual period: 1 June 1992 to 31 May 1994

Coordinator
Dr. Howard Cooke
MRC Human Genetics Unit
Edinburgh EH4 2XU
United Kingdom
Tel: 44 31 332 2471
Fax: 44 31343 2620

Participants
Dr. Christine Farr
Department of Genetics
Downing Street
Cambridge CB2 3EH
United Kingdom
Tel: 44 223 333 972
Fax: 44 223 333 992

Dr. Christine Petit
Institute Pasteur
25 Rue du Dr Roux
F-75015 Paris
France
Tel: 33 1 45 68 88 90
Fax: 33 1 45 68 8790.

Dr. Daneilla Toniolo
IGBE
Via Abbategrasso 207
I-27100 Pavia
Italy
Tel: 39 382 546340
Fax: 39 382 422286

Human Genome Analysis Programme
M. Hallen and A. Klepsch (Eds.)
IOS Press, 1995

PHYSICAL MAP OF THE 6P CHROMOSOME: DETAILED GENETIC INVESTIGATION OF THE MAJOR HISTOCOMPATIBILITY COMPLEX (MHC) REGION 6P23

F. Galibert
CNRS UPR 41, Rennes, France

The aim of this program is to draw a detailed physical and genetic map of the major histocompatibility complex (MHC) located on the human genome in 6p21-23.

The human MHC is a chromosomal region of about 5000 kb. Three sub-regions can be distinguished: the class I region encodes the transplantation antigens; the class II region encodes products which are also implicated in immunological responses; the class III region codes for proteins of the complement cascade. Other genes are present within this region such as 21 OH, TNF and numerous other genes many of which were discovered during this study.

The study of the MHC region has been chosen among many other regions of the human genome in view of:

1. its biological importance;
2. the availability of very good genetic studies of two multigenic families (important for studying the contraction-expansion phenomenon);
3. gene clustering with products implicated in different immunological processes, and with sometimes similarity in their regulation pathway (TNF and HLA-B) offers a good opportunity to understand the gene clustering within the genome (chromatin structure for example);
4. several associated diseases.

The genomic organization of the MHC region can be summarized as follows. Genes of class I are the more telomeric, genes of class II are centromeric, whereas genes of class III are in between. It is presently still difficult to give the exact number of genes encoded in this region and such knowledge will probably await complete sequencing of the whole region, since in addition to having many genes, the region also encodes many pseudogenes and genes with a high level of sequence analogy, which makes calculation through hybridization data more questionable. In fact, this sequencing strategy is one of the purposes of the following program.

The present study, which lasted two years, was initiated at the end of February 1992 and was split between seven laboratories. Three laboratories, those of Campbell - Papamatheakis and Trowsdale, are mainly working on the region encompassing class II and III genes, those of Galibert, Le Gall and Pontarotti on the region containing class I genes. Philippe Brulet, who has a large expertise in ES cells and homologous recombination, makes use of DNA fragments mapped by other contractants to search for the function of newly identifed genes.

The strategy followed by all the members of the group involves a top-to-bottom approach: YACs covering a large part of the region were first identified and characterized by restriction mapping with various rare cutting restriction enzymes, and YACs of particular interest were subsequently subcloned in more discrete entities, such as cosmid or phage recombinants.

Identification of genes by hybration of cDNA libraries with various DNA probes on the entire YAC has been done. The technique known as exon trapping was also used to identify potential new genes. In addition to this battery of techniques, DNA sequencing was also used to characterize DNA fragments subcloned from larger entities. Sequencing of large DNA fragments was also performed to elucidate the full information content of specific regions. The DNA sequence was then analyzed through various computational studies.

During the contract, several contigs have been constructed and several new genes have been revealed, either by sequence analogy to genes previously identified in other organisms, or by sequencing cDNA clones sorted out from cDNA libraries after hybridization with YAC. That will be detailed later.

Keywords: 6p; YAC contigs; cDNA; Genetic map; Physical map.

ANALYSIS OF THE CLASS II GENES REGION

Proteins of class II are expressed at the lymphocyte B surface membrane. They are essentially involved in antigens processing and presentation.

Background

It may not be fortuitous that the MHC contains a number of sets of genes with inter-related functions. This linkage may underlie co-evolution of the functions of class I and class II molecules in antigen presentation: since both types of molecule affect positive and negative selection of T cells, linkage of various alleles on a haplotype may help to maximise the T cell repertoire. Recent evidence indicates that a large proportion of peptides eluted from the grooves of class II molecules are from MHC-encoded proteins, such as peptides corresponding to class I sequences - a fact which may also impose restrictions on which alleles may be found linked together [Chicz et al., J. Exp. Med. 178, 27]. As the number of functionally related MHC genes grew, it became more apparent that identification of other genes in the region could give some insight into antigen processing and presentation.

Once the whole class II region had been cloned, we were able to concentrate on looking for novel genes in between the known loci. Initially this was achieved by probing cDNA libraries directly with genomic fragments, suitably competed with human carrier DNA. More recently we have been using other techniques, such as exon amplification or cDNA enrichment. Three new types of gene were discovered in the class II region:

1. Genes with no obvious association with the immune system. Genes in this category included the ubiquitously expressed RING1 gene, which was homologous to a family of genes with a novel type of zinc finger. Another such gene, RING3, encoded a protein homologous to the *Drosophila* maternal effect gene, *Female Sterile homoetic* or *Fsh* .

2. Novel class II genes. In 1985 we described a new class II gene, now called HLA-DNA whose product is now thought, by analogy with the mouse, to partner the product of HLA-DOB. The equivalent mouse genes, Oa and Ob, have been shown to have an interesting tissue distribution and are found on different thymus medullary cells to those expressing canonical Ia molecules, I-A and I-E [Karlsson et al., Immunol. Today 13, 469]. We were surprised two years ago to find yet another cryptic MHC class II molecule in the MHC, this time with some unique features, which were also observed in the equivalent mouse genes. The putative DM molecule is only distantly related to the other major class II loci and probably split off at around the time that class I and II diverged. DM genes are expressed in similar tissues to those expressing other class II sequences. We speculate that DM,

like CD1 or M (mta) region genes in the mouse, is dedicated to presenting particular antigens from pathogens.
3. The third group of genes, the TAPs and LMPs, have a function in antigen processing.

Four laboratories uncovered ABC (for ATP-binding cassette) transporter genes (now TAP1 and TAP2), in the class II region of the MHCs of mouse, human and rat, respectively. ABC transporters, or traffic ATPases, are found in a variety of species, from bacteria through fly, yeast and human and their known function is to transport a variety of moieties, which can include anything from small ions to peptides and large proteins such as haemolysin. The transporters generally consist of four domains, two containing multiple transmembrane stretches and two ATP binding cassettes, but can be encoded in a variety of ways. The TAP genes each contain one transmembrane and one ATP cassette domain.

Once they had been identified, the functions of the TAP genes and their products were a major priority in our laboratory. We first gathered compelling data showing that TAP1 and TAP2 products form a heterodimer. This was already likely, by analogy of the TAPs with the structures of other ABC transporter molecules, which all consist of four domains, two hydrophobic and two ATP-binding cassette. In addition, human and mouse mutant cells with a defect in a single TAP gene showed reduced class I at the cell surface, unstable class I/$\beta_2$microglobulin heterodimers internally, as well as the failure to be recognised by antigen-specific, class I restricted CTL. Most convincingly, antibodies to C-terminal peptides from TAP1 co-precipitated both proteins, confirming that they were physically associated.

A peptide transporter of the type envisaged should reside in the ER membrane. To confirm this point, the rabbit antiserum to TAP1 peptide was purified on an affinity column. The antibody revealed perinuclear staining of B cells, consistent with the endoplasmic reticulum (ER), by fluorescence microscopy. Coupling of the affinity purified antibody to gold particles and subsequent electron microscopy of ultrathin cryo-sections also revealed specific staining on the ER membrane, with evidence that the ATP cassette was oriented towards the cytoplasm. Gold particles were also found in the cis-Golgi compartment in these experiments, suggesting either that antigen loading also takes place in this compartment or that TAP gets to the Golgi and then is retrieved to the ER. Class I molecules may be continually circulated via this route.

It seems likely then that the TAP heterodimer is fulfilling the role of peptide transporter of cytoplasmically produced fragments into the lumen of the ER. Indirect evidence for this has come from a number of experiments. For example, minigenes encoding an influenza matrix protein epitope were introduced into mutant (T2, a derivative of ΦX174) cells. Only when the minigene contained an ER translocation signal sequence could the cells be sensitised to lysis by class I restricted CTL. HLA-A2 molecules escape retention in the ER and proceed to the surface in mutant cells lacking the transporter genes. Peptides eluted from these A2 molecules were shown to be derived exclusively from hydrophobic signal sequences, implying that peptides not using the co-translational route to traverse the membrane were excluded. Although these signal sequences were most likely longer than the usual 8-9 amino acids, there is some evidence, from the Rammensee laroratory, that trimming peptides normally takes place. This trimming seems to be dependent on the presence of the class I molecule.

Proteasome genes

A further clue to the workings of the antigen processing machinery also came from studying the class II region of the MHC. Intimately associated with the TAP loci were genes encoding structures related to proteasome subunits. Proteins corresponding to the equivalent mouse genes were described many years ago and were named LMP's, for low-MW polypeptides. The LMP's were initially immuno-precipitated from mouse macrophages with alloantisera and these studies established that the LMP's are components of a complex of some 15 or more subunits. This complex has many similarities with a large cytoplasmic proteolytic complex called the proteasome, an abundant structure in all eukaryotic cells which is evolutionarily highly conserved. It is probably responsible for protein turnover in the cytoplasm. The MHC-encoded LMP genes were obvious candidates for an involvement in producing peptides for transport into the ER.

There has been some recent evidence that the proteasome is not necessary for antigen processing [Arnold et al., Nature 360, 171; Momburg et al., Nature 360, 174]. We have similar unpublished data, which shows that in mutants lacking LMP2 and LMP7 genes (T2 cells transfected with TAP1 and TAP2) class I expression occurs at normal levels and some endogenous 'minor' self antigens are presented to appropriate T cells. Several explanations of the data have been suggested, including:
1. Expression of the LMP genes exerts a quantitative effect on antigen processing which is difficult to detect with a T cell readout.
2. The LMP products influence the range of peptides provided for transport in a subtle way.
3. Other proteasome subunits can substitute for LMP2 and LMP7.
4. The proteasome is not the only cytoplasmic protease that is used for antigen processing.

The complexity of the proteasome structure makes analysis of its potential role in antigen processing difficult to assess. It can exist in a number of different complexes in the cell (20S and 26S particles are the major forms and there are probably subtypes of these). There is additional complexity at the level of each individual subunit: our studies showed that the LMP7 gene product was made as a precursor protein with an extension of about 50 amino acids on its N terminus which was cleaved off after synthesis. The leader peptide could be specified by two different alternative sequences, downstream of two promoters, at the start of the LMP7 gene. Thus, although the existence of the MHC-encoded proteasome genes has provided some valuable leads to the possible mechanism of antigen processing, they have yet to be definitively implicated in the process. A convincing *in vitro* assay for protease cleavage, using proteasomes purified from different mutant cells, is essential in order to obtain evidence for their involvement.

Gene sequences

Having identified the TAP and LMP cDNA clones, we were naturally interested in their genomic organisation and sequence. Our team has collaborated with the DNA sequencing laboratory at the ICRF in these experiments. Appropriate M13 libraries were supplied to Stephan Beck's laboratory to perform complete genomic sequencing. Analysis of the sequences showed that the two TAP genes probably arose from a duplication since they have a similar exon-intron organisation. LMP2 and TAP1 start sites are separated by only ~500bp and so may share control elements, which include an ISRE, presumably involved in the transcriptional response to interferon. The LMP genes also show a similar exon/intron pattern, indicative of duplication of a single primordial gene.

Curiously, another expressed gene, RING9, mapped between the LMP7 and TAP1 genes, overlapping them at its extremities. Transcripts of this gene are differentially spliced and do not contain long open reading frames, suggesting that RING9 is a pseudogene. Another possibility is that it is involved in anti-sense regulation of expression of the genes it overlaps.

Further sequencing around the TAP and LMP genes has revealed large stretches of flanking DNA which so far do not contain any identifiable genes. Part of this material consists of repeat sequences such as Alu and part is single copy DNA.

Polymorphism

The TAP genes in the rat are highly polymorphic, alleles of TAP2 differing by up to 29 amino acids. These extraordinary variations result in differences in the profiles of peptides presented via the RT1.A product in the rodent. This finding may help to explain the location of the TAP genes in the MHC, at least in the rat, since a selective advantage could be provided by linking different TAP alleles in cis with particular class I alleles.

Surveying the degree of variation in these genes revealed a different picture in humans; the TAP1 and 2 alleles differed by only a small number of amino acids and in each case there was one major and a few minor alleles, unlike the kind of distribution seen in class I or class II genes, where there are multiple low-frequency alleles. The combinations of TAP1 and TAP2 alleles with each other were as expected from random association and there was no evidence for strong linkage disequilibrium with class I or class II variants, except in a few haplotypes, such as those containing DR3. In addition, there appeared to be a recombination hotspot between TAP1 and TAP2, not present on all haplotypes. Most likely, rat and human MHCs have evolved along different routes; TAP variation compensating for limited class I variation in rats, whereas large numbers of class I alleles at multiple class I loci may have made TAP1 variation unnecessary in humans. Our preliminary studies of some disease populations and matched controls have similarly provided little evidence for any marked involvement of the TAP genes, unlike some reports from mouse models.

Recent work

The finding of DMA and B, TNFA and B, HSP70, TAP and LMP genes within the MHC supports the tenet that the MHC contains genes with inter-related functions in antigen processing and presentation. Deletion studies by Pious and DeMars have shown that the class II region contains a gene involved in class II presentation, mutation of which affects recognition of DR3 by T cells as well as by a monoclonal antibody, 16.23 [Mellins et al., Nature 343, 71; Malnati et al., Nature 357, 702]. Surface class II molecules are unstable in mutants defective in this gene and instead of containing the usual array of peptides contain a fragment derived from the invariant chain [Riberdy et al., Nature 360, 474]. The responsible genes have now been identified as the DM genes. The DM locus is dramatically different from all of the other class II loci. The first domains of DM, α1 and ß1, share practically no sequence homology with class II. Even the normally highly conserved Ig domains are only 35 % related, at the most, to class II; almost the same level of homology to class I. DM is non-polymorphic. It is possible to model a putative DM peptide-binding groove on the class I coordinates, which we have done in collaboration with Paul Travers. The class II crystal structure has recently been published [Brown et al., Nature 364, 33] and an obvious priority is to model the DM binding domain on the DR coordinates. This may yield some information on the type of peptides that may be accommodated in the DM groove. We have studied sequence variation in DM and find little polymorphism except for a few amino acid differences in the membrane-proximal domains. For example, some class I molecules have particularly well-conserved tyrosine residues lining the pockets, particularly the B or 45 pocket, which receive a conserved arginine at position 2 of the peptide. In the mta gene product, which appears to be specialised in presenting peptides with a formylated methionine at the N-terminus, the pocket is lined with a phenylalanine. So far, peptides appear to be held in an extended linear conformation in class II molecules, protruding from the ends of the groove. The key conserved residues in the sides of the groove contacting the peptide are asparagines.

A number of MHC-associated phenotypes suggest the existence of unidentified genes involved in immune surveillance in other regions of the HLA complex. For example, the M region genes in mice have not been found in humans yet but they are probably class-I related. Other groups have also identified some interesting, polymorphic class I-related genes near the HLA-B locus with potential roles in antigen presentation [T. Spies, P. Pontarotti, personal communications]. Another clue to additional novel MHC genes is the association with certain diseases.

Some autoimmune conditions are undoubtedly influenced by the known class I and class II loci, perhaps by more than one locus linked on the haplotype. Other MHC-associated diseases, such as adrenal hyperplasia and haemochromatosis, are clearly caused by non-immune MHC-linked genes. Other MHC-disease associations hint at interesting genes remaining to be uncovered. For example, in the course of our analysis of the MHC class II region we hope to shed some light on diseases such as narcolepsy. This disease is almost exclusively associated with HLA-DR2 individuals, who have normal DQ and DR sequences. We should be able to establish whether the disease is affected by a class II locus or another linked gene.

One gene that we have not had time to focus on, but which stands out as the only non-immune system gene in the class II region is RING3. In view of the phenotype of the *Drosophila* FSH gene, it is not out of the question that RING3 is involved in an interesting developmental process in humans. The only MHC-linked phenotype in humans with a hint of any similarity with FSH so far is recurrent spontaneous abortion. In mice, there is also the interesting effect of rejection of an H-2-matched foetus which has so far defied explanation. The obvious approach to the function of RING3 is gene knockout in mice by homologous recombination.

Our experience of ten years work on the MHC class II region has entailed piecemeal compilation of bits of sequence from various cosmids; an approach which has involved a considerable investment in time and resources. In collaboration with Stephan Beck, it was decided that a more systematic approach to sequence analysis of the whole region would be cost-effective. At the same time, it would provide one of the first complete large pieces of human genomic sequence of an interesting region, for analysis of features such as gene arrangement, control regions, nucleotide distribution and repeat organization. Genomic sequencing is desirable, as opposed to cDNA sequencing, when the goal is accurate, full length sequence, sampling all genes, not just those expressed at higher levels. The full sequence is invaluable in our search for novel MHC genes and in other aspects of our work: it facilitates construction of fragments for gene knockout experiments, for example. It was agreed that, using M13 libraries from various cosmids supplied by us, Stephan Beck's laboratory would complete the sequencing of the ~800 kb class II region. ~150 kb of sequence has been completed to date, as summarised on the following Table.

MHC class II sequencing

On test runs, the GRAIL gene identification software has proved reliable in locating all or the genes we have identified by other means, except for LMP2 where the exons are smaller than 80bp. There are several sequences identified by GRAIL as genes which have yet to be characterised by other means, including some conserved exons between the DMA and DMB genes. Some of these sequences are puzzling since we can detect no cDNA clones on screening large libraries from a number of tissues.

cosmid	genes	Kbp	status
LC11	DPA and B	26239	completed, entered
U15	LMP/TAP	38899	completed, entered
U10	TAP/DOB	23831	completed, entered
HA14	DMA+B	35447	contiguous
019A		32000	4 contigs
A15		21410	2 contigs
M27B		40000	> 10 contigs

Once a single class II region sequence has been obtained we will compare some different haplotypes for variation, especially over regions such as DQ-DR where there is variation in size and gene number between haplotypes.

The function of the TAP and LMP genes

Is the low level of variation in TAP genes in man of any significance? There have been recent reports of extraordinary variation in HLA-B locus sequences in South American Indians, apparently due to reshuffling of existing sequences by recombination or gene conversion. Strong selection may have been taking place on these small populations in response to changing environmental conditions. Variation in the TAPs may have also taken place in these populations and we are investigating some of the sequences, in collaboration with Peter Parham. Having identified polymorphism of the human TAP genes we were naturally interested in seeing if this leads to any differences in function to the alleles. As a first approach, we aim to compare T cell stimulation with the 36.1 mutant cell line transfected with different TAP2 alleles. It is also necessary to cotransfect the appropriate class I allele, which include HLA-A68, HLA-B27, H-2 Db, (CTL's from Alain Townsend, Oxford), HLA-A1 restricted EBV specific T cells (Alan Rickinson, Birmingham) and two minor HLA-A restricted self antigens, HA1 and HA2, (Els Goulmy, Leiden). The second step will be to purify class I molecules from transfected cells differing only at the TAP locus (transfectants may again be best for this) and evolution of peptides for sequencing.

Although it remains the best candidate for a cytoplasmic protease complex involved in making peptides, the role of the proteasome in antigen processing has not been convincingly established. Several groups have shown that cells lacking LMP2 and LMP7 genes express class I at the cell surface at near normal levels and are capable of presenting peptides to class I restricted T cells against minor antigens. Similarly, in LMP knockout mice, class I functions are apparently almost normal, with a hint of a reduction in defences against flu infection [Tonegawa, personal communication].

These experiments have to be viewed with circumspection since there are other examples of knockout experiments with minimal phenotype, usually explained by compensation by another gene. If additional proteasome subunits are compensating for the LMP genes, then these genes may be related to the loci that have been removed.

We have explored this possibility by screening cDNA libraries with LMP2 and LMP7 probes under non-stringent conditions and in this way have cloned sequences related to both genes. The sequence most like LMP2 has already been described as the δ subunit and the sequence most like LMP7 is similar to protein sequence of a subunit called ε. Preliminary studies indicate that expression of these new proteasome subunits is downregulated by IFN. We are in the process of mapping them to a human chromosome. Antisera will be prepared to these novel ß subunits and these will be used in immunoprecipitation/Western blotting experiments to see if the presence of LMP7 and of the related subunit are mutually exclusive on proteasomes. Another goal is to remove these new genes from B cell lines by homologous recombination, or by anti-sense expression, to try to establish a role for the proteasome in antigen processing.

An alternative approach is suggested by a recent paper which identifies a yeast proteasome subunit, PRE2, closely related to LMP7 [Heinemeyer et al., J. Biol. Chem. 268, 5115]. Our novel LMP7-related gene is closer in sequence to the yeast gene than is LMP7, consistent with the notion that LMP7 is an alternative form of a constitutive gene. Inactivation of PRE2 results in accumulation of ubiquitinated proteins, enhanced sensitivity to stress and loss of chymotryptic activity of the proteasomes. It may be instructive to attempt to reconstitute the yeast cells with the different human cDNAs (LMP7 as RING10 or Y2, and the new LMP7-related sequence) and then assay any differences in phenotype.

Promoter analysis (Fig. 1 & 2)

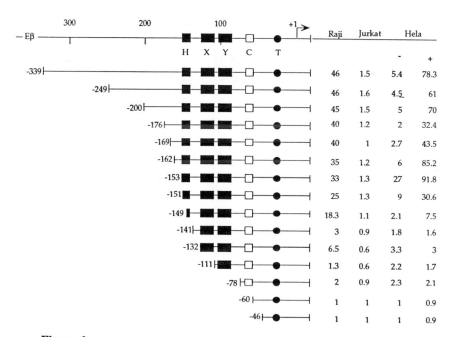

Figure 1

The best evidence for the involvement of proteasomes in antigen processing comes from assays of cleavage of substituted peptides with purified material. Cleavage takes place more after hydrophobic residues when LMP2 and 7 are present, in line with the fact that hydrophobic residues tend to be favoured at the C-terminal anchors of class I bound peptides [Goldberg, unpublished]. Gene knockout or antisense experiments may be the best approach to use here, followed by examination of substrate specificity, class I epitopes (detected with peptide-specific antibodies), or peptide occupancy of class I grooves in cells lacking one or other subunit. More evidence of proteasome involvement may be obtained by creating dominant negative mutations in the proteasome components. Some tissues other than B cells lines only express LMP2 or LMP7 after interferon induction, Hela for example, and these would be suitable recipients for transfection of individual LMP genes to monitor the effect of proteasome subunits on processing. The proteasomes lacking LMP2 or LMP7 are being examined structurally, in conjunction with LMP2 and LMP7 antisera, by electron microscopy in Richard Newman's laboratory.

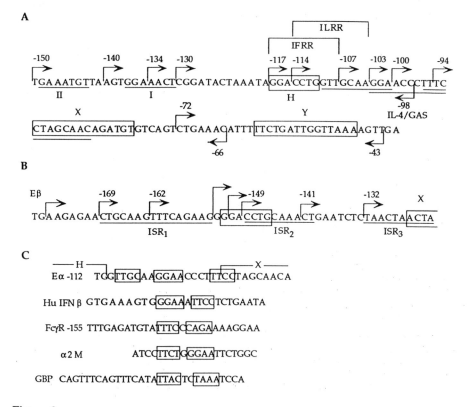

Figure 2

A: The proximal promoter area of the Eα gene. Arrows show the deletion end points. The conserved motifs are boxed. The H, X and Y boxes bind constitutive factors. In addition, an IFNγ inducible factor binds to the H box. The underlined regions I and II resemble virus / ISRE like elements. Region I is an IRF binding site and corresponds to activation by IRF. An IL-4 inducible factor binds in the area shown by bold underlines that is homologous to various GAS like sites. The boundaries for IFNγ (IFRR) and IL-4 (ILRR) response are shown by brackets. Elimination of the IFRR coincides with loss of most of the B lymphoid activity of the promoter.

B: The organization of the Eß regulatory region. The IFN elements IRS1, 2, 3, are underlined.

C: GAS like homologies in various elements. Note the divergent orientation of the half sites.

Emphasis during this program was placed on the functional characterization of several DNA elements that determine B cell and cytokine regulation of MHC class II genes. These studies included the mouse Eα and Eß and the human DRα and more recently DM genes. By cloning corresponding areas of genes in front of suitable reporter plasmids, and using CAT assays and RNA blots, we have determined that the similarity in regulation between human and mouse genes resides mostly in their promoter areas, where all share conserved regulatory elements known as H, X, and Y boxes. The promoter area comprising these boxes is necessary and sufficient for proper regulation and expression of class II genes. However, deletion and point mutations have shown that either conserved motif in isolation, even when multimerised, is unable to confer regulated expression on surrogate promoters. These studies indicate that the class II gene promoters are complex, and require the synergistic collaboration of multiple regulatory elements for their proper regulation. Interestingly, elements and regions involved in B cell expression are also required for cytokine induction, with some exceptions that will be discussed below.

Site directed, point and 5' deletion mutants in the critical Eß regulatory region show that the H box area is mostly involved in B cell specific expression of this gene. The same results have been obtained recently with the Eα promoter. In the Eß, sequences both 5' and 3' of the H box are required for IFNγ induction. Thus, we have defined novel elements, designated Interferon stimulated region 1, 2, and 3 (lSR1, 2, and 3) that are also recognized by IFN inducible factors (see below) and show similarities to other IFN regulated elements. ISR1 is located between -162 and -153. lSR2 is located between -151 and -141 and overlaps with the 3' part of the H box. In the Eα, the contribution of sequences 5' of the H box is minor in comparison to the Eß promoter, as studied by 5' deletions. This region in Eα(-150 to -130) carries some homologies to the ISRE/VRE and one of those is a putative IRF binding site. In agreement with this, expression of IRF by transfection, increases CAT activity in the presence but not in the absence of the type I VRE site in the promoter context. The H box of Eα, which seems to be functionally related to the ISRs of Eß, is of major importance for INFγ response. As in view of this and of results showing that the combined H and X boxes of Eß respond better than the corresponding region of Eα, it is assumed that i) sequences either 5' or 3' of the H+X are also important for full IFN response and IRF may be one of the contributing mediators; ii) in spite of obvious similarities, the H boxes of Eα and Eß perform distinct functions. In the case of the Eß gene, mutations on the Y box have small effect on IFNγ inducibility, whereas in the Eα, inclusion of the Y box increases response of heterologous promoters substantially, and its elimination in the context of the Eα promoter is deleterious. This difference may be due to the presence of an additional CAT box further downstream in the Eß promoter.

We have studied in parallel the regulation of the Eα by IL-4 and shown that a region including X and Y is also important for this type of regulation in B lymphoid cells. These studies indicate that in addition to the above the region between H and X (-114 to -103) is required. This is the first instance to our knowledge of two regulatory regions in the class II genes showing clear topological distinction. Interestingly, the region required for IL-4 response (ILRR), shows important similarities to a subfamily of IFNγ activated sequences (GAS).

Taken together, these results show that in addition to the common X and Y elements, different class II genes have or use different elements for regulation, which is in agreement with other observations pointing to the role of distinct elements such as the octa (DRα) and the X2 (Aα and DRα). More specifically, we have shown that the H box seems to be involved in B lymphoid expression for both the Eα and Eß genes and in IFNγ regulation for the Eα only. Conversely, IFNγ response in Eß is mediated by the strong ISR1 and weak ISR0 sequences located upstream and downstream of the H box respectively. Finally, we have defined another region, ILRR, involved in IL-4 response, situated 3' of the H box of Eα. These results provide a more integrated view of the functional anatomy of class II promoters and set the basis for further studies on regulation.

To obtain more information on class II gene regulation, we have extended our studies to include the DMα and DMβ genes, provided by Dr. J. Trowsdale. These genes have interesting characteristics in antigen presentation. We have subcloned the promoter area of these genes immediately 3' of the initiation ATG and extending 1.9 and 3 Kb for the DMα and DMβ respectively. We have then constructed reporter fusions. To delimit their functionally important regions, we are currently carrying out transfection assays.

Signal transduction and gene regulation

Inhibitor studies

We have studied the effect of various kinase and phosphatase inhibitors on class II expression. In human Hela cells, staurosporin at concentrations that affect several kinases inhibits IFNγ response as evaluated by both CAT and RNA analysis. The same effect was observed by genistein, an inhibitor of tyrosine kinases. Theophyline (calcium/calmodulin kinase inhibitor) reduces induction levels to about 60% of the control whereas other substances such as inhibitors of PKC (sphingosine) or G proteins (mevalonate) were inactive. In contrast, sphingosine was active in suppressing both IL-4 and IFNγ response in mouse cells. The serine type phosphatase inhibitor okadaic acid was inactive, but the tyrosine phosphatase inhibitor vanadate was a potent inhibitor of the IFNγ but not IL-4 response. Staurosporine also strongly inhibited IL-4 response in mouse cells. This indicates that various regulatory kinases are involved in class II induction exhibiting cell type and or cytokine specific preferences. In addition, IFNγ response is regulated by both tyrosine phosphatases and kinases. Interestingly, genistein and vanadate also inhibit IFN induction of the STAT 91 and subsequent transcriptional activation of GAS elements. These results are in line with biochemical data that show inactivation of cytokine-induced, DNA-binding regulatoty factors (see below) and may help to link initial transduction events with end promoter effects.

Another aspect of this line of work has been the study of cytokine induced differentiation of the human myeloid leukemia HL60. We have shown that in addition to other known inducers such as IFNγ, IL-4 is able to induce differentiation in HL60 cells. This is accompanied by induction of class II expression which is regulated by distinct mechanisms: calcium/calmodulin kinase inhibitors suppress IFN-γ response, whereas IL4 response is abolished by G protein antagonists. Differentiation induced by TNF-α, which is accompanied by the induction of NFkB (both at the RNA and posttranslational levels), does not permit expression of class II genes. These data indicate that alternative pathways can be used for differentiation and that class II expression does not always accompany this process.

Cognate nuclear factors (Fig. 3)

We have defined various nuclear factors that bind to the elements described above using electrophoretic mobility shift, competition and methylation interference assays. Some of these are expressed constitutively in many cell types regardless of their classs II phenotype, whereas others are expressed either in B cells or are activated by cytokines.

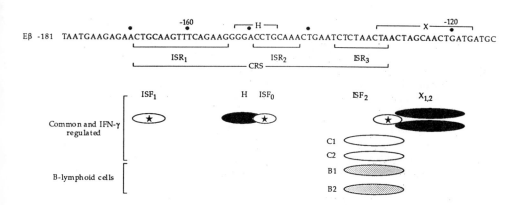

Figure 3

1. Common factors: The H, X, and Y elements bind to ubiquitous factors as they have been observed by many groups. In addition, we have described factors that bind in the IRS3 of Eß, immediately 5' of the X box and in the region 5' of the H box of Eα.

2. Lymphoid factors: Two such factors bind in the IRS3, one present in B and the other both in B and T cells.

3. Inducible factors: Three IFN inducible factors (ISF1, 0, and 2) bind in the IRS1, IRS2, and IRS3 of the Eß promoter and are involved in IFNγ control. Another factor which is constitutively expressed in B cells, binds in the H box of Eα following IFNγ treatment (ISFH). Competition analysis indicated that those factors are related to each other as well as to factors that bind to other IFN regulated elements such as ISRE and the GAS of the GBP gene. UV cross-linking experiments show that the ISFH has MW similar to the STAT 91 protein which is involved in activation of the GAS element. Anti-phosphotyrosine antibodies and phosphatase treatment show that ISFH is tyrosine phosphorylated in residue(s) critical for binding. We are currently investigating the possibility that ISFH is immunologically related to STAT91 by using antibodies. Furthermore we are using vectors expressing wt or mutant forms of the JAK2 and STAT 91 proteins to access their importance in IFNγ mediated expression.

Another line of work, yet to be exploited, is the detection of a retinoic acid inducible factor in embryonic stem cells that binds at around -130 bp of the Eα promoter. Antibodies against the Drosophila steroid receptor, like factor CF-1, inactivate the binding of this factor.

Similar analysis has led to the identification of IL-4 activated factors in the ILRR of the Eα. In spite of extensive information on various effects of IL-4 on its cellular targets, little is known about the underlying molecular events. MHC class II genes are induced transcriptionally by IL-4 and provide an interesting system to address this problem. We have determined the critical area in the proximal promoter region of the Eα class II gene that is required for IL-4 regulalion. This is composed of the X and Y class II motifs as well as of sequences extending to -114. We have identified a novel factor (NFIL-4) which is activated upon treatment of B and T lymphoid lines (as well as B and T spleen cells) by IL-4 and binds to the ILRR at a site that resembles the core consensus of the IFNγ activation sequence (GAS). Binding and competition assays demonstrated that similar IL-4 inducible complexes bind to an INFNß promoter site overlapping the PRDII/NFkB element as well as to the Interferon-γ response element of the Fcγ receptor (GRR) and the acute phase response element (APRE) of the a 2 macroglobulin promoters. Interestingly, competition assays indicate that NFIL-4 sites define a group of cytokine response sites distinct than the prototype GBP /GAS or the ISRs of Eß.

Using antibodies and shift assays we have shown that this factor is immunologically unrelated to NFkB or STAT91 proteins that also recognize the above element following activation by their proper inducers. Activation of NFIL4 occurs rapidly (within 5 min) in the absence of protein synthesis, from an inactive cytoplasmic pool. Removal of IL-4 leads to fast inactivation of the factor, a process that is partly inhibited by vanadate, a tyrosine phosphatase inhibitor. The importance of phosphorylation is further demonstrated by abolition of binding by the kinase inhibitor staurosporine, and either tyrosine phosphatase or anti-phosphotyrosine antibody. UV cross-linking experiments indicate that a protein species of about 45 kDa is in direct contact with the DNA, a situation that is reminiscent of the GRR where a 45 kDa seems to participate along with the STAT91 in the complex formed following IFNγ. Methylation interference shows protection of guanine residues contained in the region homologous to the pseudodyad symmetry of the GAS i.e. TTCCNNNAA. Inspection of the sequences under study allows the classification of these elements into two groups in relation to the orientation of the half site, i.e. 5' GGAA--TTCC 3' or 5' TTCC--GGAA 3'. The GAS of GBP and some other genes, as well as PRDII fall into the former category whereas GRR and APRE into the latter category. In the Eα-ILRR we have noted the presence of two neighbour sites that belong to the former category although the two central half sites may be combined to form a site of the former class. Since differential response to cytokines and lack of cross competition between some GAS member sites has been demonstrated, this observation may have important functional implications. Because of its quick activation by tyrosine kinase(s) and binding similarities to the STAT proteins, we suggest that NFIL-4 represents an antigenically divergent member of this family regulated by distinct kinase(s). These characteristics place NFIL-4 in the category of transducers, targeted to diverse promoters which are regulated by multiple cytokines and may help to elucidate the IL-4 pathway and its functional interrelation to other signalling pathways.

In order to clone regulatory factors of the H box region, we have developed a one - hybrid yeast system using Eα elements that will be able to drive a minimal promoter when the cognate transactivators become available by co-transformation with a Hela cDNA library fused to the activation domain of VP16. This system is now complete for the genetic selection.

Suppression of class II expression by adenovirus oncogenes (Fig. 4 & 5)

Earlier observations have shown that adenovirus infection and/or transformation had profound effects in cellular functions. The activity of various cellular genes was altered following adenoviral gene expression. MHC gene expression is also deregulated depending on the virus strain and the host cell type combination. Suppression of MHC class I or II gene expression that will lead to inability for proper antigen presentation, is of major importance in determining the fate of virally infected cells and immune control of tranformed cells. Past studies have established that the major mediator in adenoviral infection is the oncoprotein E1A which by itself can stimulate or suppress gene expression. Mutational analysis demonstrated that suppression and activation reside in distinct regions of the molecule, namely the conserved region I and II are responsible for suppression and the conserved region III for activation. Although

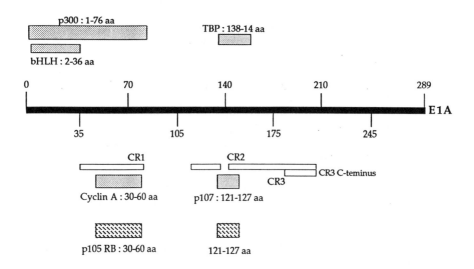

Figure 4

Map of the E1A protein, showing the conserved regions and their overlap with deletion boundaries shown to be neccesary for interaction with celular proteins. Missing amino acids in mutants are: CR1: 38-65, CR2: 125-133, CR3: 140-185. Mutant proteins are expressed under the control of the LTR of RSV.

activation by E1A is better understood and involves the interaction between the CRIII and components of the transcription machinery such as the TBP and or upstream activator factors, much less is known about the molecular basis of suppression. Such understanding is important towards the development of strategies for reversing the effects of E1A. We have been using transient transfection assays, andshown that E1A is able to suppress class II promoters. This effect is mediated by the CRI domain and affects all aspects of class II regulation, namely B lymphoid expression, IFNγ and IL-4 response. Blocking of the IFN pathways has been shown before for ISREs and attributed to the inactivation of the IFN inducible, cognate factor involved, i.e. ISGF3. We have extended these data to demonstrate that the core GAS of GBP, that is presumably regulated solely by STAT91, is also blocked. This is accompanied by inability to induce STAT91 binding. This effect is also observed with the IFNγ factor that bind to the GRR element. Our analysis further demonstrates that not only cytokine response but also the constitutive expression of the class II regulatory region is blocked by E1A. This results indicate that a common key regulatory mechanism such as proper function of the X or Y factors, is affected by E1A. Alternatively different regulatory steps may be affected. In an initial attempt to study the molecular basis of this effect, we have used various promoter constructs and demonstrated that the proximal regulatory region of class II genes is itself the target for suppression. Further delimitation of the element involved was not feasible due to the combinatorial nature of the promoter, that requires the presence of an array of elements for proper regulation. However we have determine that the cytokine inducible factor NFIL-4, is also inactivated following adenovirus infection in a manner similar to the effect of E1A on ISGF3 and STAT91. Since the H box associated, B lymphoid function in Eα can be distinguished from the ILRR, it is reasonable to conclude that, at least in this case, the effect of E1A on basal promoter activity is distinct from its effect on IL-4 response. To better establish the role of E1A in this blockade (indicated initially by transient transfection) we have tried to isolate stably transformed Hela cells, expressing high levels of E1A, but without success. We finally managed to isolate clones from similarly tranfected COS monkey cells which we currently analyse. Inactivation of the cytokine induced factors by E1A may be due to a) direct physical association and sequestration b) inactivation of upstream regulatory events such as kinase activation and transduction or c) activation or inactivation by E1A of another putative gene that is involved in the cascade. In all these cases the role of the CRI domain is implicit. To test these possibilities we have developed the following systems:

1. To study direct interaction of the E1A with cellular proteins we have developed a bacterial expression system that allows both pseudo-affinity purification (Histidine modified protein) and in vitro labeling of the protein by γ-ATP (HMK modified) and we soon expect to carry out mixing experiments and shift assays.

2. The kinase and factor activation steps will be studied by standard procedures using antibodies and western blots.

3. The possibility of sequestration by the CRI will also be independently studied by the yeast two hybrid system using LexA-E1A (or E1A mutants) fusions. The preparatory work necessary for the yeast two hybrid screening have been completed.

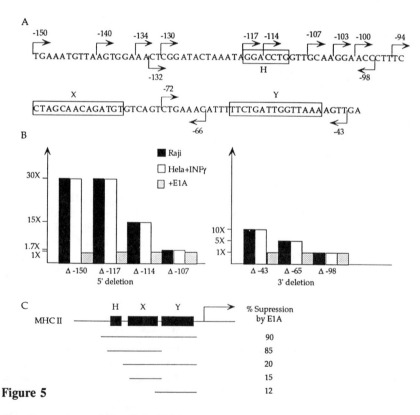

Figure 5

Class II promoters and the effect of E1A.

A: The proximal regulatory region of the Eα promoter showing some of the succesive deletions used and the limits of the conserved motifs H, X and Y.

B: The effect of E1A on various constructs transfected in Raji B lymphoid and in Hela cells with or without IFNγ.

C: Summary of the supression mediated by E1A to different combinations of regulatory class II elements. The activity in the presence of the vector alone or the CR1 mutant is 100 %.

THE CLASS III REGION

Evidence for a new gene between the G7a and G7 genes

A 10 kb genomic DNA fragment separating the G7a and G7 genes (Fig. 6) was used in zoo blot analysis and was found to be conserved between species. Exon trapping analysis of part of this region has resulted in the isolation of two discrete exons that have been shown to correspond to part of the conserved sequences identified by zoo blot analysis. The presence of these exons indicate the location of a previously undescribed gene that we have labelled G7c. Translation of the DNA sequences of the exons in three phases has revealed the presence of two potential open reading frames. The nucleotide sequences of the exons, and the translated protein sequences, do not show homology with any other known sequences in the databases. Screening of cDNA libraries by PCR, and RT-PCR analysis of RNA samples derived from a variety of cell lines, using oligo-nucleotide primers that hybridise to the trapped exons, has subsequently indicated that G7c is expressed in cultured B lymphocyte cell lines. An 8.8 kb genomic probe corresponding to the G7c gene has been used to screen a B lymphoblastoid cell line cDNA library and 7 duplicating positive clones have been detected. These have been rescreened and a clone with a 1.3 kb cDNA insert has been isolated. This clone has been sequenced though the DNA or derived amino acid sequences have so far failed to reveal homologies with other known sequences.

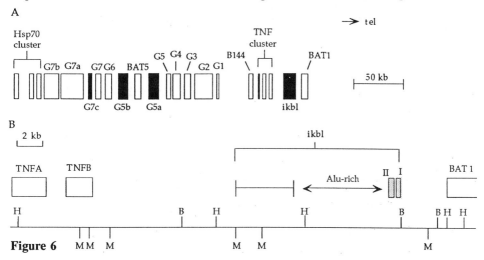

Figure 6

A: Molecular map of the MHC class III region between the BAT1 and HSP70 genes indicating the location of new genes (black boxes) defined in this study.

B: An expanded view of the BAT1/TNF region showing a restriction map of the cosmid TN62, containing the ikbl gene. The open boxes indicate the boundaries of genes. The double-headed arrow indicated the large intron containing the 13 Alu repeats demonstrated by Iris et al. The filled boxes represent the positions of the first exons of ikbl, while the limits of the remainder of the ikbl gene are indicated centromeric of the Alu-rich region by a bar. Sites are shown for the restriction enzymes HindIII (H), BamHI (M) and BglII (B).

Evidence for a new gene between BAT1 and the TNF cluster

A 25 kb region between BAT1 and TNFB was isolated from the cosmid TN62, in the form of 3 contiguous BamHI fragments of 13.6 kb, 2.1 kb and 9.4 kb in size (Fig. 6). Each of these fragments was used to probe a "zoo blot" of genomic DNA from human, sheep, rabbit and shark. The 13.6 kb and 2.1 kb probes hybridised to specific bands in the sheep and rabbit tracks, indicating cross-species conservation of sequence within these fragments, and constituting evidence for the presence of a novel gene within this region.

Northern blot analysis using the BamHI fragments as probes revealed faint signals in total RNA from the cell lines U937 and HepG2, corresponding to a mRNA of ~1.6 kb.

```
CCGAGCTTCTTAAACACAGGCCTTGGGCTACGGCTCTGGGGGTACTTGGGGGGGCGGGGG        60
CAGGTCTGATGAGTAACCCCTCCCCCCAGGTTCCAGAGGAAGAAGCCTCCACATCTGTCT       120
         M  S  N  P  S  P  Q  V  P  E  E  E  A  S  T  S  V        17

GCCGGCCCAAGAGTTCCATGGCCTCCACTTCCCGCCGCCAACGCCGAGAACGTCGCTTTC       180
 C  R  P  K  S  S  M  A  S  T  S  R  R  Q  R  R  E  R  R  F       37

TCCGTCGTTACTTGTCTGCAGGACGGCTGGGGGCCCAGGCCCTCCTCCAGCGACACCCAG       240
 R  R  Y  L  S  A  G  R  L  V  R  A  Q  A  L  L  Q  R  H  P       57

GCCTCGATGTAGATGCTGGGCAGCCCCCACCACTGCACCGGGCCTGTGCCCGCCACGATG       300
 G  L  D  V  D  A  G  Q  P  P  P  L  H  R  A  C  A  R  H  D       77

CCCCTGCCCTGTGCCTGCTGCTTCGGCTCGGGGCTGACCCTGCCCACCAGGACCGCCATG       360
 A  P  A  L  C  L  L  L  R  L  G  A  D  P  A  H  Q  D  R  H       97

GGGACACGGCACTGCATGCTGCTGCCCGCCAGGGCCCAGATGCCTACACCGATTTCTTCC       420
 G  D  T  A  L  H  A  A  A  R  Q  G  P  D  A  Y  T  D  F  F      117

TCCCGCTGCTAAGCCGCTGTCCCTCTGCCATGGGAATAAAGAATAAGGATGGGGAGACCC       480
 L  P  L  L  S  R  C  P  S  A  M  G  I  K  N  K  D  G  E  T      137

CTGGCCAAATTTTGGGCTGGGGACCCCCCTGGGATTCTGCTGAAGAGGAGGAAGAAGATG       540
 P  G  Q  I  L  G  W  G  P  P  W  D  S  A  E  E  E  E  E  D      157

ATGCCTCCAAGGAGCGGGAATGGAGACAGAAGCTCCAGGGTGAGCTGGAGGACGAGTGGC       600
 D  A  S  K  E  R  W  R  Q  K  L  Q  G  E  L  E  D  E  W       177

AGGAAGTCATGGGGAGGTTTGAAGGTGATGCCTCCCATGAAACCCAGGAACCTGAGTCCT       660
 Q  E  V  M  G  R  F  E  G  D  A  S  H  E  T  Q  E  P  E  S      197

TCTCAGCCTGGTCAGATCGCCTGGCCCGGGAACATGCCCAGAAGTGCCAGCAGCAGCAGC       720
 F  S  A  W  S  D  R  L  A  R  E  H  A  Q  K  C  Q  Q  Q  Q      217

GAGAAGCAGAGGGATCCTGTCGACCCCCACGTGCTGAGGGCTCCAGCCAGAGCTGGCGAC       780
 R  E  A  E  G  S  C  R  P  P  R  A  E  G  S  S  Q  S  W  R      237

ACGAGGAGGAGGAGCAGCGGCTCTTCAGGGAGCGAGCCCGGGCCAAGGAGGAAGAGCTGC       840
 H  E  E  E  Q  R  L  F  R  E  R  A  R  A  K  E  E  E  L       257

GTGAGAGCCGAGCCAGGAGGGCGCAGGAGGCTCTAGGGGACCGAGAACCCAAGCCAACCA       900
 R  E  S  R  A  R  R  A  Q  E  A  L  G  D  R  E  P  K  P  T      277

GGGCCGGGCCCAGGGAAGAGCACCCCAGAGGAGCGGGGAGGGGCAGCCTCTGGCGATTTG       960
 R  A  G  P  R  E  E  H  P  R  G  A  G  R  G  S  L  W  R  F      297

GTGATGTGCCCTGGCCCTGCCCTGGGGGAGGGGACCCAGAGGCCATGGCTGCAGCCCTGG      1020
 G  D  V  P  W  P  C  P  G  G  G  D  P  E  A  M  A  A  A  L      317

TGGCCAGGGGCCCCCCCTTTGGAGGAACAGGGGGCTCTGAGGAGGTACTTGAGGGTCCAGC      1080
 V  A  R  G  P  L  E  E  Q  G  A  L  R  R  Y  L  R  V  Q       337

AGGTCCGCTGGCACCCTGACCGCTTCCTGCAGCGATTCCGAAGCCAGATTGAGACCTGGG      1140
 Q  V  R  W  H  P  D  R  F  L  Q  R  F  R  S  Q  I  E  T  W      357

AGCTGGGCCGTGTGATGGGAGCAGTGACAGCCCTTTCTCAGGCCCTGAATCGCCATGCAG      1200
 E  L  G  R  V  M  G  A  V  T  A  L  S  Q  A  L  N  R  H  A      377

AGGCCCTCAAGTGACCCTAGGGAAGAAGCAAGAAACTTCGGGGCTGCAGCCTCAGGATGA      1260
 E  A  L  K  *                                                   381

GGCAGAAGGAAGGGTAAGGGAAAGGATGGGGACCACAAGGAAGAGCCAGGTGCTGCTCAG      1320
CAGAGGATATGGGTGGGAGCGAAAGTTGTAACAAGTGGGGGTGGGGGGTGCGGGCCGCCA      1380
CCACTGCTCCTTGACTCTGCCGTTTCCTAATAAGACCTGGTTCCACATCTCAAAAAAAAA      1440
AAAAAAAAAAAAAAAAAAAA                                            1459
```

Figure 7

The nucleotide and predicted amino acid sequences of ikbl. (These sequences have been deposited in the EMBL, GenBank and DDJB databases under the accession number X77909). The putative translation initiation site ATG, and the polyadenylation signal are underlined in the DNA sequence. Potential casein kinase II phosphorylation sites are underlined in the amino acid sequence and potential protein kinase C phosphorylation sites are overlined. The first ANK repeat is located between amino acids 60 and 92; the second between amino acids 93 and 123; and the incomplete repeat between amino acids 124 and 150. The acidic region is located between amino acids 152 and 164, and the leucine-rich heptad repeat between amino acids 359 and 381.

Isolation and characterisation of cDNA clones for the novel gene

A premonocytic leukaemic cell line (U937) cDNA library was screened using the 2.1 kb BamHI genomic fragment as a probe. Three overlapping cDNA clones were isolated with inserts of 600 bp, 1350 bp, and 1500 bp (designated 1U1, 1U2, and 3U1, respectively). The three clones were restriction mapped to determine the extent of overlap and it was found that the 1U1 and 1U2 cDNA inserts were completely contained within the 3U1 cDNA insert. The insert from the 3U1 cDNA clone was used to probe a Northern blot of total and poly (A) + RNA from a variety of cell lines. In all cell lines examined this probe hybridised to a single band of ~1.6 kb in size, in addition to a second band comigrating with the 28S RNA. Comparison of the relative intensity of the two bands between total and poly (A) + RNA revealed a substantial decrease in the intensity of the upper band in the poly (A) + lanes, indicating that this upper band was a result of cross-hybridisation with the 28S RNA. Since clone 3U1 contains an insert that is very similar in size to the mRNA as estimated by Northern analysis, it was selected for sequencing.

The complete sequence of the 3U1 cDNA insert was determined on both strands, with a degeneracy of 5.78, revealing it to be 1459 bp in length (Fig. 7). An unusual polyadenylation signal (AATAAG) 17 nucleotides upstream of a short (28 bp) poly (A) + tail defined the 3' end of the cDNA. Assuming that the mRNA contains an average length poly (A) + tail (~150 bp) this would indicate that the 3U1 cDNA is near full length.

The longest open reading frame, of 1143 bp, is initiated by the ATG start codon closest to the 5' end of the cDNA sequence at nucleotide 69 and terminates at the stop codon (TGA) at nucleotide 1212. Although there is no in-frame stop codon upstream of the ATG codon in the 3U1 cDNA sequence, an in-frame stop codon is found 162 bases upstream of this candidate ATG, according to the genomic sequence.

The derived amino acid sequence of ikbl

The predicted protein encoded by the 3U1 cDNA is 381 amino acids in length (Fig. 7), with an Mw of 43214. The hydropathy profile of the polypeptide demonstrates that it is notably hydrophilic, and does not contain hydrophobic domains that would indicate the presence of a signal peptide or potential transmembrane regions. There is a very basic domain near the N-terminus of the protein (amino acids 29-39) of unknown functional significance. A motifs search performed on the predicted amino acid sequence of the cDNA revealed the presence of two potential casein kinase II and five potential kinase C phosphorylation sites (Fig. 7).

The predicted amino acid sequence was screened against the NBRF and SwissProt protein databases to search for similarities with known protein sequences. This search revealed the presence of two full and one partial copies of a 33 amino acid repeat known as the ANK repeat (also ankyrin repeat, cell cycle repeat, Notch repeat and CDC10/SW16 repeat) between amino acids 60 and 151 (Fig. 8B). The greatest sequence identity of the ANK repeats was the IκB family of proteins and particularly those of the p100 NFκB variant (also lyt10; 14). The first and second full ANK repeats of ikbl closely resemble the second and third repeats of the IκB family, and together are 44% identical and 58% similar to these repeats in NFκBp100. Immediately following these two well conserved repeats is a third repeat that corresponds poorly to the consensus sequence (Fig. 8A & 8B), and a short region rich in acidic amino acid (9 glutamic and aspartic acids over a 13 residue stretch between residues 152 and 164). This pattern of several ANK repeats followed by a poorly fitting incomplete repeat and an adjacent acidic domain is highly redolent of the IκB family with the exception of Bcl3 which lacks the acidic region (Fig 9).

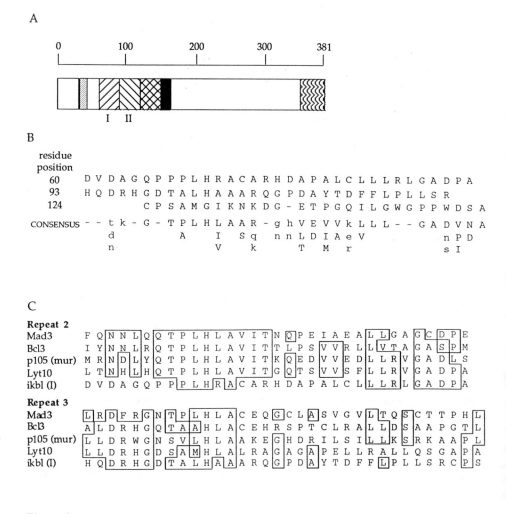

Figure 8

Analysis of the ANK repeat regions encoded by ikbl.

A: Schematic representation of the predicted protein structure of ikbl. The two full ANK repeats are indicated by diagonal lines, and the third incomplete repeat by the hatched area. Roman numerals indicate the order of the repeats. The acidic region is indicated by the black box, the short basic region by the dotted area and the putative leucine zipper by the wavy lines.

B: Alignment of the tree ANK repeats present in ikbl. A consensus sequence for all ANK repeats is indicated below (adapted from 13). The lower case letters represent frequently occuring amino acids, and the upper case letters represent core elements of the repeat.

C: Alignment of the complexe ANK repeats of ikbl with other members of the IκB family. Residues that are conserved in at least three members of the family are boxed. Repeat numbers refer to the order of the repeats in IκBα. The first repeat of ikbl is aligned with the second repeat of the members of the IκB family, and the second repeat of ikbl with the third repeat of the other family members.

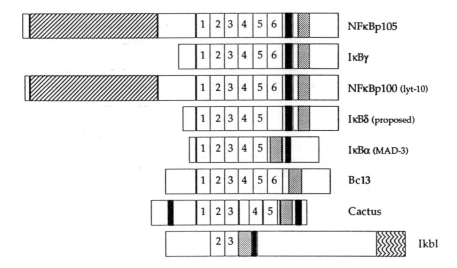

Figure 9

The IκB family of proteins. The proteins are aligned by their ANK repeats, with conserved repeats indicated by numerals. Incomplete repeats are indicated by dotted boxes, acidic regions by black boxes, the rel homology domains of NFκBp105 and p100 by hatched boxes, and the putative leucine zipper of ikbl by the wavy lines. The sizes of these molecules are not to scale.

Multiple alignments of the three ANK repeats of ikbl with the individual repeats of the IκB proteins IκBα (MAD3), NFκBp105, NFκBp100 and Bc13 by the AMPS program, revealed that the first and second ANK repeats of ikbl are most similar to the second and third repeats of NFκBp100 (ALIGN scores of 6.40 and 4.78 SD units respectively Fig. 8C) and that the third incomplete repeat of ikbl is most similar to the fourth repeat of NFκBp100 (ALIGN score 2.35 SD units as compared to 1.97 for the next most significant score) and probably represents a degenerated form of this repeat. In a similar manner, the final incomplete repeat of IκBα could represent a degenerated form of the sixth repeat of NFκBp105 (ALIGN score 5.85 SD units compared with 4.27 for the next most significant similarity).

No other significant similarities were detected for the rest of the ikbl protein sequence, although there is a region at the C-terminus that has a heptad repeat of three leucines (residues 359, 373 and 380) and one valine (at residue position 366) that is reminiscent of a leucine zipper.

The genomic localisation of the ikbl gene

Most of the 90 kb between the BAT1 and G2 genes has been sequenced by Iris et al. (Nature Genetics 1993, 2, 137). Computer analysis predicted the presence of 3 exons in the region containing ikbl, one of which demonstrated similarity with the ANK repeats of NFκB. Comparison of this partial genomic sequence with the ikbl cDNA has allowed us to assign the positions and boundaries of the first two exons of ikbl, and to read upstream of our clone. Nucleotides 7446-7170 of the genomic sequence are complementary to nucleotides 126-402 of the ikbl cDNA (exon 2 of ikbl in our nomenclature) and encode the one and a half ANK repeats described by Iris et al. Our first exon could represent one of the telomeric exons of Iris et al., although their data suggests that both telomeric exons lie outside the 5' limits of ikbl. Downstream of the second exon of ikbl lies a dense cluster of Alu repeats (Fig. 6B) that interrupt the gene for at least 7 kb. No further genomic sequence is available to allow elucidation of the position and size of the downstream exons of ikbl.

The 3U1 cDNA insert probe was hybridised to Southern blots of cloned DNA from cosmid TN62 and uncloned genomic DNA from the HLA-homozygous cell line ICE5, which was used to construct the cosmid library from which cosmid TN62 was isolated. The hybridisation pattern obtained from the cosmid TN62 blot localised the 3' end of the gene to a 2.1 kb BamHI fragment. Given that the location of the 5' exons has been mapped precisely by DNA sequence analysis, this indicates that the ikbl gene spans ~13.5 kb of DNA. The pattern of hybridisation of the 3U1 cDNA insert probe on the genomic Southern blot corresponded exactly with that of the blot of cosmid TN62, indicating that ikbl is a single copy gene.

Other genes in the class III region

Cross-hybridisation of genomic DNA fragments derived from the gaps between the G6 and BAT5 genes, and the BAT5 and G5 genes, in zoo blot analysis has indicated that these two segments of DNA may contain addition novel genes. Recently, cDNA clones have been isolated from a U937 cDNA library using an 18 kb BssHII fragment separating the BAT5 and G5 genes. These cDNA clones which correspond to at least one novel gene located between the BAT5 and G5 genes and this is being characterised further.

ANALYSIS OF THE CLASS I REGION

As for the other region this study involves a structural analysis through the cloning of the entire region into YACs and cosmids and the screening of several cDNA libraries followed by the identification of various mRNA by hybridization and sequencing.

Cloning and map of the human MHC class I region and the distal part

We have partially cloned the human MHC class I region into Yeast Artificial Chromosome (YAC) [Chimini et al., Immunogenetics 1990, 32, 419-426], and in addition we have the YACs covering the MHC class I region isolated at the CEPH.

Using probes from these YACs and cosmids, we have achieved a continuous map from HLA-E to HLA-F genes [El Kalhoun et al., Immunogenetics 1992, 35-3, 153-159]. We have then localized several markers telomeric to the MHC class I region: butyrophiline, Ret Finger Protein and Myeline Oligodendrocyte Glycoprotein [Pham-Dinh et al., Proc. Natl. Acad. Sci. USA 1993, 90, 7990-7994 ; Vernet et al., J. Mol. Evol. 1993, 37-6, 600-612]. In addition, we have localized the OTF-3 gene within the MHC class I region 100 kb telomeric to HLA-C [Guillaudeux et al., Cytogenet. Cell Genet. 1993, 63, 212-214 ; Crouau-Roy et al., Genomics 1994, 21, 241-243]. These gene sequences and also sequence from genes probably mapping within this region were used to design STS (sequence tagged site) primers. STS primers were used to screen the CEPH YAC library. The positive clones allowed us to construct a YAC contig covering the distal part of the MHC class I region, a map was then realized at YAC and Genomic level [Amadou et al., submitted].

Search for recombination hot spot and meiotic map

The meiotic map was facilitated by the fact that the region contains many polymorphic markers that allow to identify families with members with recombinant chromosomes. Using these families we have precized the localization of OTF-3 gene [Crouau-Roy et al., Genomics 1994, 21, 241-243], furthermore the localization of several recombinations points was clarified [Crouau-Roy et al., Human Immunology 1993, 38, 132-136]. In addition, we have localised and identified several polymorphic microsatellites within this region [Crouau-Roy et al., in preparation].

Search for new coding sequences

We have identified several coding sequences by different technics:
1. Screening of cDNA libraries;
2. Synteny analysis;
3. Sequencing of genomic fragments conserved between species and informatic analysis;
4. Localization of paralogous genes;
5. Identification of conserved sequences between species.

Screening of cDNA libraries:

MMRI and HSRI: These genes have been isolated by direct screening of cDNA libraries using whole YAC as probe. MMRI mouse gene and its human equivalent: IISRI are highly conserved. They show sequence similarity with a subclass of GTP binding protein [Denizot et al., Genomics 1992, 14, 857-862 ; Vernet et al., Mammalian Genome 1993, 5, 100-105].
   P5-1: This sequence is specifically transcribed in B cells, it maps between HLA-C and HLA-A [Vernet et al., Immunogenetics 1993, 38, 57-53]. We have finally showed that P5-1 corresponds to a hybrid sequence formed of the 5' part of an MHC class I gene fused *de novo* to an unrelated sequence [Avoustin et al., submitted].

Synteny analysis

Otf3 is a POU domain gene involved in the early embryonic development. It was first cloned in the mouse genome and localized to the mouse MHC class I region. We first localized its human equivalent, OTF3, by in situ hybridization to the 6p21.3-6p22 chromosome band [Guillaudeux et al., Cytogenet. Cell Genet. 1993, 63,212-214]. We then refined its localization by meiotic and physical mapping [Crouau-Roy et al., Genomics 1994, 21, 241-243].

Sequencing of genomic fragments conserved between species and informatic analysis, Localization of paralogous genes

B30.2 sequence and its multigenic family: The B30.2 exon has been identified using a strategy consisting in the sequencing of genomic fragments that are conserved between human and pig. This gene belongs to a multigenic family including genes coding for zinc finger protein. This family is composed of at least 4 members. We have localized these members by in situ hybridization. Two of these were localized close to the MHC [Vernet et al., J. Mol. Evol. 1993, 37-6, 600-612]. These genes are coding for butyrophiline and RFP. Furthermore, the C terminal domain of butyrophiline shares sequence similarity with the C terminal domain of MOG. We have localized the MOG gene to the 6p21.3-6p22 chromosome band [Pham-Dinh et al., Proc. Natl. Acad. Sci. USA 1993, 90, 7990-7994]. We have recently refined their localization by pulsed field gel analysis on genomic human DNA and YAC [Amadou et al., submitted]. We have also localized the other members of this multigenic family [Frank et al., Am. J. Hum. Genet. 1993, 52, 183-191].

Identification of sequences conserved between species

Sequences TU42, D6S131, Tctex5, GRC: These sequences have been mapped in the mouse MHC. We have shown that they are conserved in human and that they map also in the MHC [Amadou et al., submitted].

Analysis of the conserved syntenic unit UA, UB in man and mouse. Cloning of an evolutionary breakpoint

The 6p21.2-6p22.1, 6p22.2-6p23 regions are respectively homologuous to two regions localized to the mouse chromosome 17 and 13, and correspond to two conserved synteny units. The synteny unit corresponding to the 6p22.2-6p22.1 region is named UA. In mouse, this synteny unit was analyzed in collaboration with K. Fisher-Lindal and K. Artzt (USA). They have mapped the murine equivalents of R1, B30.2 and MOG (Pham-Dinh et al., 1993, non published results). At the same time we have localized human equivalents of mouse genes present in the syntenic region [Amadou et al., submitted]. This allowed us to show the conservation of the gene order between the two species [Amadou et al., submitted].

The second conserved synteny unit corresponding to the 6p22.2-6p23 region is named UB. Its equivalent is localized to mouse chromosome 13. Genes in mouse were localized by in situ hybridization (col MG Mattei) [Amadou et al., submitted] and genetic analysis (col N Jenkins) [Amadou et al., submitted]. The murine equivalent of butyrophiline and RFP genes have thus been mapped to the mouse chromosome 13. The comparison between man and mouse shows that the gene order is conserved [Amadou et al., submitted] in this synteny unit.

During this work, with the help of the mapping of paralogous genes we have showed that the human UA/UB organization: UA close to UB, represent the human/mouse ancestral one [Amadou et al., submitted]. We have furthermore pinpointed the localization of the UA/UB breaking-point. The human genomic region corresponding to the breaking-point was cloned into YAC, in order to analyse its structure. We have also shown that this breaking-point is recurrent during the evolution as it corresponds to the distal inversion point found in the mouse haplotype [Amadou et al., submitted].

Gene duplications and exon shuffling in the 6p21.2-6p22 region

The B30.2 family

The B30.2 exon presents sequence similarity with 3 genes: butyrophiline, RFP and 52 kD SSa/Ro. We have localized butyrophiline and RFP in the same genomic region as B30.2. We can postulate that these three genes arose by duplication and that they were not separated. Furthermore butyrophiline shows sequence similarity with the other only in its C terminal part. The N terminal part of butyrophiline shows sequence similarity with the Ig-like domain of MOG. Strikingly, MOG was localized to the same region as RFP and butyrophiline. From these data we postulate that an exon shuffling event occurred between MOG and RFP genes ancestor, giving rise to butyrophiline gene. These genes were not separated in human [Vernet et al., J. Mol. Evol., 1993, 37-6: 600-612].

MHC class I genes duplication

We have shown that the MHC class I gene family stemmed from duplication of a DNA fragment of 20 kb including an HLA-A like gene and an other class I gene. We could furthermore show that several non homologous recombinationl events occurred within this duplication unit [Avoustin et al., submitted].

The P5-1 gene

We have shown that P5-1 is a new type of hybrid gene. It was indeed created de novo by fusion of two non mobile sequences, the 5' part of an MHC class I gene (promotor, first exon and the first part of intron I) and an unrelated sequence. Furthermore, this fusion event occurred in the primate lineage, i.e. late in evolution. Finally, we have found that the MHC class I truncated genes could serve as promotor pool and thus participate in the creation of new genes [Avoustin et al., submitted].

DETAILED ANALYSIS OF THE REGION CENTERED AROUND HLA-A

The hemochromatosis gene (HFE) maps to 6p21.3 and is less than 1 cM from the HLA class I genes; however, the accurate physical location of the gene has remained elusive and controversial. The unambigous identification of a crossover event within hemochromatosis families is very difficult. It is particulary hampered by the variability of the phenotypic expression as well as by the sex- and age-related penetrance of the disease. For these practical considerations, traditional linkage analysis could prove of limited value for refining further the extrapolated physical position of HFE. We therefore embarked upon a linkage-disequilibrium analysis of HFE and normal chromosomes from the Britain population. Sixty-six hemochromatosis families yielding 151 hemochromatosis chromosomes and 182 normal chromosomes were RFLP-typed with a battery of probes, including two newly derived polymorphic markers from the 6.7 and HLA-F loci located 150 and 250 kb telomeric to HLA-A, respectively. The results suggest a strong peak of existing linkage disequilibrium focused within the i82 to 6.7 interval (approximately 250 kb). The zone of linkage disequilibrium is flanked by the i97 locus, positioned 30 kb proximal to i82, and the HLA-F gene, found 250 kb distal to HLA-A, markers of which display no significant association with HFE. These data support the possibility that HFE resides within the 400 kb expanse of DNA between i97 and HLA-F. Alternatively, the very tight association of HLA-A3 and allele 1 of the 6.7 locus, both of which are comprised by the major ancestral or founder HFE haplotype in Brittany, support the possibility that the disease gene may reside immediately telomeric to the 6.7 locus within the linkage-disequilibrium zone. Additionally, hemochromatosis haplotypes possessing HLA-A11 and the low-frequency HLA-F polymorphism (allele 2) are supportive of a separate founder chromosome containing a second, independently arising mutant allele. Overall, the establishment of a likely "hemochromatosis critical region" centromeric boundary and the identification of a linkage-disequilibrium zone both significantly contribute to a reduction in the amount of DNA required to be searched for novel coding sequences constituting the HFE defect.

To further refine the analysis of the region centered around the HLA-A locus two overlapping yeast artificial chromosomes named B30 which has an insert of 320 kb, and E5 with an insert of 450 kb, were used to make cosmid libraries. These libraries were then organized to obtain a contig nearly achieved at the present time. These two contigs are made of cosmids the integrity of which was assessed by parallel restriction enzyme digestion and comparison with the digestion pattern of the whole YAC will be used in the following program for the entire sequencing of that region along with exon trapping and bioinformatic search.

In addition to this the YAC B30 was used to screen a cDNA library of human duodenal mucosa where the biochemical defect of the hemochromatosis gene should be expressed. Through hybridization 8 independent cDNA clones were isolated and sequenced. Comparison sequences with data bank revealed no matching for 7 new genes expressed in the duodenal mucosa. These new genes are located within a region that may well contain the gene responsible for hemochromatosis and have therefore been named HCG I-VII (Hemochromatosis Candidate Gene). HCG I, III, V and VI are probably single copy genes, situated at 180, 155, 140 and 230 kb centromeric to HLA-A, respectively. HCG II, one of HCG IV and one of HCG VII are centromeric to HLA-A (at 30, 70 and 100 kb respectively). Another copy of HCG IV is 20 kb telomeric to HLA-A. Each of the genes localized on the YAC B30 is associated with an CpG/HTF island.

CONCLUSION

Through this collaboration study of the whole MHC region substantial results were obtained corresponding to the preparation of a whole battery of reagents YACs -cosmid contig- cDNA probes enabling to pursue the establisment of a physical and genetic map of the region which is far from complete but well engaged.

In addition, several genes worth recalling were identified and more or less characterized such as:
1. RING 3, which is related to the Drosophila gene "female sterile homeotic".
2. DM only distantly related to other class III products.
3. ABC transporter or TAPS and the proteasome component.
4. A gene sharing a substantial homology with SUP 45, a gene previously identified in yeast. This new gene has been identified and located in the class I regions.
5. Several genes whose cDNA map to the class I region were also identified and sequenced. One of them corresponds to a gene previously identified in yeast and call SUP 45. It appears very interesting and promising.

Of course, an important work still needs to be clone before a complete knowledge of this very important region is gained. However, the prospect to get it is good and in the coming years interesting results should come up.

Contract number: GENO-CT91-0026
Contractual period: 1 February 1992 to 31 January 1994

Coordinator
Dr. Francis Galibert
Laboratoire de Biochimie et Biologie Moléculaire
UPR 41 CNRS "Recombinaisons Génétiques"
Faculté de Médecine
2 av du Pr Léon Bernard
F-35043 Rennes Cedex
France
Tel: 33 99 336 216
Fax: 33 99 336 200

Participants
Dr. Philippe Brulet
URA 1148 CNRS
Institut Pasteur
Bâtiment de Biologie Moléculaire
25 rue du Docteur Roux
F-75724 Paris Cedex 15
France
Tel: 33 1 4061 3051
Fax: 33 1 4306 9835

Dr. Robert Ducan Campbell
MRC Immunochemistry Unit
Department of Biochemistry
University of Oxford
South Parks Road
UK-Oxford OX1 3QU
United Kingdom
Tel: 44 865 275 354
Fax: 44 865 275 729

Professor Jean-Yves Le Gall
Laboratoire de Biochimie et Biologie Moléculaire
UPR 41 CNRS "Recombinaisons Génétiques"
Faculté de Médecine
2 av du Pr Léon Bernard
F-35043 Rennes Cedex
France
Tel: 33 99 336 820
Fax: 33 99 336 898

Dr. Joseph Papamatheakis
Foundation for Research & Technology-Hellas
Institut of Molecular Biology & Biotechnology
P.O. Box N° 1527
GR-711 10 Heraklion
Crete
Tel: 30 81 210 079
Fax: 30 81 230 469

Dr. Pierre Pontarotti
CRPG - UPR 8291 CNRS
Université Toulouse 3, CHU Purpan
Avenue de Grande Bretagne
F-31300 Toulouse
France
Tel: 33 6 1499 414
Fax: 33 6 1499 036

Dr. John Trowsdale
Imperial Cancer Research Fund
Human Immunogenetics Laboratory
P.O. Box N° 123
UK-Lincoln's Inn Fields
London WC2A 3PX
United Kingdom
Tel: 44 71 269 3209
Fax: 44 71 831 6786

Human Genome Analysis Programme
M. Hallen and A. Klepsch (Eds.)
IOS Press, 1995

DEVELOPMENT AND IMPROVEMENT OF TECHNOLOGY FOR GENOME ANALYSIS OF THE X CHROMOSOME

G. Romeo
Istituto Giannina Gaslini, Genova, Italy

1. Background information

The main goal of our project was to implement a new procedure to clone some of the genes included in microdeletions of the chromosome X present in patients with contigous gene deletion syndromes. This procedure aimed at the construction of genomic libraries highly enriched in sequences corresponding to those that are deleted. It relied on the use of a modification of the PERT technique (Kunkel et al., Proc. Natl. Acad. Sci. USA, 1985, 84, 6521-6525; Nussbaum et al., Proc. Natl. Acad. Sci. USA, 1987, 84, 6521-6525), the PERT reassociated sequences being selected through several cycles of non-specific PCR (Kinzler and Vogelstein, Nucleic Acids Res., 1989, 17, 3645-3653).

To optimise the conditions for sequence enrichment, we designed several modifications of the PERT protocol. We first set up the conditions allowing to obtain a first enrichment of X chromosomes by Fluorescence-Activated Chromosome Sorting (FACS). Subsequently, a further enrichment in target sequences was obtained using the PERT technique in combination with the Alu-PCR amplification technique described by Nelson et al. (Proc. Natl. Acad. Sci. USA, 1991, 86, 6686-6690). This method allows selective amplification of genomic regions comprised between Alu sequences. We also used as a starting material several appropriate somatic cell hybrids with the idea of extending the method to the cloning of regions deleted in autosomal deletions. During the first 18 months of the project, we have subsequently worked out and mastered:
1. The conditions for reassociation of chromosome X-enriched DNA by PERT.
2. The specific amplification of the products obtained in these experiments; this required to test the efficacy of various adapter molecules and the conditions of PCR.
3. Finally, the experimental conditions for Alu-PCR amplification of somatic cell hybrids having retained the human X chromosomes.

Despite the large amount of work invested in this project, we were unable to clone the DNA sequences generated by PERT with a sufficient efficacy and reproducibility. Among the technical difficulties we encountered, the poor efficiency of the cloning of the PCR products was further diminished by the small proportion of these products in the final reaction. The additional experiments which we designed to circumvent these problems (reduction of the rate of complexity of the genomic sequences to clone using highly enriched chromosome preparations, alternative methods of enrichment based on a biotin/avidin system) did not improve the quality of the results. After 18 months of efforts, we concluded that the success of the planned protocol was hampered by unsolvable technical difficulties and we abandoned this approach. Nevertheless, Lisitsyn et al. seemed to have been successful (with a procedure similar to that we had designed) in a work published in January 1993 (Cloning the differences between two complex genomes, Science, 1993, 259, 946-951).

While trying to develop this completely new technological approach, the two participant laboratories were exchanging traditional techniques which became instrumental in reaching the results described in the following sections.

Among these results, the mapping and identification of the gene for Hirschsprung disease (HSCR) has a general interest because it opened the way to the delineation of a new concept in the study of the molecular basis of genetic diseases namely that of phenotypic diversity due to allelic series (Romeo and McKusick, Nature Genetics 7:451-453, 1994 and see section of Results and Discussion).

Key words: Psoralen-modified oligonucleotide primers; DGGE; Hirschsprung; Phenotypic diversity; Allelic series.

2. Objectives and primary approaches

The main objective of this project was to develop new technology useful for the study of inherited diseases with particular emphasis on X linked disorders. This objective was essentially achieved through the transfer of technology between the 2 participating laboratories which has been particulary productive in the fields of genetic mapping and of the identification of mutations. The main results in this respect are represented by the identification of candidate genes for the recessive forms of dystrophic epidermolysis bullosa and epidermolysis bullosa simplex (in the French laboratory) by the localization on the X chromosome of a new form of hypophosphatemic rickets and by the identification of the gene for autosomal dominant Hirschsprung disease (HSCR) on chromosome 10 (in the Italian laboratory).

3. Results and discussion

3.1 Genova Group

All the technology developed during the initial period of the project was used in the attempt to clone an important X-linked gene causing Menkes disease. The physical mapping of the gene reported at the end of 1992 (Consalez et al., [1]), led however to the cloning of a gene closely linked but not identical with the Menkes gene.

The same type of technology developed for the Menkes project (production of particular somatic cell hybrids, use of YACs and preparations of cosmid libraries from YAC human inserts etc) was used to physically map in a 250 Kb region the gene for HSCR (also called congenital megacolon). This is a relatively frequent intestinal malformation found in 1 every 5000 newborns, genetically mapped on chromosome 10 using 15 pedigrees with recurrence of the disease, 12 of which were French [2,3].

Both the genetic and the physical mapping of this disease gene were greatly facilitated by the analysis of a large deletion of chromosome 10 observed in a patient with HSCR at the Gaslini Institute in Genoa before the starting of this project (Martucciello et al. Pediatr. Surg. Int. 7:308-310, 1992).

The technique which allowed to isolate in somatic cell hybrid the deleted chromosome 10 from this patient was also developed in the laboratory of Molecular Genetics of the Gaslini Institute (Puliti et al. Cytogenetic Cell Genet 63:102-106, 1992) and was repeatedly used to isolate other deletions from HSCR patients [3]. In brief this technique was developed in order to select human-hamster somatic cell hybrids which retained a human chromosome 10 (either deleted or non-deleted) from these patients. The technique is explained in the scheme of figure 1.

The physical mapping of the HSCR gene was made possible by the availability of the above technique and of lymphoblastoid cell lines from 3 HSCR patient showing

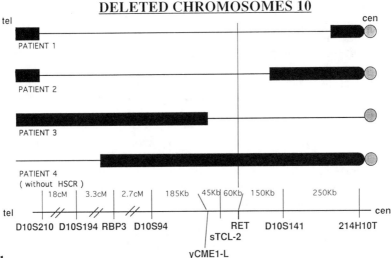

Figure 1
Enrichment for hybrid clones retaining human chromosome 10 (from Puliti et al. Cytogenetic Cell Genet. 63: 102-106, 1992 and Yin L. et al. Human Molec. Genetics 11: 1803-1808, 1993). A mouse monoclonal antibody (Mab) against the β subunit of the human fibronectin receptor (Hβ-FNR) was used against cultured human- hamster somatic cell hybrids which might or might not have retained the gene for Hβ-FNR, located on human chromosome 10. Only hybrid cell retaining human chromosome 10 were therefore able to react with Dynabeads coated anti-mouse IgG, which allowed therefore the separation of positive (for human chromosome 10) and negative cells.

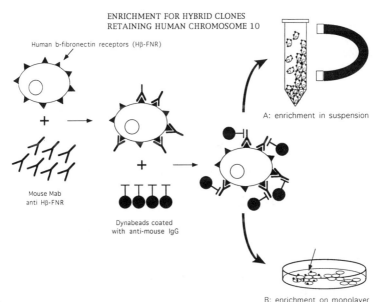

Figure 2
Deleted chromosome 10 (from Yin L. et al Human Molec. Genetics 11: 1803-1808, 1993). Patients 1, 2 and 3 (affected with HSCR) showed a deleted chromosome 10 which was isolated in somatic cell hybrids (as described in figure 1) and characterized for different genetic markers. This allowed to estimate the extent of each deletion and, more important, to define the Smallest Region of Overlap (SRO) among them (approximately 250 Kb) which contains the RET protooncogene.

different deletions of chromosome 10 which defined a Smallest Region of Overlap (SRO) [3]. In this SRO (spanning about 250 Kb of genomic DNA) the RET protooncogene was identified as the most likely candidate for being responsible of HSCR. In spite of the fact that RET had been known for 10 years, its genomic organization and number of exons werenot known. The work performed in Genoa by Ceccherini et al. [4,5] not only allowed the delineation of the exact structure of the gene, but also made it possible to identifiy several point mutations of RET whcih documented the causative role of this gene in HSCR [6].

While the mutations of RET observed in HSCR patients are spred through the different domains of the gene, 3 other inherited disorders namely Multiple Endocrine Neoplasia type 2A (MEN 2A), type 2B (MEN 2B) and Familiar Medullary Thyroid Carcinoma (FMTC) are characterized by mutations in specific domains of RET. As an example a single mutation in exon 16 of RET (namely Met 918->Thr) is present in 95% of the patients with MEN 2B studied so far in the Genoa laboratory (Hofstra et al. Nature 367: 375-376, 1994) as well as in other laboratories.

In some very rare pedigrees patients affected with more than one neurocristopathy can be observed (e.g. HSCR and MEN 2B or HSCR and MEN 2A). The observation that these different phenotypes in a single pedigree are associated with the same mutation of RET led to the development of the concept of phenotypic diversity,a phenomenon which might find an explanation (among others) in the action of modifier genes (Romeo and McKusick Nature Genetics ibidem). The phenotypic diversity of the mutations of RET was exemplified by the study carried out in Genoa of an interesting pedigree showing Multiple Endocrine Neoplasia type 2A with localized Lychen Amyloidosis [7].

The activity of the Italian laboratory along this line of research is now continuing with the aim of studying the biological differences among the different mutations of RET, which are being studied in appropriate expression systems.

Other results in traditional fields of interest of the Italian laboratory, namely in the fields of gene mapping [8], of the population genetics of CF [9] and of the functional study of the CFTR gene (10) were also reported by the Italian laboratory as part of the present project.

3.2 Creteil Group

Among the cell lines obtained by the Creteil group from patients with contiguous gene deletions syndromes (with the aim of using them in the framework of the technical developments described under Background) one concerned a patient having X-linked agammaglobulinemia in association with growth hormone deficiency. This syndrome was believed to be possibly caused by a sub- microscopic deletion of the X chromosome in the region Xq21.3- Xq22. During the course of the present project, the agammaglobulinemia gene (btk) was cloned, and this prompted us to analyse this gene in the relevant patient. Contrary to our expectations, we did not find any deletion but were able to show that an intronic mutation of the btk gene (1882+5G>A) results in an abnormal splicing of the gene in the tyrosine-kinase domain of the brk protein [1].

In parallel to these efforts, our laboratory has been successful in developing or improving new methods for genome analysis, particularly with regard to the detection of nucleotide variability in human health and disease. In particular, to improve the denaturing gradient gel electrophoresis technique (DGGE), a gene scanning procedure efficient in mutation detection that uses PCR primers with long tails of GC (GC-clamps), and is therefore tedious and expensive, we have designed a new approach to GC-clamping based on the use of psoralen-modified oligonucleotide primers. These primers introduce in the amplified molecule an efficient chemical clamp since the psoralen can be activated by UV light to induce cross-linking between the two DNA strands to be analysed. We have applied this technique to the analysis of cystic fibrosis and hemogloninopathies mutations, using the CFTR and Globin genes as model systems in comparative experiments [12]. The technique is now widely used as an alternative to GC-clamped DGGE, and has recently shown its efficacy in the detection of CFTR and RET gene mutations by several groups.

These and other developments have been applied with success in our laboratory in the study of several genetic disorders such as epidermolysis bullosa, retinitis pigmentosa, retinoblastoma and growth hormone receptor deficiencies. We have described the molecular basis for several forms of epidermolyis bullosa by using a combination of linkage analysis studies and molecular testing of possible candidate genes [13-15]. A novel mutation (ask) was found in a case of autosomal recessive retinitis pigmentosa (in press). Finally, we have described the spectrum of mutations altering growth hormone receptor function in a group of patients affected with a growth hormone insensitivity syndrome (Laron syndrome) [16] and shown how some of these mutations affect receptor homodimerization [17].

4. Major scientific breakthroughs

The identification of the RET protooncogene as responsible for Hirschsprung (HSCR) was commented by News and Views article in Nature with the title: One gene four syndromes (Nature 367: 319- 320, 1994). While the mutations of RET observed in HSCR patients are spred through the different domains of the gene, 3 other inherited disorders namely Multiple Endocrine Neoplasia type 2A (MEN 2A), type 2B (MEN 2B) and Familiar Medullary Thyroid Carcinoma (FMTC) are characterized by mutations in specific domains of RET. As an example a single mutation in exon 16 of RET (namely Met 918->Thr) is present in 95% of the patients with MEN 2B.

5. Major cooperative links

As a result of this project a close collaboration has been established in Europe whith different laboratories working on the RET protooncoge like the laboratory of Dr. Bernard Rossi (Unité de Recherche en Immunol. Cell. et Mol. - Avenue de Valombrose - 06107 Nice cedex 02, France) and that of Dr. Vassili Pachnis (MRC, - Mill Hill, London).

References

[1] Consalez G.G., Gecz J., Stayton C.L., Dabovic B., Pasini B., Pezzolo A., Bicocchi P., Fontes M. and Romeo G.: Fine mapping and cloning of the breakpoint associated with Menkes syndrome in a female patient. Genomics 14:557-561, 1992. (*)
[2] Lyonnet S., Bolino A., Pelet A., Abel L., Nihoul-Feketé C., Briard M.L., Mok Sui V., Kaariainen H., Martucciello G., Lerone M., Puliti A., Yin L., Weissenbach J., Devoto M., Munnich A. and Romeo G.: A gene for Hirschsprung disease maps to the proximal ong arm of chromosome 10. Nature Genetics 4: 346-350, 1993. (*)
[3] Yin L., Ceccherini I., Pasini B., Matera I., Bicocchi M.P. Barone V., Bocciardi R., Kääriäinen Helena, Weber D., Devoto M., Romeo G.: Close linkage with the RET proto-oncogene and deletion mutations in autosomal dominant Hirschsprung disease. Human Mol. Genet. vol 2, 11:1803-1808, 1993. (*)

[4] Ceccherini I., Bocciardi R., Luo Y., Pasini B., Hofstra R., Takahashi M., Romeo G.: Exon structure and flanking intronic sequences of the human RET proto-oncogene. Bioch. Bioph. Res. Comm 196:1288-1295, 1993. (*)

[5] Romeo G., Ronchetto P., Yin L., Barone V., Seri M., Ceccherini I., Pasini B., Bocciardi R., Lerone M., Kaariainen H., Martucciello G.: Point mutations affecting the tyrosine kinase domain of the RET protooncogene in Hirschsprung patients. Nature, 367:377-378, 1994. (*)

[6] Bolino A., Devoto M., Enia G., Zoccali C., Weissenbach J., Romeo G.: Genetic Mapping in the Xp11.2 region of a new form of X-linked hypophosphatemic rickets. Eur J Hum Genet, 1:269-279, 1993. (*)

[7] Morral N., Bertanpetit J., Estivil X., Nunes V., Casals T., Giménez J., Reis A., Varon-Meteeva R., Macek Jr. M., Kalaydjieva L., Angelicheva D., Dancheva R., Romeo G., Russo M.P., Garnerone S., Restagno G., Ferrari M., Magnai C., Clausters M., Desgeorges M., Schwartz M., Scharz M., Dallapiccola B., Novelli G., Ferec C., de Arce M., Nemeti M., Kere J., Anvret M., Dahl N., Kadasi L.: Tracing the origin of the major cystic fivrosis mutation (deltaF508) in European populations. Nature Genetics 7:169-175, 1994. (*)

[8] Ceccherini I., Romei C., Barone V., Pacini F., Martino E., Loviselli A., Pinchera A. and Romeo G.: Indentification of the Cys634->Tyr mutation of the RET proto-oncogene in a pedigree with multiple endocrine neoplasia type 2A and localized cutaneous lichen amyloidosis. J. Endocrinol. Invest. 17:201-204, 1994. (*)

[9] Galietta L.J.V., Zagarra-Moran O., Mastrocola T., Wöhrle C., Rugolo M., Romeo G.: Activation of Ca^{2+}-dependent K^+ and Cl^- currents by UTP and ATP in CFPAC-1 cells. Pflügers Arch. Vol. 426:534-41, 1994 (*)

[10] Ceccherini I., Hofstra R.M.W., Yin Luo, Stulp R.P., Barone V., Stelwagen T., Bocciardi R., Nijveen H., Bolino A. Seri M., Ronchetto P., Pasini B., Bozzano M., Buys H.C.M. and Romeo G.: DNA polymorphisms and conditions for SSCP analysis of the 20 exons of the RET proto-oncogene. Oncogene, in press. (*)

[11] Duriez B., Duquesnoy P., Dastot F., Bougneres P., Amselem S. and Goossens M.: An exon shipping mutation in the BTK gene of a patient with X-linked agammaglobulinemia and isolated hormone deficiency. FEBS Letter 346: 165-170, 1994. (*)

[12] Costes B., Girodon E., Ghanem N., Chassignol M., Thuong N.T., Dupret D. and Gossens M.: Psoralen-modified oligonucleotide primers improve detection of mutations by denaturing gradient gel electrophoresis and provide an alternative to GC-clamping. Hum. Mol. Genet. 2: 393-397, 1993.

[13] Hovnanian A., Duquesnoy P., Blanchet-Bardon C., Knowlton R., Amselem S., Lathrop M., Dibertret L., Uitto J., Goossens M.: Genetic linkage of recessive dystrophic epidermolylis bullosa to the type VII collagen gene. J. Clin. Invest. Invest. 90: 1032- 1036, 1992.

[14] Hovnanian A., Pollack E., Hilal L., Rochat A., Prost C., Barrandon Y. and Goossens M.: A missense mutation in the rod domain of keratin 14 associated with recessive epidermolysis bullosa simplex. Nature Genet. 3: 327-332, 1993.

[15] Hilal L., Rochat A., Duquesnoy P., Blanchet-Bardon C., Wechsler J., Martin N., Christiano A., Barrandon Y., Uitto J., Goossens M., and Hovnanian A.: A homozygous insertion-deletion in the type VII collagen gene (COL7A1) in Hallopeau-Siemems dystrophic epidermolysis bullosa. Nature Genet. 5: 287-293, 1994. (*)

[16] Amselem S., Duquesnoy P., Duriez B., Dastot F., Sobrier M.L., Valleix S. and Goossens M.: Spectrum of growth hormone receptor mutations and associated haplotypes in Laron syndrome. Hum. Mol. Genet. 2: 355-359, 1993.

[17] Duquesnoy P., Sobrier M.L., Duriez B., Dastot F., Buchanan C.R., Savage M.O., Preece M.A., Craescu C.T., Blouquit Y., Goossens M. and Amselem S.: A single amino acid substitution in the exoplasmic domain of the human growth hormone (GH) receptor confers familial GH resistance (Laron syndrome) with positive GH- binding activity by abolishing receptor homodimerization. EMBO J., 13: 1386-1395, 1994.

Publications in which the financial contribution is acknowledged: (*)

Contract number: GENO-CT91-0027
Contractual period: 1 March 1992 to 30 September 1994

Coordinator
Prof. Giovanni Romeo
Lab. di Genetica Molecolare
Istituto G. Gaslini
Largo G. Gaslini, 5
I-16147 Genova-Quarto
Italy
Tel: 39 10 563 6400-370
Fax: 39 10 391 254
E-mail GENETICA@IGECUNIV.CISI.UNIGE.IT

Participant
Prof. Michel Goossens
University of Paris XI
Med. School-Hôpital Henri Mondor
INSERM U91
F-94010-Creteil
France
Tel: 33 1 498 128 60
Fax: 33 1 498 128 42

No. of publications: No. 10 from Prof. Romeo's group and no. 7 from Prof. Goossen's group (see list).

Human Genome Analysis Programme
M. Hallen and A. Klepsch (Eds.)
IOS Press, 1995

IMPROVEMENT OF HIGH RESOLUTION IN SITU HYBRIDIZATION MAPPING OF DNA SEQUENCES AND NEW APPROACHES TO DETECT SPECIFIC CHROMOSOMAL ABERRATIONS BY MULTIPROBE MULTICOLOR IN SITU HYBRIDIZATION

P. Lichter
Deutsches Krebs-Forschungs-Zentrum (DKFZ), Heidelberg, Germany

1. Background information

Fluorescence in situ hybridization (FISH) with selected DNA probes allows to delineate specific DNA regions in cellular preparations and can therefore be used for the physical mapping of DNA fragments. The fact that the DNA of each chromosome can be recognized as a distinct entity in the cell nucleus offers the opportunity to exploit in situ hybridization also for the evaluation of chromosome aberrations not only in mitotic cells, but also in interphase nuclei. The concept of analyzing chromosome aberrations in interphase nuclei has become increasingly important for prenatal diagnostics and tumor cytogenetics. This approach is especially suitable for the analysis of human malignancies, where the preparation of metaphase spreads is, in general, rather difficult (if not impossible), because the cultured cells have only small proliferative activity. Interphase cytogenetics is highly dependent on the availability of physically mapped genomic DNA probes and therefore, its clinical applications are advancing in parallel to the human genome project.

Comparative genomic hybridization (CGH) is a FISH method that allows to detect chromosomal imbalances in a comprehensive manner by comparing the hybridization patterns of whole genomic DNA from normal and tumor cells.

Key Words: High Resolution FISH Mapping; Diagnostic DNA Probes; Recurrent Chromosome Aberrations; Multicolor In Situ Hybridization; Comparative Genomic Hybridization.

2. Objectives and primary approaches

Development of new diagnostic tools for the detection of tumor associated chromosomal aberrations as a spin off from improved physical maps in the corresponding regions of the human genome. These objectives require new methodological developments of DNA hybridization techniques, primarily of FISH protocols.

Our collaborative study is aiming on the methodological development of FISH protocols that are especially designed to meet clinical requirements. Thus, sets of DNA probes are generated allowing the routine diagnosis of the most common cytogenetic abnormalities. Furthermore, multicolor FISH protocols are established for the simultaneous diagnosis of the most important chromosomal changes in certain types of leukemias.

3. Results and discussion

1) Assessment of the practicability and resolution of various new techniques for high resolution mapping by FISH and their application for the generation of a physical map of 17q11. 2) Characterization of specific chromosomal aberrations associated with leukemias and optimization of protocols to detect these aberrations by FISH using genomic DNA probes; these chromosomal aberrations include translocations and deletions involving 11q23, translocation t(9;22)(q34;q11) and trisomy 12 in lymphoid leukemias, as well as translocations t(9;22)(q34;q11), t(8;21) and t(3;21) in myeloid leukemias. 3) Detection of new recurrent aberrations in chronic lymphocytic leukemias and optimization of DNA probe sets for their clinical diagnosis; these include deletion of the RB-1 gene and the TP53 gene. 4) Assessment of the practicability of multicolor probe sets in hematological diseases. 5) Establishment and further development of the new approach of comparative genomic hybridization (CGH):

3.1 Development and assessment of improved techniques for the linear mapping of DNA probes (Lichter)

Premature chromosome condensation

In order to improve the resolution of mapping DNA segments located close to each other, several techniques were investigated which all include preparations of long chromosome structures. Prematurely condensed chromosomes, so-called "PCCs" (premature chromosome condensation) were prepared by the fusion of primary human fibroblasts with mitotic Hela cells (in cooperation with Prof. Sperling, Berlin). Using two color in situ hybridization with probe pairs from closely spaced cosmids (of chromosome 8 and 11), we were able to get a resolution which was superior to the resolution obtained when using metaphase chromosomes. However, a particular difficulty is provided by the fact that the chromosomes of the Hela cells also contribute to the formation of PCCs. Since Hela chromosomes are rearranged multifold, it is not suitable to use Hela as mitotic fusion partner. In order to circumvent this difficulty, mitotic cells of mice and hamsters were used as fusion partners. However, the success rate in obtaining human PCCs after the fusion of primary human fibroblasts with rodent cells was low. Accordingly, we feel it is not advisable to use PCC preparations for the routine mapping of large numbers of probes.

Inhibitors of DNA-Condensation

In parallel, we explored new methods for the preparation of decondensed chromosomes. One approach was to inhibit chromatin-condensation using topoisomerase-II inhibitors. By applying etoposide as inhibitor we obtained chromatin structures, which allow the ordering of differentially labeled probes with a resolution superior to the PCCs (see Joos et al. 1994). Heng et al. (Proc Natl Acad Sci USA 89, 9509-9513, 1992) demonstrated a significantly improved resolution using the topoisomerase-II inhibitor VM26. Treatment with this substance yields - under suitable conditions - to extended fibers of free chromatin. These can be used for the high resolution mapping of closely spaced DNA sequences (≤100 kb).

Mapping by interphase in situ hybridization

The approach of interphase in situ mapping is based on the high degree of chromatin decondensation in the cell nucleus allowing to establish high resolution physical maps of the genome. However, the order of the probes is concluded indirectly from the average distances measured between two hybridization signals. To evaluate this approach, we used a set of probes from human chromosome 17 (and not 11 as originally planned). Since it was impossible to order the gene for vitronectin and NF1 (neurofibromatosis I) on 17q11 using prometaphase chromosomes (Fink et al. Hum. Genet. 88, 569-572, 1992), a number of cosmids from this region was isolated in collaboration with D. Jenne (München). Using these probes we established a map shown in Table 1, which localizes the vitronectin gene proximal to NF1. Our probe collection on 17q11 provides a tool for the determination of the resolution of other mapping procedures (Fink et al., 1993). In our hands the approach of interphase mapping yielded a mapping resolution of approximately 100 kb.

- Fink T.M., Ohl S., Hoffmeyer S., Jenne D.E., Lichter P. (1993) Construction of a physical map in the region 17cen-q11.2 by in situ interphase mapping. Conference of the Society of Human Genetics (Würzburg).

Range of Mapping Resolutions

A new method for high resolution in situ hybridization was reported by Wiegant et al.. (Hum Mol Genet 1, 587-592, 1992). Hybridization against DNA Halo preparations allowed to order probes with a resolution of ≤ 10 kb. We have performed multicolor in situ hybridization with cosmid probes from chromosome 8q24 to Halo preparations (see Joos et al. 1994) to establish the methodology for analyses regarding the three dimensional genome organization. Our evaluation of the various mapping approaches as well as a summary of the resolution to be achieved was recently published (see Joos et al 1994).

Figure 1
Comparison of the mapping resolution achieved by using various molecular cytogenetic techniques

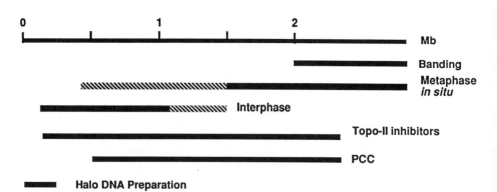

Physical map of 17cen-17q11 generated by in situ interphase mapping

cen ... tel

	D17Z1	CRYB1	D17S33	5'-NF1					3'NF1	D17S145
HGML ID:	D17Z1	→ CRYB1	→ D17S33	→ 5'-NF1	→	→	→	→	3'NF1 →	D17S145
synonym/clone	p17H8	pbeta8-2	HHH202							2B/B35
primer:				NF-FH-1-1	NF-FH-2-1	NF-FH-2-2	NF-FH-1-3	NF-FH-2-3	NF-FH-1-4	
nucleotide:				(1-1000)	(900-1935)	(2361-3735)	(3583-4718)	(4634-5365)	(5618-6877)	
cosmids:	D07191 H02115		H127 E0981 E0557 C07130 A04136 F06111 D04178	A04138 A06105 F0790	H10189	A1062 C06107 H10189 C10105	D02134	C0861 D1048	E05164 H0410 E09186 G11176 A04176	C1280 F1166

Table 1

Summary of the physical map of 17cen-q11 generated by applying the in situ interphase mapping approach. The order and orientation of gene loci in 17q11 is indicated. Cosmids isolated for the corresponding loci are listed in the lower part of the columns. They were isolated from a chromosome 17 specific cosmid library (H. Lehrach, ICRF, London) in collaboration with Dieter Jenne (München). For in situ hybridization, only cosmids were used whose identity was confirmed by hybridization to specific DNA fragments (D17Z1, CRYB1, pHHH202) or by specific primers (all NF1 cosmids, D17S145).

3.2 Establishment of in situ hybridization probe sets for detecting structural aberrations in leukemias (Lichter, Hagemeijer, Döhner)

In order to design multiprobe sets for the multicolor detection of chromosomal aberrations in leukemias, three lines of research were followed for the definition of in situ hybridization probes optimal to detect single chromosome aberrations: i) conventional cytogenetic analysis was performed to further elucidate recurrent chromosome aberrations in acute and chronic leukemias, in particular with regard to chromosome 11q; ii) in situ hybridization analysis was performed on preparations of B-cell chronic lymphocytic leukemias (B-CLL) with probes from chromosome 12 and chromosome 11q in order to characterize the capability of the corresponding probes to detect trisomy 12 or the disease specific deletions in chromosome 11q, and subsequently similar studies were carried out for other relevant breakpoints in leukemias; iii) in situ hybridization was used to detect new recurrent chromosome aberrations in B-cell lymphoproliferative diseases resulting in new probes to be included in the disease specific multicolor probe set (such as for chromosomes 10, 13 and 17).

Chromosome 12, B-CLL (Döhner, Lichter)

The alphoid DNA probe of chromosome 12 proved to be a highly efficient probe for the detection of trisomy 12 in B-CLL. Performing interphase analysis with this probe revealed a higher percentage of trisomy 12 cases as compared to the data obtained by chromosome banding analysis (see Döhner et al. 1993). This is most likely due to difficulties in adequate stimulation of the B-cells during short term culturing. However, it was also found that in the cells of a few patients the centromere region of chromosome 12 was highly decondensed, causing difficulties in enumerating the interphase signals of the alphoid DNA probe. This becomes a problem in the diagnosis of cases where only small percentages of the analyzed cell population exhibit a trisomy. Therefore, additional probes of chromosome 12 - as e.g. probes from 12q13 covering a region of partial trisomy in B-CLL - are currently tested with regard to their efficiency in detecting the numerical chromosome 12 aberrations.

Chromosome 11q, B-CLL (Lichter, Hagemeijer, Döhner, Zaccaria)

A number of cosmids mapping along the long arm of chromosome 11 were used in a blind experiment to investigate their diagnostic potential for the detection of 11q deletions in B-cell lymphoproliferative diseases (01 and 03). As outlined in table 2, 24 patients with previously diagnosed cytogenetic aberrations were probed with 4 different cosmid probes. By this analysis three 11q deletions could be confirmed (see table 2). This study is currently being completed for all five probes listed in order to cover the major chromosome bands in this analysis and to characterize the extension of the various deletions in more detail. Since the deletion areas need to be further characterized, sets of YACs from these region - including a contig of 12 YACs - have been obtained, which are currently being tested on a large series of patients. Such analyses are also carried out on acute leukemia patients by Dr. Hagemeijer.

Summary of Interphase Screening for Deletions in 11q in B-CLL/B-PLL

Patient Codes	cen : XB-10	: 3.16	: 23.20	: 4.13	: 5.8	: tel
90 PB 68	-	-				
90 PB 76				-		
90 PB 78	-	del		del	-	
90 LK 79	-	del		-	-	
90 PB 89	-				-	
90 PB 91	-	-			-	
90 PB 103	-					
90 LK 137	-					
91 LK 1				del	-	
91 PB 23		-				
91 PB 24	-	-		-	-	
91 PB 69	-					
91 PB 73	-	-		-	-	
91 PB 76	-			-		
91 PB 88	-	-		-	-	
91 Spl 123	-					
92 PB 4	-	-				
92 PB 14	-			-		
92 PB 15	-			-	-	
92 LK 18	-			-		
92 PB 23	-	-		-	-	
92 PB 25	-	-		-		
92 PB 26	-			-	-	
92 Pl 56	-					

Cosmid probes mapping along chromosome 11q

Table 2
Interphase Screening for Deletions in 11q in B-CLL/B-PLL
- = two copies; **del** = one copy

Chromosome 11q, Acute leukemias (Hagemeijer)

In Rotterdam the project effectively started on July 1st 1992 with the engagement of Berna Beverloo, a postdoctoral fellow with experience in different kinds of luminescence and advanced forms of microscopy. The first months were dedicated to basic training in cytogenetics, applied to leukemia, molecular genetics, in particular labeling, fluorescent in situ hybridization (FISH) as well as amplification of probes. She stayed in Heidelberg (with Dr. Lichter) for two weeks, where she was trained in multicolor FISH using chromosome 11q specific probes. These probes and others are being used for the characterization of leukemic material.

Characterization of breakpoints on chromosome 11q in leukemia. (The description of this study is more extensive, since it has so far been published only as an abstract)

11q23 abnormalities are frequently observed in acute lymphoid leukemia as well as in acute myeloid leukemia (see Beverloo et al. 1994). These abnormalities occur in 5-10% of all leukemias, especially AML (acute myeloid leukemia) of the FAB-M4/M5 type and the null- or biphenotypic ALL (acute lymphoblastic leukemia). The cytogenetic incidence, however in childhood leukemia within 12 months of age is approximately 50%. Patients having an 11q23 translocation in general have a very poor prognosis and require aggressive treatment. Cytogenetic analysis of abnormalities in which 11q23 is involved, is difficult.

Since the beginning of this EC project, the gene on 11q23 involved in the above mentioned translocations was cloned by two independent groups. This gene, known as ALL-1, MLL, Htrx or Hrx, is a gene sharing high homology to the Drosophila trithorax gene. It is thought to play a role in differentiation and regulation. Analysis of these translocations showed the formation of chimeric genes, so that both hybrid genes are transcribed actively. The breakpoints in the MLL gene seem to cluster in a region of approximately 8.4 kb (exon 5 until exon 11), occurring mostly in introns localized between the exons 6 and 7, 7 and 8, and 8 and 9. Rearrangements of this gene were studied using three techniques: first by Southern blot analysis with a cDNA probe spanning the major breakpoint cluster region, secondly by RT-PCR (this approach is, however only feasible when the fusion partners of the MLL gene has been cloned), and at last by fluorescent in situ hybridization (FISH).

Patients were analyzed by FISH using cosmid probes (provided by the coordinator 01 and by Dr. L. Selleri, San Diego) and YAC probes (provided by Prof. Dr. B.D. Young, UK) spanning and flanking the 11q23 breakpoint. With this set of probes, 11q23 abnormalities were detected in several lineages of leukemias. So far 25 patients (suspected of) having 11q23 abnormalities were studied. Breakpoint heterogeneity was observed in two patients. In cooperation with the Dutch Childhood Leukemia Study Group (SNWLK), 26 patients with congenital leukemias (below 1 year of age) of both the ALL and AML type were studied. Leukemic cells were collected and stored in the cellbank of the SNWLK from 1979 until now. The material was analyzed by Southern Blotting, and RT-PCR. If enough material was available, cells were cultured for performing FISH. In this group of patients 42% cytogenetically showed an 11q23 abnormality (ALL: 56%, AML: 20%). Using Southern blot hybridization 81% showed an 11q23 abnormality (ALL: 94%, AML: 60%). Currently we are analyzing these samples by RT-PCR to figure out if a known translocation caused the rearrangement. From those patients of which cultured material is available, FISH studies are being performed. This approach was also used for investigation of 11q23 rearrangements in adults and children >1 year of age. Several patients have been identified that show a normal karyotype but an MLL rearrangement on the DNA level (table 3).

Table 3

Number of patients analyzed for 11q23/MLL rearrangements using various techniques

Indication	type	number of patients with 11q23 abnormalities in karyotype		Number of patients showing an MLL rearrangement by Southern blot analysis	Number of patients analyzed by RT-PCR showing a fusion product
Congenital leukemia	AML	yes	3	3/3	
	n=9	no	6	5/6	1
	ALL	yes	9	9/9	6
	n=18	no	9	6/9	
	AUL	yes	0	0/0	
	n=2	no	2	2/2	
Adults/children	AML	yes	17	15/17	5
> 1 yr	n=37	no	21	1/21	
	ALL	yes	10	10/10	8
	n=16	no	6	6/6	
	AUL	yes	2	2/2	2
	n=2	no	0	0/0	
	other	doubt on 11q	6	0/6	

Our results so far indicate that the t(11q23) rearrangements are more frequent in leukemia than originally suspected by cytogenetics alone. The results also indicate that abnormalities of chromosome 11q attributed to other regions than band 11q23 can in fact be complex rearrangements (deletions, translocations, inversion) also implicating the MLL gene. The t(11q23) is particularly frequent in some subgroups of leukemia that we set out to screen systematically, retrospectively for some, and prospectively for all e.g. patients having AML-M4/M5 and ALL with null-phenotype.

Optimization of the detection of the t(9;22)(q34;q11) translocation in CML and ALL (Lichter, Hagemeijer, Döhner)

The Ph^1 translocation is highly characteristic for CML and its presence is an absolute requirement for a patient to be eligible for interferon (IFN) therapy protocols. Using 2 breakpoint flanking cosmid probes in two color combinations, the Ph^1 translocation can be detected on metaphase spreads as well as in interphase nuclei. The same two cosmid probes have proved to be effective at diagnosing $Ph^1(+)$ALL. The latter is frequently occurring in adult ALL (30% or more) and is an indicator of very poor outcome. Whereas Dr. Hagemeijer has tested the practicability of this probe set and showed some applications (see Hagemeijer et al. 1993), Dr. Döhner and Dr. Lichter redesigned the probe set for this translocation in order to optimize it with regard to higher detection sensitivities (see Bentz et al., 1994). That probe set was now provided to Dr. Hagemeijer. In Rotterdam as well as in Heidelberg clinical screening tests will be performed using these probes.

Detection of t(8;21) and t(3;21) (Hagemeijer)

t(8;21) is found in more than 10% of the AML, and the t(3;21) is rare and associated with myeloid blast crisis of CML, MDS or (secondary) AML. Both translocations involve the AML-1 gene located on 21q22. Molecular characterization of the gene and development of useful probes occurred in collaboration with N. Sacchi, University of Milan, Italy.

Two cosmid probes spanning the breakpoint on AML-1 were used for FISH analysis of 13 cases of AML t(8;21) and a variant as well as to 7 cases of t(3;21) in parallel with RT-PCR or molecular analysis (de Greef et al., Leukemia, in press). Due to the variability of the breakpoint in a large intron, more complex probes are needed which are currently being tested. The results with new probes - one P1 from the ETO(CDR) gene and one cosmid of the 5' region of the AML-1 gene - are very promising although this has not yet been applied to a series of patients having this type of translocation. Probes containing larger inserts (YAC, P1) spanning the breakpoint of AML-1 are also being tested for the detection of this translocation in interphase nuclei.

Diagnostic tools for 17p (Lichter, Fontes)

Michael Fontes sent a co-worker to the coordinator's laboratory in order to train in fluorescence in situ hybridization techniques using YAC probes. In the course of this lab visit several YACs derived from 17p were successfully used as in situ hybridization probes. However, it became clear that these YACs produce interphase signals, which are too disperse to allow an accurate enumeration of hybridization signals. Thus, they are not suitable for the detection of deletions, duplications or partial trisomies of the corresponding chromosomal region. However, in the laboratory of Dr. Fontes other YACs were successfully used to characterize 17p microdeletions in Smith-Magenis syndrome patient material by FISH (see Chevillard et al., 1993). The method was also used within other EC funded projects regarding the establishment of physical maps and the extension of contigs along human chromosome 17p.

3.3 New Recurrent Chromosome Aberrations

Chromosome 13q14 in B-CLL (Lichter, Döhner)

Chromosome regions suspicious for disease specific genomic changes have also been investigated by in situ hybridization using suitable DNA probes. Using the genomic probe of the RB-1 locus we could establish a high frequency of RB-1 deletions in B-CLL patients (see Stilgenbauer et al. 1993, Döhner et al. 1994). In about 20 - 30% of the patients a monoallelic deletion of RB-1 was observed shedding a new light on the pathogenetic role of RB-1 for B-CLL and demonstrating the need to include a RB 1 probe into the multicolor disease specific in situ hybridization probe set. We also found aberrations of chromosome 10q in a region, where we could previously map the gene for apoptosis 1 (Lichter et al. Genomics 14, 179-180, 192).

Chromosome 17p13 in B-CLL (Lichter, Döhner)

Based on this finding, the relevance of still another tumor suppressor gene, the p53 gene, was studied. Again in 20-25% of all patients a deletion was found. In addition to that, patients bearing a p53 deletion within the leukemic cell clone had a significantly poorer prognosis than the group without p53 deletion (see Döhner et al, Blood 1994). *This is to our knowledge the first time, that a significant prognostic correlation with a cytogenetic feature was found by FISH!*

The fact that new genomic regions could be found as regions involved in recurrent chromosome aberrations in B-CLL (despite the large amount of cytogenetic data available for this disease) clearly demonstrated the need for new techniques allowing for the sensitive and comprehensive detection of chromosomal aberrations.

3.4 Disease-specific Multicolor Probe Sets (Lichter, Hagemeijer, Döhner, Zaccaria)

A disease specific multiprobe set should allow to simultaneously detect the chromosomal aberrations relevant for a particular disease. At a meeting of the project management group in Rotterdam, priority lists were developed to define which aberrations, targets and probes should be included in such probe sets. Strategies were developed for B-CLL and various acute leukemias.

Whereas the multicolor probe sets are currently being put together in the group of Dr. Lichter, preparations of cytogenetically characterized chromosome aberrations in chronic and acute leukemias have been prepared in the groups of Drs. Hagemeijer, Döhner and Zaccaria. Dr. Zaccaria prepared a large panel of metaphase chromosomes containing 11q23 aberrations. In a newly funded EC project multicolor probe sets will be sent from the coordinator (Dr. Lichter) to Dr. Hagemijer in order to evaluate the diagnostic potential of the probe sets in Rotterdam in a blind study. Simultaneously, this study will be carried out in the laboratory of the coordinator using preparations provided by Dr. Hagemeijer and Dr. Döhner.

3.5 Establishment and further Development of Reverse Painting and Comparative Genomic Hybridization (Lichter)

Based on the need for such a new technique we established and further developed a new approach called reverse chromosome painting in the course of this EC funded project (see Joos et al. 1993). The approach, presented first by Kallioniemi, Pinkel and coworkers in 1992, is based on the hybridization of whole genomic DNA from a tumor cell population to normal human chromosomes. Under in situ suppression hybridization conditions, this results in a more or less general staining of the normal chromosomes. However, sequences overrepresented in the tumor cells generate a stronger signal and sequences underrepresented a weaker signal along the corresponding region. For an internal standard normal genomic DNA is cohybridized and visualized in a different color. This allows to assess chromosomal imbalancies by comparing the images generated by tumor cell DNA and normal genomic DNA as probes. The procedure has been termed comparative genomic hybridization, CGH (Kalliomeni et al. Science 258, 818-821, 1992), and was established at a very early time and in the group of Dr. Lichter in collaboration with the group of Dr. T. Cremer (see du Manoir et al. 1993) and since then further developed. Applying CGH to a T-PLL patient we identified a clonal aberration which was not found when following the standards of a tumorcytogenetic analysis (see du Manoir et al. 1993). Thus, further studies are needed in order to assess possible artefacts produced by cell culturing, which affect the data obtained by chromosome banding analysis. CGH is currently being applied to gain further insight into leukemia-specific chromosomal imbalancies. CGH analysis of AML patients showed virtually no discrepancy to the data obtained by chromosome banding (see Bentz et al., Genes, Chromosomes & Cancer 1994). Thus, AML provides tumor material well suited for testing new developments in the CGH evaluation procedure. A recent study in B-CLL, however, revealed a considerable amount of discrepancies between CGH and chromosome banding. This study contributes to a newly funded EC project (PL930055).

4. Major scientific breakthroughs and/or industrial applications

- Assessment of mapping strategies - Clinical evaluation of genome data -
- Definition of several *new diagnostic probe sets* for routine applications (e.g. for the Philadelphia chromosome translocation and for TP53): The corresponding publications set standards for industrial companies developing such diagnostic probes.
- New recurrent aberrations in B-CLL: in contrast to previous assumptions - tumor suppressor genes, in particular *RB1* and *TP53*, are frequently inactivated in chronic lymphocytic leukemia, possibly playing a pathogenetic role in this disease.
- As an alternative to multicolor hybridization probe sets, the new approach of *CGH* - a major breakthrough for the analysis of genomic imbalances in tumors - could be established at a very early time. In addition, important further developments of CGH as well as applications of CGH in hematological diseases were performed within this project.

5. Project Management

In order to manage the project it was necessary - in addition to the lines of communication by telephone and fax - to arrange the following lab visits or meetings:

a) Edith Passage from the lab of INSERM visited the lab of the coordinator at DKFZ to learn the multicolor in situ hybridization technique. She successfully transfered the technology by establishing the procedure back in Marseille (March 16-28, 1992).

b) Berna Beverloo from Rotterdam visited the lab of the coordinator for training in multicolor fluorescence in situ hybridization using 11q specific DNA probes (October 5-16, 1992). She also took probes from Heidelberg to Rotterdam in order to characterize leukemia patient material using these probes.

c) The coordinator Peter Lichter and Hartmut Doehner traveled to Anne Hagemeijer in Rotterdam for a management meeting (March 11-12, 1993). This meeting was necessary to review the current data, to establish a priority list of probes to be included in the multicolor probe set, and to exchange diagnostic DNA probes.

Large quantities of patient specimen preparations were provided to the coordinator by Hagemeijer, Döhner and Zaccaria. DNA Probes were exchanged between Lichter and Fontes, Lichter and Hagemeijer as well as Lichter and Döhner.

Technology was transfered mainly from Lichter to Hagemeijer, Döhner and Fontes.

Joint Publications

- Bentz M., Cabot G., Moos M., Speicher M.R., Ganser A., Lichter P., Döhner H. (1994) Detection of chimeric BCR-ABL genes on bone marrow samples and blood smears in chronic myeloid and acute lymphoblastic leukemia by in situ hybridization. Blood 83, 1922-1928.
- Bentz M., Döhner H., Huck K., Schütz B., Ganser A., Joos S., du Manoir S., Lichter P. (1994) Comparative genomic hybridization in the investigation of myeloid leukemias. Genes Chromosomes & Cancer (in press)
- Döhner H., Pohl S., Bulgay-Mörschel M., Stilgenbauer S., Bentz M., Lichter P. (1993) Trisomy 12 in chronic lymphoid leukemias - a metaphase and interphase cytogenetic analysis. Leukemia 7, 516-520.
- Döhner H., Fischer K., Bentz M., Hansen K., Benner A., Cabot G., Diehl D., Schlenk R., Coy J., Stilgenbauer S., Volkmann M., Galle P.R., Poustka A., Hunstein W., Lichter P. (1994) p53 gene deletion predicts for poor survival and non-response to therapy with purine analogs in chronic B-cell leukemias. Blood (in press).
- Döhner H., Pilz T., Fischer K., Cabot G., Diehl D., Fink T., Stilgenbauer S., Bentz M., Lichter P. (1994) Molecular cytogenetic analysis of RB-1 deletions in chronic B-cell leukemias. Leuk. Lymphoma (in press).
- Stilgenbauer S., Döhner H., Bulgay-Mörschel M., Weitz S., Bentz M., Lichter P. (1993) High frequency of monoallelic retinoblastoma gene deletion in chronic lymphoid leukemia revealed by interphase cytogenetics. Blood 81, 2118-2124.

Individual Publications

- Beverloo H.B., Wijsman J., Smit E.M.E., de Klein A., Hagemeijer A. (1994) Detection of 11q23 abnormalities in acute leukemias of different lineages using RT-PCR, Southern blot analysis and FISH. Br. J. Haem. 87 suppl. 1, 120.
- Darfler M., Magnani I., Kearney L., Wijsman J., Hagemeijer A., Sacchi N. (1994) Interphase cytogenetics of the t(8;21)(q22;q22) associated with acute myelogenous leukemia by two-color fluorescence in situ hybridization. (submitted).

- De Greef G.E., Hagemeijer A., Morgan R., Wijsman J., Hoefsloot L.H., Sandberg A.A., Sacchi N. (1994) Identical fusion transcript associated with different breakpoints in the AML-1 gene in simple and variant t(8;21) acute myeloid leukemia. Leukemia (in press).
- Joos S., Scherthan H., Speicher M.R., Schlegel J., Cremer T., Lichter P. (1993) Detection of amplified genomic sequences by reverse chromosome painting using genomic tumor DNA as probe. Hum. Genet. 90, 584-589.
- Joos S., Fink T.M., Rätsch A., Lichter P. (1994) Mapping and chromosome analysis: the potential of fluorescence in situ hybridization. J Biotech 35, 135-153.
- Fink T., Lichter P., Ohl S., Assum G., Jenne D.E. (1994) Construction of a physical map in the region 17cen-q11.2 by in situ interphase mapping. (manuscript prepared).
- Hernandez J.M., Mecucci C., Beverloo H.B., Wlodarska I., Stul M., Michaux L., Verhoef G., van Orshoven A., Hagemeijer A., van den Berghe H. (1994) Characterization of translocation t(11;15)(q23;q14) in acute non-lymphoblastic leukemia (ANLL). (manuscript prepared).

Closely related publications of the participants

- Bentz, M., Döhner, H., Cabot, G., Lichter, P. (1994) Fluorescence in situ hybridization in leukemias: "The FISH are spawning". Leukemia 8, 1447-1452.
- Chevillard, C., Le Paslier, D., Passage, E., Ougen, P., Billault, A., Boyer, S., Mazan, S., Bachellerie, J.P., Vignal, A., Cohen, D., Fontes, M. (1993) Relationship between Charcot-Marie-Tooth 1A and Smith-Magenis regions. snU3 may be a candidate gene for the Smith-Magenis syndrome. Hum. Mol. Genet. 2, 1235-1243.
  (in the above paper the interaction with the coordinator is acknowledged, but unfortunately it was forgotten to explicitly refer to the EC grant).
- Du Manoir S., Speicher M.R., Joos S., Schröck E., Popp S., Döhner H., Kovacs G., Robert-Nicoud M., Lichter P., Cremer T. (1993) Detection of complete and partial chromosome gains and losses by comparative genomic in situ hybridiyzation. Hum. Genet. 90, 590-610.
- Hagemeijer A., Buijs A., Smit E., Janssen B., Creemers G.-J., van der Plas D., Grosveld G. (1993) Translocation of Bcr to chromosome 9: a new cytogenetic variant detected by FISH in two Ph-negative, Bcr-positive patients with chronic myeloid leukemia. Genes, Chromosomes & Cancer 8:237-245.
- Sacchi N., Nisson P.E., Wations P.C., Faustinella F., Wijsman J., Hagemeijer A. (1994) AML-1 fusion transcripts in t(3;21) positive leukemia: Evidence of molecular heterogeneity and usage of splicing sites frequently involved in the generation of normal AML-1 transcripts. Genes, Chromosomes & Cancer (in press).
- Van Lom K., Hagemeijer A., Smit E.M.E., Löwenberg B. (1993) In situ hybridization on May-Grünwald Giemsa-stained bone marrow and blood smears of patients with hematologic disorders allows detection of cell-lineage-specific cytogenetic abnormalities. Blood 82, 884-888.
- Van Ooteghem R.B.C., Smit E.M.E., Beishuizen A., Lambrechts A.C., vd Blij-Philipsen M., Smilde T.J., Hagemeijer A. (1994) A new B-cell line showing a complex translocation (8;14;18) and Bcl2 rearrangement. Cancer Genet. Cytogenet. 74, 87-94.

Contract number: GENO-CT910013

Contractual period: 1 November 1991 to 31 October 1993

The work of this project started within the group of the coordinator Peter Lichter (participant 01) in February 1992 by the appointments of the undergraduate student Stephan Stilgenbauer (from February 1st to October 31st, 1992), the graduate student Ulrike Mathieu (since April 1st, 1992), and the postdoc Dr. Martin Bentz (from April 1, 1993 to September 30, 1993) and within the group of Anne Hagemeijer (participant 02) with the engagement of the postdoctoral fellow Berna Beverloo (since July 1st 1992). Participants 03, 04, and 05 did not receive funding for personnel by the EC.

Coordinator
Dr. Peter Lichter (01)
Abt. 0675
DKFZ
Im Neuenheimer Feld 280
D-69120 Heidelberg
Germany
Tel: 49 6221 424 609
Fax: 49 6221 424 639

Participants
Dr. Anne Hagemeijer (02)
Faculty of Medicine
Dept. of Cell Biology and Genetics
Erasmus Universiteit
Molewaterplein 50
NL-3000 DR Rotterdam
The Netherlands
Tel: 31 10 408 1111
Fax: 31 10 436 0225

Dr. Hartmut Döhner (03)
Medizinische Klinik und Poliklinik V
Universität Heidelberg
Hospitalstr. 3
D-69115 Heidelberg
Germany
Tel: 49 6221 568 033
Fax: 49 6221 563 813

Dr. Alfonso Zaccaria (04)
Istituto di Ematologia
Università di Bologna
Policlinico S. Orsola
Via G. Massarenti 9
I-40138 Bologna
Italy
Tel: 39 51 6363 680
Fax: 39 51 3989 73

Dr. Michel Fontes (05)
Institut National de la Santé et
de la Recherche Médicale
Institut de Pédiatrie
INSERM U242
F-13385 Marseille
France
Tel: 33 91 784 477
Fax: 33 91 494 194

Human Genome Analysis Programme
M. Hallen and A. Klepsch (Eds.)
IOS Press, 1995

REAGENTS AND METHODS FOR HUMAN GENOME ANALYSIS

G. Schmitz-Agheguian
Boehringer Mannheim, Penzberg, Germany

1. Background information

In order to analyse the structure of the human DNA and to clarify the mechanism of specific human diseases many laboratories have focused on the development of a complete physical map of the human chromosomes with the ultimate goal to sequence the entire human genome. Megabase maps are crucial for human genome analysis since they fill the gap between the fine resolution physical map in the kilobase range, and the low resolution genetic map (linkage map) in the centimorgan range. Megabase mapping has been limited so far by the low number of rare cutter nucleases which allow to fragment human DNA at sites of 8 bp length or longer. Thus, success of the human genome mapping project will strongly depend on new tools for megabase mapping.

2. Objectives and primary approaches

The goal of the cooperative work was to develop new tools for cutting DNA in the megabase range in order to improve the physical mapping of the human genome and to get access to specific regions (genes) of the human genome. Two major objectives were proposed:

1. *New cleavage techniques which cut DNA at sequences greater than 12 base pairs in order to create tools to cut the human genome at any desired site.* This goal should be reached by development of an insertion technique using the intron encoded rare cutter endonuclease I-SceI, by purifying and analysis of another intron encoded rare cutter endonuclease I-CsmI (see report from Dujon laboratory) and by development of artificial nucleases (see report from Schmitz laboratory).

2. *New nucleases which recognize DNA sequences up to 12 base pairs.* This goal was planned to be reached by screening for new restriction endonucleases recognizing 8 bp sequences (see reports from Bouriotis and Brown laboratories) and by modification of restriction endonuclease activity by methylation of the substrate DNA (see reports from Schmitz and Brown laboratories).

Publications

1. A. Thierry and B. Dujon. Nested chromosomal fragmentation in yeast using the meganuclease I-Sce I: a new method for physical mapping of eukaryotic genomes. Nuc. Ac. Res. (1992) 20, 5625-5631.
2. A. Perrin, M. Buckle and B. Dujon. Asymmetrical recognition and activity of the I-Sce I endonuclease on its site and on intron-exon junctions. EMBO J.(1993) 12, 2939-2947.
3. L. Colleaux, C. Rougeulle, P. Avner, B. Dujon. Rapid physical mapping of YAC inserts by random integration of I-Sce I sites. Human molecular genetics (1993) 2, 265-271.
4. C. Rougeulle, L. Colleaux, B. Dujon and P. Avner. Generation and characterisation of an ordered lambda clone array for the 460 kb region surrounding the murine Xist sequence. Human Molecular Genetics (1994, in press).

5. H. Tettelin, A. Thierry, C. Fairhead, A. Perrin, B. Dujon. In *vitro* fragmentation of yeast chromosomes and YACs at artificially inserted sites and applications to genome mapping. Methods in Molecular Genetics (K. W. Adolph, Ed.) Academic Press (1994, in press).
6. N. Storm, T. Walter, K. Mühlegger and G. Schmitz. An Enzymatic Way of Artificial Nuclease. Poster presentation at Conference "Tools for Genome Mapping" Institute Pasteur, January 1994.
7. M. Rina and V. Bouriotis Cloning, purification and characterization of the BseC I DNA methyltransferase from B. *stearorthermophilus*. (1993) Gene: 133, 91-94.
8. M. Rina, M. Markaki and V. Bouriotis Sequence of the cloned bseCIM gene: M. BseCI reveals high homology to M.BanIII. (1994) Gene: In press.
9. A. Reiser, W. Ankenbauer, N. Brown, R. Schmitt and G. Schmitz. "Achilles Heel Cleavage of DNA using Oct2A, *Raf* repressor or MerR as protecting proteins". Poster presentation at Conference "Tools for Genome Mapping" Institut Pasteur, January 1994.
10. Two additional publications are planned from Brown laboratory. One describing the new restriction endonucleases from *Helicobacter pylori* and
11. one in collaboration with Beohringer Mannheim describing the use of MerR in 'Achilles heel' cleavage of DNA.

FINAL REPORT FROM B. DUJON LABORATORY

Project: Application of the rare cutter endonuclease I-Sce I for genome mapping and development of a new rare cutter endonuclease I-Csm I.

Key Words: Intron encoded endonucleases; I-SceI; I-CsmI; insertion vectors; insertion mapping.

1. Background information

Intron encoded endonucleases were discovered in my lab several years ago with the demonstration of the endonucleolytic activity of I-Sce I (Colleaux et al., Cell (1986) 44, 521-533). The much higher specificity of such nucleases compared to the rare cutter bacterial restriction enzymes was also discovered in my lab by analysis of the I-Sce I site by systematic in vitro mutagenesis (Colleaux et al., PNAS (1988) 85, 6022-6026). Several other intron encoded endonucleases have now been characterized from a variety of organisms (reviewed by Dujon, Gene (1989) 82, 91-114). Cleavage specificities are different from one another. Some endonucleases are highly specific, like I-Sce I, others tolerate very degenerate sites and cleave DNA frequently. The basic enzymatic properties of I-Sce I had just been characterized at the start of this program (Monteilhet et al., Nuc.Ac Res. (1990) 18, 1407-1413). Finally an artificial gene had been constructed in my lab to allow overexpression of I-Sce I from E. coli cells (the natural intronic ORF cannot be used, due to the non-universal genetic code in yeast mitochondria) and a preparation of I-Sce I made out of this gene had just been commercialised by Boehringer Mannheim at the start of this program.

The sequence of many other group I introns from a variety of organisms is now available and a significant fraction of them contain long open reading frames that are good candidates for encoding site specific endonucleases. One such case, I-Csm I, had just been described in my lab at the start of this program (Colleaux *et al.*, Mol. Gen. Genet. (1990) 223, 288-296). It is encoded by the mobile group I intron of the apocytochrome b gene of *Chlamydomonas smithii* mitochondria. The advantage of I-CsmI was double: first, the genetic code of Chlamydomonas mitochondria is universal, allowing direct expression of the intronic ORF in *E. coli* or other heterologous expression systems; second, I-Csm I is a member of the same structural subfamily as I-Sce I, suggesting that it may also have a high recognition specificity.

2. Objectives

Two major objectives were proposed by the Institut Pasteur participant:
1. application of the rare cutter endonuclease I-Sce I for genome mapping
2. development of a new rare cutter endonuclease I-Csm I.
    The first objective included the construction of a variety of vectors aimed at inserting artificial I-Sce I sites in different eucaryotic genomes.

3. Work performed and results

First objective: construction of several vectors and their applications to assess their properties.
    1. *Insertion vectors containing I-Sce I cassette*: Plasmid vectors have been constructed for yeast (pAF100, pAF101, pAF107 and pAF109) and for YAC inserts containing mouse DNA (pAF123) or human DNA (pAF131). Their maps and properties are described in publications 1, 3, 4 and 5. The purpose of these vectors is to insert artificial I-Sce I sites for genome mapping.
    Other insertion vectors have been developed for mouse cells from a defective retrovirus in which the I-Sce I site was placed in the LTR. The purpose of these vectors is to insert artificial I-Sce I sites for in *vivo site* specific gene replacement (Choulika et al.,Nature (1994, submitted).
    Cutting bacterial, yeast and mouse DNAs with I-Sce I at artificially inserted sites has been achieved. Detailed mapping by secondary partial digest with a frequent cutter endonuclease has been tried on DNAs from transgenic yeast and mouse strains. Fragments were revealed by indirect end-labelling.
    2. *A new mapping strategy has been developed*: It consists of building artificial I-Sce I maps by inserting I-Sce I sites at a variety of places along a given yeast chromosome. Nested chromosomal fragments can then be prepared and used as probes to locate genes, cosmids or lambda clones. The strategy, which makes use of site specific homologous recombination in yeast, has been adapted to mapping YAC inserts containing mouse or human DNA. The feasibility and usefulness of this method were determined on mapping the chromosome X inactivation center in mouse (publication 4), and on mapping two different human YAC inserts.

Second objective: development of I-Csm I as a site specific endonuclease.

Several *E.coli* vectors expressing the rare cutter endonuclease I-Csm I have been constructed. Preparations of the enzyme have been made from induced *E.coli* cells containing these vectors. Antibodies have been raised against I-Csm I. The enzymatic activity of I-Csm I has been studied in different conditions but proved to be very weak, if any. Thus the enzyme preparations made until now are not directly applicable for mapping purposes.

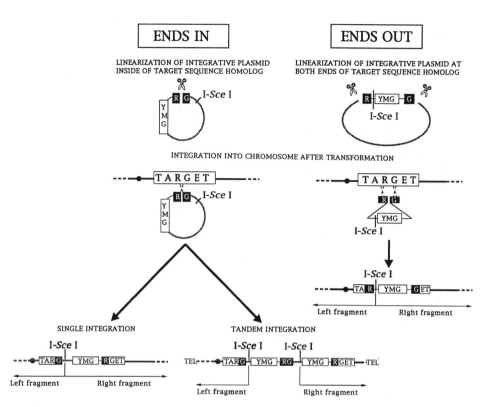

Figure 1

Topologies used for yeast integrative transformation using an I-*Sce* I cassette. Yeast chromosomes are shown in bold lines with a black circle to represent the centromere. The targetted sequence is boxed. Transforming DNA is shown with "YMG": Yeast Marker Gene and "RG": target sequence homolog.

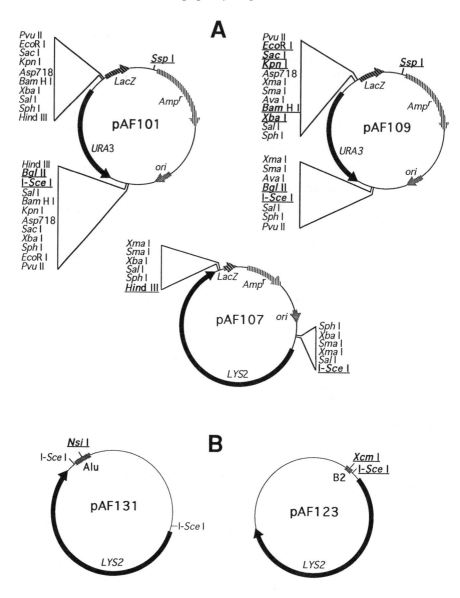

Figure 2

Maps of basic integrative vectors.
2a. Vectors for integration of the I-*Sce* I- *URA3* or I-*Sce* I- *LYS2* cassettes. All vectors
are pUC19 derivatives. Unique sites are bold-underlined. Duplicated sites available to
prepare the cassettes are also indicated. Absent sites from pAF101 and pAF109 are *Bcl*
I, *Cla* I, *Eag* I, *Hpa* I, *Nhe* I, *Nru* I, *Sac* II, *Sna* BI and *Xho* 1, and from pAF107: *Apa*
I, *Cla* I, *Eag* I, *Mlu* I, *Not* I, *Nsi* I, *Pac* I and *Xcm* I.

2b. Vectors for multiple integration of the I-*Sce* I- *LYS2* cassette into YACs. All vectors
are pBluescriptSK+ derivatives. Unique sites are bold-underlined. pAF123 contains the
B2 repetitive element from mouse DNA, pAF131 contains the Alu repetitive element
from human DNA in which an *Nsi* I site has been inserted by *in vitro* mutagenesis.

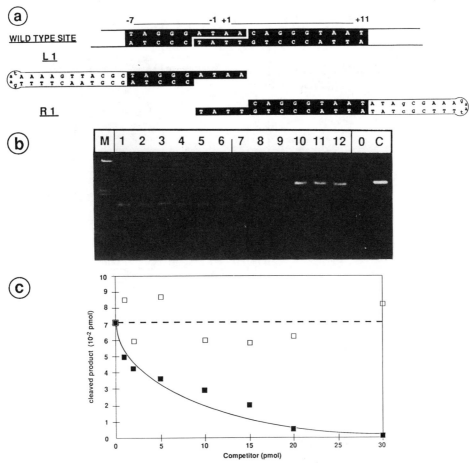

Figure 3
Effects of the two reaction products on enzyme activity

3a. Top: Sequence of the wild type recognition site of I-*Sce* I in the intron less gene. Bottom: Oligonucleotides L1 and R1. Each oligonucleotide has been synthesised as a hairpin with 3'OH overhangs identical to the cleaved products. Capital, lower case letters and black box as in figure 1.

3b. 0.14 pmoles of *Dra* I digested plasmid pSCM522 (used as wild-type substrate) were mixed with various amounts of the oligonucleotides L1 (lanes 1 to 6) or R1 (lanes 7 to 12) at 0°C in standard incubation buffer and 1 unit of I-*Sce* I was added in a total reaction volume of 20 μl. Reactions were started by addition of 0.005 M MgCl^2 and transferred at 37°C. Subsequent steps as in 2a with 30 min. of incubation time.

Lanes 1 to 6: 0.4, 2, 4, 200, 400 and 800 pmoles of L1, respectively. Lanes 7 to 12: 0.4, 2, 4, 200, 400 and 800 pmoles of R1, respectively. Lane 0: control without oligonucleotide, lane C: control without enzyme, lane M: molecular weight marker (λ *Mlu* I digest).

3c. 5 pmoles of 5' end labelled FF3 were mixed with various amounts of the oligonucleotides L2 ($\square$) or R2 ($\blacksquare$) at 0°C in standard incubation buffer and 0.1 unit of I-*Sce* I was added in a total reaction volume of 10μl. The reactions were started by addition of 0.008 MgCl$_2$ and transfer at 37°C. Subsequent steps as in 2a with 30 min. incubation time.

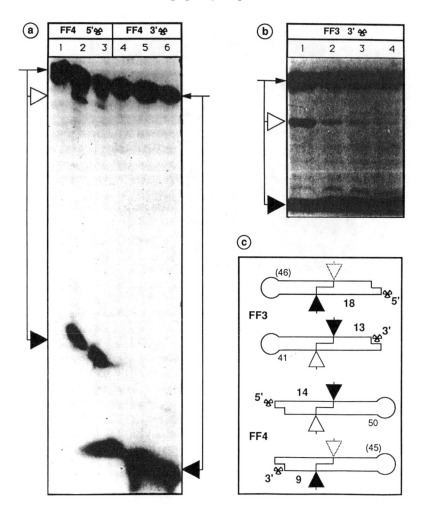

Figure 4
Asymmetrical nicking activity of I-*Sce* I

4a. 4 pmoles of 5' end-labelled (lanes 1 to 3) or 3' end-labelled (lanes 4 to 6) of FF4 oligonucleotide, were mixed with 1 unit of I-*Sce* I at 0°C in standard incubation buffer. Reactions were started by addition of 0.008 M of $MgCl_2$ (except lane 4: 0.002 M $MgCl_2$). Subsequent steps as in 2a. Lane 1: control without Mg^{++}, incubation 15 min.; lanes 2 and 5: incubation for 2 min.; lanes 3, 4 and 6: incubation for 15 min. Thin arrows indicates uncleaved substrate, black arrows indicates cleaved product and white arrows, nicked fragment.

4b. 5 pmoles of 3' end labelled FF3 oligonucleotide were mixed with 5 units of I-*Sce* I at O°C in standard incubation buffer. Subsequent steps as in figure 2a except for incubation times (lanes 1 to 4, 0.25, 0.5, 1 and 2 min., respectively). Arrows as in 4a.

4c. Summary of 5' and 3' end-labelling of oligonucleotides FF3 and FF4. Black arrows indicate first cleavage from the label: cleavage corresponding to double strand break or to nick cannot be distinguished. White arrows indicate the second cleavage from the label correspond to nick (dashes: nick are not observed). Size of labelled products corresponding to each possible cut are indicated.

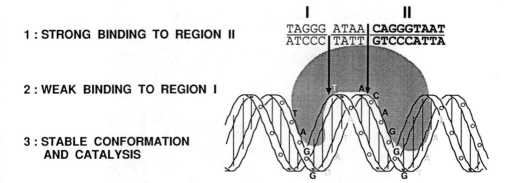

1 : STRONG BINDING TO REGION II

2 : WEAK BINDING TO REGION I

3 : STABLE CONFORMATION AND CATALYSIS

Figure 5
A two step recognition model for I-*Sce* I.

Two recognition regions (I and II) are identified. Binding of the enzyme is assumed to take place in region II, followed by binding to region I, if present. After tight binding occurred, catalysis takes place as indicated by arrows. The catalytic domain of the enzyme is likely to face the minor grove while recognition domains could face the flanking major groves in regions I and II.

4. Coordination and cooperation

There have been three joint meetings of the subcontractors. The last one, held at Institut Pasteur in January 1994, also included a selected list of invited speakers from various parts of the world and was attended by a group of ca. 80 external participants.

The Institut Pasteur group has benefited greatly from the preparations of I-Sce I enzyme made at Boehringer Mannheim GmbH. On the other hand, our expertise with yeast mapping and sequencing has been determinant in developing the vectors and methods for the new mapping procedure with rare cutter endonucleases.

Publications

1. A. Thierry and B. Dujon. Nested chromosomal fragmentation in yeast using the meganuclease I-Sce I: a new method for physical mapping of eukaryotic genomes. Nuc. Ac. Res. (1992) 20, 5625-5631.
2. A. Perrin, M. Buckle and B. Dujon: Asymmetrical recognition and activity of the I-Sce I endonuclease on its site and on intron-exon junctions. EMBO J. (1993) 12, 2939-2947.
3. L. Colleaux, C. Rougeulle, P. Avner, B. Dujon and P. Avner: Rapid physical mapping of YAC inserts by random integration of I-Sce I sites. Human molecular genetics (1993) 2, 265-271
4. C. Rougeulle, L. Colleaux, B. Dujon and P. Avner: Generation and characterisation of an ordered lambda clone array for the 460 kb region surrounding the murine Xist sequence. Human Molecular Genetics (1994, in press).
5. Tettelin, A. Thierry, C. Fairhead, A. Perrin, G. Dujon: *In vitro* fragmentation of yeast chromosomes and YACs at artificially inserted sites and applications to genome mapping. Methods in Molecular Genetics (K.W. Adolph, Ed.) Academic Press (1994, in press).

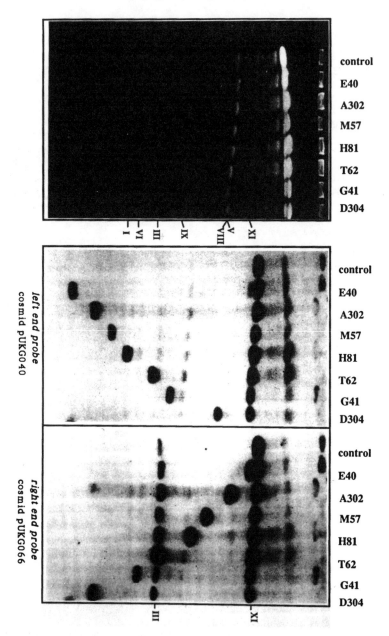

Figure 6
Mapping the I-*Sce* I sites of transgenic yeast strains by hybridization with left end and right end probes of chromosome XI.

Chromosomes from FY1679 (control) and the seven transgenic yeast strains were digested with I-*Sce* I under conditions described in Materials and Methods. Transgenic strains were placed in order as explained in figure 3. Electrophoresis conditions were as in figure 2. ^{32}P labelled cosmids pUKG040 and pUKG066 were used as left end and right end probes, respectively.

Table 1
Set of transgenic strains with I-*Sce* sites used for genome mapping

Chr.	Strain	Integrative vector	Disrupted gene	Ref.
IV	FY23/RD112			
	FY23/RD248			
XV	FY23/RO181 (*)			
	FY1679/O321	pAF412		
	FY1679/O272	pAF403		
	FY1679/O471	pAF421		
	FY1679/O306	pAF411		
	FY1679/O477	pAF426		
	FY1679/O491	pAF430		
	FY1679/O323	pAF416		
	FY1679/O497	pAF435		
VII	FY23/RG007			
	FY23/RG162			
	FY1679/G05	pAF453	cdc43::URA3- I -*Sce* I	
	FY1679/G06	pAF454	cdc20::URA3- I -*Sce* I	
	FY1679/G11	pAF460	dst1::URA3- I -*Sce* I	
	FY1679/G09	pAF457	pdr1::URA3- I -*Sce* I	
	FY1679/G12	pAF461	gcd2::URA3- I -*Sce* I	
	FY1679/G13	pAF462	spt6::URA3- I -*Sce* I	
	FY1679/G15	pAF465	hip1::URA3- I -*Sce* I	
	FY1679/G19	pAF471	mes1::URA3- I -*Sce* I	
XVI	FY23/RP142			
	FY23/RP270			
XIII	FY23/R255			
II	FY23/RB231 (*)			
XIV	FY23/RN208 (*)			
X	FY1679/JC41	pC41		(1)
	FY1679/JC82	pC82		(1)
	FY1679/JT21	pAF304	tif2::URA3- I -*Sce* I	
XI	FY1679/KA302	pAF302	fas1::URA3- I -*Sce* I	(2)
	FY1679/KD304	pAF304	tif1::URA3- I -*Sce* I	(2)
	FY1679/KE40	pAF305		(2)
	FY1679/KG41	pAF306	mak11 or cdc16::URA3- I -*Sce* I	(2)
	FY1679/KH81	pAF021		(2)
	FY1679/KM57	pAF307		(2)
	FY1679/KT62	pAF308		(2)
V	FY23/R216 (*)			
VIII	FY23/R165			
IX	FY23/RI117			
	FY1679/I20	pAF473	suc2::URA3- I -*Sce* I	

Table 1 (continued)

Chr.	Strain	Integrative vector	Disrupted gene	Ref.
III	FY23/CC6	pAF201	ycr521::URA3- I -Sce I	(3)
	FY73/CC11	pAF201	ycr521::URA3- I -Sce I	(3)
	FY1679/CC14	pAF201	ycr521::URA3- I -Sce I	(3)
	FY1679/CC23	pAF202	ycr522::URA3- I -Sce I	(3)
	FY1679/CA34	pAF228	ycr524::URA3- I -Sce I	(3)
VI	FY23/RF222 (*)			
I	FY23/RA170			

-Yeast chromosomes carrying I-Sce I cassettes are listed in order of decreasing size (chromosome XII is omitted).
-Transgenic strains nomenclature indicates transformed host strain (refer to table I) followed, after the slash, by a combination of letters and numbers to specify the integrated site. Cassettes inserted at random are indicated by R as the first letter.
-(*) indicates reduced mobility on PFGE.
-Integrative vectors are derived from pAF101 or pAF109 (see figure 2).

(1)   M.-E. Huang, J.-C. Chuat, A. Thierry, B. Dujon and F. Galibert, DNA Sequence (in press).
(2)   A. Thierry, A. Perrin, J. Boyer, C. Fairhead and B. Dujon, Nucl. Ac. Res. 19, 189 (1991).
(3)   A. Thierry, C. Fairhead and B. Dujon, Yeast 6, 521 (1990).

FINAL REPORT FROM G. SCHMITZ LABORATORY (T. WALTER LAB)

Project: Development of artificial nucleases for genome mapping.

Key Words: Artificial nuclease; ortho-phenanthroline; enzymatic synthesis; oxidative cutting; triple helix.

1. Background information

Currently, fragmentation of nucleic acids for cloning and analysis is performed with naturally occurring restriction enzymes with a recognition sequence of 4 - 8 base pairs (bp). More recently intron encoded sequence specific nucleases (transposases) which cut less frequent and recognise 15 to 18 bp have also been applied. An alternative technology for less frequent cutting is the combined use of site specific DNA methylases and restriction endonucleases which reduce the specificity to 10 - 12 bp. Drawback of these methods are the availability of only a few specificities.

Several groups have investigated methods to create artificial nucleases which use the inherent specificity of nucleic acid hybridization of synthetic oligonucleotides. Thus the specificity of the synthetic nuclease can be designed by the nucleotide sequence and the length of the oligonucleotide according to the experiment. Subsequently to the oligonucleotide synthesis reactive moieties have been coupled to the oligonucleotide by chemical means. These artificial nucleases display indeed a high specificity, however, the overall cutting efficiency is low. In addition the preparation of these reagents is very laborious which has limited practical application in the past.

2. Objectives and primary approaches

The objective of this project was the development of artificial nucleases which allow the researcher to design the target recognition sequence and the frequency of cutting according to the needs of the experiments mainly for rare cutting of complete genoms. Our strategy utilises the ultimate specificity of nucleic acid hybridization either by Watson / Crick base paring or triple helix formation for target recognition and the introduction of a small chemical group, ortho-phenanthroline (OP), which executes the cutting function. We have chosen well established enzymatic nucleic acids modification methods for incorporation of OP since the acceptance of new technologies is highly dependent on the ease and convenience of its application. Both, RNA and DNA with incorporation of several OP were planed to allow for wide variability and more efficient cutting due to multiple reaction centres.

3. Results and discussion

Using conventional and established nucleotide chemistry different nucleotide triphosphates coupled to OP via a spacer arm have been synthesized. The length of the spacer arm has been varied in order to achieve optimal incorporation and cutting. The following substances have been produced during the course of this project:
* phenanthrolineamido-5-[(2-thia)-butylamido (4,9,-dioxa)-dodecylamido-vinyl]-UTP (OP-24-UTP),
* phenanthrolineamido-5-[(2-thia)-butylamido (4,9,-dioxa)-dodecylamido-vinyl]-dUTP (OP-24-dUTP),
* phenanthrolineamido-5-[(2-thia)-butylamido-allyl]-UTP (OP-11-UTP),
* phenanthrolineamido-5-[(2-thia)-butylamido-allyl]-dUTP (OP-11-dUTP)

The structure was analysed and confirmed by NMR and mass-spectroscopy. The synthesis of phenanthrolineamido-5-vinyl-dUTP (OP-4-dUTP) failed. Also the synthesis of ^{14}C labelled OP-24-UTP was unsuccessful due to impurities in the purchased radiolabled chemicals.

Reaction conditions for enzymatic incorporation of the various OP-derivatised nucleotide triphosphates have been optimised for the following labeling enzymes: terminal transferase (EC 2.7.7.31), Klenow-enzyme (DNA-polymerase I, "large fragment", EC 2.7.7.7), Taq DNA-polymerase (EC 2.7.7.7), SP6 RNA-polymerase and T7 RNA-polymerase (EC 2.7.7.6).

Ultimately, the conditions for the target recognition and the cutting reaction have been varied for single and double stranded nucleic acids.

1. Synthesis and functionality of OP modified nucleotides: The synthesis of OP-24-(d)UTP and OP-11-(d)UTP (Fig. 1) was performed with 50 % yield, respectively. The structure was proofed by ^{1}H- ^{31}P-NMR and mass spectroscopy. The synthesised OP modified nucleotide triphosphates were active in our activity test were the substance (e.g. OP-24-dUTP) is incubated with substrate DNA, CuSO$_4$, and mercaptopropionic acid (MPA) under cutting reaction conditions (Fig. 2). The confirmed reaction was pH independent. The ccc-form of the employed pBR 322 DNA converted to the oc-form after 5 minutes. A small amount of linear DNA was observed after 15 minutes. Longer incubation resulted in complete degradation of the DNA.

2. *Incorporation efficiency of the synthesised derivatised nucleotides*: The tailing reaction was performed with OP-11-(d)UTP and OP-24-(d)UTP. The incorporation rate of modified dUTP is in the range of 4-6 nucleotides after 60 minutes incubation. With OP-UTP only two residues were incorporated as was expected from the known preference of terminal transferase for deoxynucleotide-triphosphates (Fig. 3).

OP-dUTP was also accepted by the Klenow enzyme. However the reaction rate is much slower than with unmodified nucleotides. The primer oligonucleotide was annealed to single stranded M13 DNA and extended to the double stranded oc-form. The reaction is retarded by increasing the amount of OP-dUTP. After 4 hours the starting DNA is shifted to a higher molecular weight by 50% . After over night incubation the single strand was almost completely filled in to the double stranded form.

The attempt of RNA synthesis by *in vitro* transcription failed using an amount of 100 % OP-UTP in the reaction mixture. Even with lower amounts of OP-UTP down to 30 % of total UTP the RNA synthesis rate was dramatically decreased.

3. *Target recognition*: OP derivatised nucleic acids were hybridized to single strand and partially denatured ds DNA targets under various stringency conditions. Specificity of target recognition and the hybridisation efficiency was confirmed by trial hybridisation with digoxigenin (DIG) labeled probes and anti-DIG-AP detection and was found to be almost quantitative. In a second approach triple helix formation with poly-pyrimidine oligonucleotides has been performed. Triple helix formation was confirmed by application of biotin and OP double-labeled oligonucleotides. Thus, the triple helix complex can be separated with magnetic forces and be quantitated. Approximately 10 % of the target DNA was found to be in a triple helix complex.

4. *Scission results*: An OP-end labeled 30mer oligonucleotide was used from an equal molar ratio to a 200 fold excess over the homologue target DNA. With low amounts of the oligonucleotide only inefficient scission was observed. Increasing the concentration of the modified oligonucleotide induced degradation of the target DNA after 120 minutes incubation (Fig. 4).

The filled in double stranded M13 DNA was completely degradated after 5 minutes cleavage reaction.

Triple helix complexes of super coiled plasmid DNA formed with OP-labeled poly-pyrimidine oligonucleotides were quantitatively converted to the oc form. Thus we conclude that only one strand was cut by the OP directed scission reaction.

4. Major scientific breakthroughs and/or industrial applications

The synthesis of various OP derivatised nucleotidetriphosphates has been successfully been performed for the first time. Enzymatic incorporation has been established with several DNA and RNA polymerases. However, no future work is planned on this project. Due to the low efficiency of the cleavage reaction and detection of rather nicking of one strand than double strand cleavage there is at present no practical use of this technology.

5. Major cooperative links

Valuable input was given and suggestions were made for the progress of the project by all participants during the regular project meetings. There was no direct interrelation due to the specific objectives and aspects of the artificial nuclease project which did not overlap with work done by other participants.

Publications

"An Enzymatic Way of Artificial Nuclease Synthesis." N. Storm, T. Walter, K. Mühlegger and G. Schmitz. Poster presentation at Conference "Tools for Genome Mapping" Institute Pasteur, Paris, January 16 - 18.1994.

The work was performed by N. Storm.

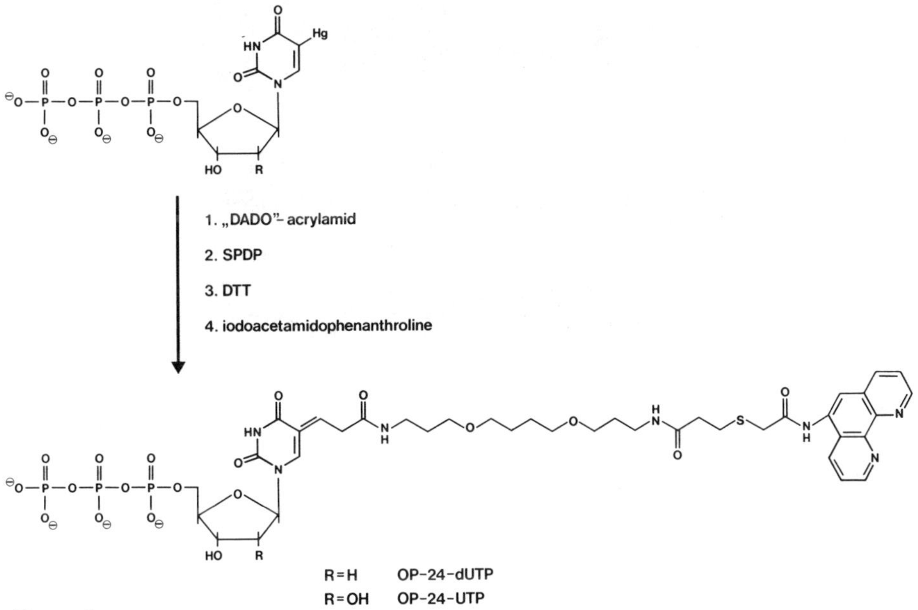

1. „DADO"- acrylamid
2. SPDP
3. DTT
4. iodoacetamidophenanthroline

R=H   OP-24-dUTP
R=OH   OP-24-UTP

Figure 1

Reaction scheme of the o-phenanthroline-24-(d)UTP synthesis (OP-24-(d)UTP). OP-11-(d)UTP was synthesised in a similar way. The starting material was 5-(3-aminoallyl)-(d)UTP. It was coupled with SPDP, reduced with DTT and reacted with iodoacetamidophenanthroline in the same way.

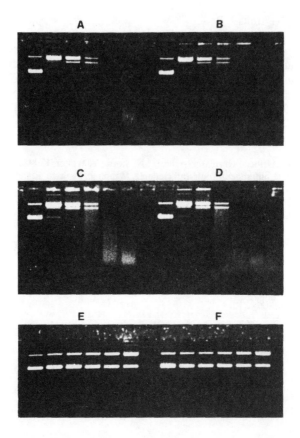

Figure 2

Activity test of the unincorporated OP-11-dUTP at different pH. Reaction conditions:
~ 5 μg DNA (pBR 322 ccc), 5mM Tris-HCl, 10 mM MgCl$_2$, 100 mM KCl, 0.2mM OP-11-dUTP, 9 μM CuSO$_4$. Start with 6mM 3-mercaptopropionic acid (3-MPA).
Stop with 17mM neocuproine.

Samples were taken after 0, 5, 15, 30, 60, 120 minutes.

Series:	A B	C	D	E		F
		without Cu^{2+}		without 3-MPA		
pH	6.0	7.0	8.0	9.0	7.0	7.0

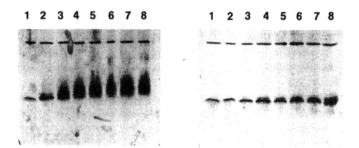

Figure 3

Tailing reaction of a 30mer oligonucleotide with OP-11-UTP and -dUTP Reaction conditions: 200mM K-cacodylate, 25mM Tris-HCl pH 6.6, 0.25 mg/ml BSA, 5mM CoCl$_2$, 1mM OP-11-UTP or dUTP, 250 pmol 30mer, 500 U terminal transferase incubation at 37o C.

lane:	1	2	3	4	5	6	7	8
reaction time:	0	5	15	30	45	60	75	90 min

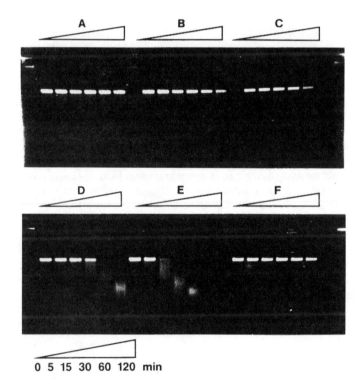

Figure 4

Cleavage reaction under conditions shown in figure 2 at p 7.0 after hybridisation of the tailed 30mer to OP-11-dUTP.

FINAL REPORT FROM V. BOURIOTIS LABORATORY

Project: Screening for novel restriction endonuncleases and strategies for producing infrequent cleavage sites in DNA.

Key Words: Restriction endonucleases; methyl transferases; screening; cloning; RE/ME rare cutting.

1. Objectives

1. Screening of procaryotic strains for the identification of new restriction endonucleases including rare cutters.
   2. Cloning, purification and characterization of the BseCI DNA methyltransferase from *Bacillus stearothermophilus*. Sequence of the cloned bseCIM gene.
   3. Application of M.BseCI in combination with restriction endonuclease DpnI for genome mapping.

2. Results

1. 242 procaryotic strains were screened and 31 restriction endonucleases were identified. Six restriction endonucleases were purified from contaminating nuclease activities and their recognition sequences and cleavage sites were identified. The enzymes are isoschizomers of NaeI, BstNI, Sau3AI, AgeI, NarI and Sau96I.
   2. The gene (bseCIM) encoding the BseCI DNA methyltransferase from *a Bacillus stearothermophilus* species was cloned and expressed in *E. Coli* using plasmid vector pBR322. The Mtase was purified to homogeneity and further characterized. Its size as determined by SDS and gel filtration was 68 kDa, suggesting that the enzyme exists as a monomer. When lambda DNA was used as substrate the optimum temperature for Mtase activity was determined to be 50-55°C and the optimum pH to be ~7.4. M.BseCI is inhibited by concentrations of NaCI and KCI greater than 50 mM. It does not require Mg^{2+} for activity and methylates the 3' adenine residue in the sequence 5'-ATCGAT-3' similarly to its isoschizomer M.ClaI. The nucleotide (nt) sequence of a 2357 bp BspMII-EcoRI fragment encoding the bseCIM gene was determined. The sequence predicts a methyltransferase of 579 aa, Mr 66700. Comparison of the deduced aa sequence of M.BseCI with sequences of various Mtases revealed a significant homology of M.BseCI to m6A-MTases especially to its isoschizomer MBanIII *from Bacillus aneurinolyticus*.

3. Cooperation

Ms. A. Christodoulidou was trained at Boehringer Mannheim on the use of Pulsed Field Gel Electrophoresis.

4. Future goals

The very limited knowledge of 3D structures of DNA Mtases makes the crystallographic analysis of the BseCI Mtase an interesting undertaking. The protein has been purified in mg quantities and crystallization experiments are in progress.

Publications

1. Cloning, purification and characterization of the BseC I DNA methyltransferase from *B. stearothermophilus*. M. Rina and V. Bouriotis (1993) Gene: 133,91-94.
2. Sequence of the cloned bseCIM gene: M. BseCI reveals high homology to M.BanIII M. Rina, M. Markaki and V. Bouriotis (1994) Gene: In press.

FINAL REPORT FROM N.L. BROWN LABORATORY

Project: Isolation of novel restriction endonucleases and strategies for producing infrequent cleavage sites in DNA.

Key Words: Restriction endonucleases; screening; RE/ME rare cutting; Achilles Heel; MerR.

1. Objectives and primary approaches

The immediate objectives of the Birmingham laboratory and the approaches used were:
1. *The isolation of novel restriction endonucleases.* Standard methods of screening bacterial strains were to be used to identify bacterial strains containing type II restriction endonucleases; those strains in which endonucleases which cleaved small bacteriophage DNAs were not detected were to be screened for rare-cutting endonucleases.

2. *Strategies for producing infrequent cleavage sites in DNA.* The main strategy for producing rare cleavage was through the modification of restriction endonuclease activity by methylation of the substrate DNA. Attempts were to be made to purify a modification methylase and use it to modify the recognition sequences of a second restriction-modification systems, such that the recognition site of the second system could not be modified by the second modification enzyme, but could be cleaved by the second endonuclease. Other strategies were expected to evolve in collaboration with the other participants.

2. Results and discussion

1. *Novel restriction endonucleases.* A preliminary screen of 15 strains of bacteria has been completed. The following enzymes have been identified:

Source Strain	Enzyme	Recognition Site
Anabaena berrow	*Abe*I	GG/WCC (AvaII)
	*Abe*II	TGC/GCA (MstI)
Aphanizomenon flos-aquae CCAP 1401/1	*Aph*I	?
	*Aph*II	?
Nostoc muscorum PCC6719	*Nmu*(6719) I	C/YCGRG (AvaI)
	Nmu(6719) II	GG/WCC (AvaII)
Helicobacter pylori (Roberts)	*Hpy*I	GT/AC (RsaI)
	*Hpy*II	GTN/NAC (NEW)
Helicobacter pylori (type strain)	*Hpy*AI	GAT/ATC (EcoRV)
	*Hpy*AII	? (NEW)
	*Hpy*AIII	?

Of these, AphI and AphII proved to be too unstable to characterise further; HpyII and HpyAII are new specifications, but the latter is contaminated with HpyAIII (specificity unknown). HpyAII and HpyAIII are still therefore being characterised. One of the HpyAII cleavage sites is in the sequence CCGCG/GTGG. The remaining enzymes are isoschizomers of known enzymes.

The optimum reaction conditions for the Hpy enzymes were determined to be:

Source Strain	Enzyme	Recognition site	pH opt.	[KCl] mM	T°C
Helicobacter pylori (Roberts)	*Hpy*I	GT/AC (RsaI)	7.5	100	55
	*Hpy*II	GTN/NAC (NEW)	7.5	100	55
Helicobacter pylori (type strain)	*Hpy*AI	GAT/ATC(EcoRV)	7.5	0	37
	*Hpy*AII	?CCGCG/GTGG (NEW) in Bluescript polylinker			
	*Hpy*AIII	?	?	?	?

The new specificities add to the armoury of available restriction endonuclease specificities for the digestion of DNA, but - with the possible exception of *Hpy*AII - will cut too frequently to be of use in obtaining specific large fragments of genomic DNA. No restriction endonucleases of rare specificity were found by this random screening approach.

2. *Strategies for producing rare cleavage of DNA* have been done in two ways:
a. Combinations of restriction endonucleases and modification methylases to generate high specificity combinations of enzymes have been investigated.

A potentially useful line of enquiry using the restriction/modification enzymes from *Enterobacter aerogenes* (recognition sequence 5'YGGCCR), *Streptomyces fimbriatus* (5'-GGCCNNNNNGGCC) and *Rhodopseudomonas spheriodes* (5'GTAC) proved intractable. This was due to the difficulty in obtaining active modification methylases from the last two of these strains. We purified the *R.Eae*I restriction endonuclease and

M.EaeI modification methylase from *E. aerogenes* PW201. *S. fimbriatus* and *R. spheroides* biomass provided by Boehringer Mannheim GmbH allowed us to attempt a large number of different purification methods. This line of investigation was abandoned due to the difficulty in isolating some of the required enzymes.

b. Protection of selected sites by DNA-binding proteins (the 'Achilles heel' method) has been performed in collaboration with Boehringer Mannheim GmbH, using the MerR regulatory protein purified and provided by my laboratory. We constructed an expression vector in my laboratory that allowed overproduction of the MerR protein, and we established conditions for storing MerR in stable, active form. The 'Achilles Heel' methylation protection experiments were performed at Boehringer-Mannheim, and the results of the experiments are reported elsewhere.

3. Scientific and industrial applications

The programme of research was intended to supply underpinning technology for the human genome project. The isolation of two new restriction endonucleases provides further useful additions to the available enzymes for dissecting DNA. The use of MerR in the 'Achilles Heel' approach is promising and may develop further when mutant MerR proteins have been produced in the Birmingham laboratory.

4. Major cooperative links

Collaboration between the Birmingham laboratory and Boehringer-Mannheim GmbH allowed the following activities in the programme, which would have not been possible in the absence of this collaboration. The provision of biomass of *S. fimbriatus* and *R. sheroides* by Boehringer-Mannheim enabled the Birmingham group exhaustively to test methods for stable preparation of modification methylases from these two strains. The overexpression and purification of the MerR protein by the Birmingham laboratory allowed Boehringer-Mannheim to undertake a successful series of 'Achilles heel' experiments. Further work on the latter approach is planned should the Birmingham group be successful in obtaining DNA binding of lower specificity but high affinity with some of their mutant MerR proteins.

Publications

1. "Achilles Heel Cleavage of DNA using Oct2A, Raf repressor or MerR as protecting proteins." A. Reiser, W. Ankenbauer, N. Brown, R. Schmitt and G. Schmitz. Poster presentation at Conference "Tools for Genome Mapping" Institut Pasteur, January 1994.
2. Two publications are planned. One describing the new restriction endonucleases from *Helicobacter pylori* and
3. one in collaboration with Boehringer-Mannheim GmbH describing the use of MerR in "Achilles heel" cleavage of DNA.

FINAL REPORT FROM G. SCHMITZ LABORATORY
(W. ANKENBAUER LAB)

Project: Achilles Heel Cleavage of DNA by combining the activities of sequence specific DNA binding proteins with DNA Methylase and Restriction Endonuclease.

Key Words: Achilles Heel cleavage; MerR; Raf repressor; OctA; restriction endonucleases; DNA methylases.

1. Background information

Mapping and manipulation of very large genomes would be faciliated by the availability of DNA cleavage methods with very high site specifity which cut chromosomal DNA into a small number of fragments. It was shown by Koob *et al.* (Koob, M.; Grimes, E. and Szybalski, W. (1988) Science **241**, 1084-1086.) that the combination of a sequence specific DNA binding protein, a DNA methylase and a restriction endonuclease can be used to create a "cleavage sequence", which is a combination of the recognition sites of these proteins. With this technique any restriction site that can be selectively protected from methylation can be made unique. This approach was called Achilles Heel Cleavage. Koob *et al.* used the combined activity of three proteins:
1. a repressor, which specifically binds to very rare sites (operators) of about 20 bp in length.
2. a modification methylase, which methylates all corresponding restriction sites with the exception of those protected by the repressor, and
3. a restriction endonuclease with the same specificity as the modification methylase.

2. Objectives and primary approaches

Cleavage at a 20 bp sequence, used in primary studies, should statistically give fragments of 1×10^{12} base pairs. The aim of our project was to develop cleavage reagents which cleave more frequently and therefore we analysed other DNA binding proteins, which protect smaller recognition sequences.
  Three combinations of proteins were tested:

1. The eucaryotic transcription factor Oct2A in combination with M.NlaIII and R.NlaIII

The octamer sequence ATGCAAAT is a functional element in the promotors of immunoglobulin heavy (IgH) and light-chain (IgL) genes and in the heavy chain enhancer. This motif also appears in the promotors of the ubiquitously expressed snRNA and histone H2B genes. The lymphoid cell-specific octamer transcription factor Oct 2A interacts specifically with this conserved sequence element (Kemler, I.; Schreiber, E.; Müller, M. M.; Mathias, P. and Schaffner, W. (1989) EMBO J. **8**, 2001-2008.).
  For the Achilles Heel Cleavage we combined Oct2A with the restriction/modification system NlaIII of Neisseria lactamica which recognizes the sequence CATG. *M.NlaIII*

is adenine-specific.

With this combination a final cleavage sequence of 9 bp would be created which gives statistically one cut per 262 144 base pairs.

```
ATGCAAAT          binding site of Oct2A
CATG              recognition sequence of M.NlaIII
CATG              recognition sequence of R.NlaIII
```
```
CATGCAAAT         Achilles Heel Cleavage sequence
```

2. MerR protein in combination with M.SssI and R.MaeII

The metal-sensing regulatory protein MerR controls the transcriptional regulation of mer, the bacterial operon encoding resistance to inorganic mercury. In the absence of Hg(II) MerR represses, in the presence of Hg(II) MerR activates the transcription of the mer operon. MerR binds as a dimer to a seven bp dyad symmetrical repeat located between the -10 and -35 hexamer of the mer promotor (Livrelli, V.; Lee, I.W. and Summers, A.O. (1993) J. Biol. Chem. **268**, 2623-2631.).

For the Achilles Heel Cleavage the MerR protein was combined with the CpG DNA methylase *SssI* and the restriction endonuclease *MaeII*, which recognizes the sequence ACGT. *M.SssI* methylates completely and exclusively all cytosine residues within the dinucleotide recognition site 5' CG 3'.

This approach gives a cleavage sequence of 16 bp with a statistic occurrence of once per $4,3 \times 10^9$ bp.

```
TCCGTACNNNNGTACGGA     binding site of MerR protein
    CG   CG            recognition sequence of M.SssI
    ACGTACGT           recognition sites for R.MaeII
```
```
TCCGTACGTACGTACGGA     Achilles Heel Cleavage sequence
```

3. Raf repressor in combination with M.SssI and R.MaeII

The initial plans to use Oct2A and MerR proteins for Achilles Heel Cleavage were realized. In addition to these systems another protein was analyzed, the Raf repressor.

The Raf repressor negatively regulates the transcription of the plasmid borne Raf operon consisting of three genes encoding enzymes required for uptake and hydrolysis of Raffinose in *E.coli*. Raf repressor binds to an operator with two 18 bp palindromic nucleotide sequences that flank the -35 Raf promotor box. But as gel shift assays revealed, only one 18 bp palindrome is necessary for a specific and stable repressor binding (Aslanidis, C; Muiznieks, I. and Schmitt, R. (1990) Mol. Gen. Genet. **223**, 297-304.).

Like MerR, Raf repressor was combined with *M.SssI* and *R.MaeII*.

This combination should give a final cleavage sequence of 18 bp. The statistic cleavage frequency would be one cut per $6,8 \times 10^{10}$ base pairs.

```
AACCGAAACGTTTTGGTT     binding site of Raf repressor
   CG     CG           recognition sequence of M.SssI
       ACGT            recognition site of R.MaeII
```
```
AACCGAAACGTTTTGGTT     Achilles Heel Cleavage sequence
```

3. Work performed

1. DNA binding proteins

Transcription factor Oct2A was purified in our laboratory. The expression clone was made available by W. Schaffner, Universität Zürich.

Purified MerR protein was kindly provided from Prof. N. L. Brown, Birmingham together with detailed information about the binding conditions.

The Raf repressor expression clone was kindly provided from I. Muiznieks, Universität Köln, exact information about purification and binding conditions was obtained from Prof. R. Schmitt, Universität Regensburg. The repressor was purified in our laboratory.

The binding affinity, specifity and conditions of the three purified DNA binding proteins were tested by gel shift assays with Digoxigenin[11]-dUTP labelled oligonucleotides containing the different specific binding sequences of the proteins.

2. DNA methylases

The gene for the methylase *NlaIII* was overexpressed in *E.coli*. Three clones were constructed initially. Two of them contain a $(His)_3$-fusion at the 3'-end and 5'-end, respectively, to allow purification by zinc chelate affinity chromatography. The enzymes expressed from all three clones were purified in our labratory.

3. Test substrates

Oligonucleotides containing the sequences to be cleaved by the Achilles Heel Cleavage were introduced into plasmids.

4. Achilles Heel Cleavage

Achilles Heel Cleavage was performed with all three systems.

4. Results and discussion

1. Achilles Heel Cleavage with Oct2A as binding protein

Gel shift assays showed that bound Oct2A was completely displaced by subsequent methylation using *M.NlaIII* derived from the original clone (without a $(His)_3$-fusion) and the clone with a $(His)_3$-fusion at the 3'-end. Therefore, Achilles Heel Cleavage could only be performed using the M.NlaIII clone with the $(His)_3$-fusion at the 5'-end, which only partly displaced bound Oct2A. As figure 1 shows using the combination Oct2A, *M.NlaIII*-5'-$(His)_3$ and *R.NlaIII* the test DNA was cleaved partially at the expected site and in addition at several other sites of the plasmid. It seems that the affinity of Oct2A is not high enough to protect the binding site completely from methylation. Increasing concentrations of Oct2A result in nonspecific binding to the DNA. Further optimization of assay conditions and modifications of *M.NlaIII* did not significantly improve the cleavage specifity. Therefore, this system is not suitable for the "Achilles Heel Cleavage" method.

2. Achilles Heel Cleavage with MerR as binding protein

With the combination of MerR, *M.SssI* and *R.MaeII* the plasmid DNA containing the binding sites for MerR, *M.SssI* and *R.MaeII* was specifically cleaved at the expected site (Fig. 2).

3. Achilles Heel Cleavage with Raf repressor as binding protein

The third combination using Raf repressor as protecting protein, *M.SssI* and *R.MaeII* also gave promising results. The binding site of Raf repressor was specifically protected from methylation by *M.SssI* and cleaved by *R.MaeII*. All other sites for the restriction endonuclease *MaeII* in the test plasmid were completely methylated (Fig. 3).

From the three DNA binding proteins examined, two - MerR protein and Raf repressor - were shown to be suitable for the Achilles Heel Cleavage method. Due to their length of 16 respectively 18 bp the binding sites of MerR and Raf repressor rarely occur and usually have to be artificially introduced by homologous or site-specific recombination. However, these systems could be new tools for the mapping and precise molecular dissection of large genomes. For example they could provide a unique cleavage and labeling site suitable for the subsequent use of the Smith and Birnstiel strategy for mapping other restriction sites (Smith, H.O. and Birnstiel, M.L. (1976) Nucleic Acids Res. **3**, 2387-2398.).

5. Major cooperative links

Boehringer Mannheim received overexpressed highly purified MerR protein from Prof. N. Brown, Birmingham. If Prof. Brown will be successful in obtaining DNA binding mutants of MerR with shorter recognition sequences and high affinity, another collaboration is planned to exploit the system commercially.

Publications

1. "Achilles Heel Cleavage of DNA using Oct2A, Raf repressor or MerR protein as protecting proteins." A. Reiser, W. Ankenbauer, N. Brown, R. Schmitt and G. Schmitz. Posterpresentation at Conference "Tools for Genome Mapping" Institut Pasteur, January 1994.
2. One publication is planned from this work in collaboration with Prof. N. Brown describing the use of MerR in "Achilles Heel" cleavage of DNA.

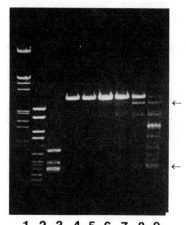

Figure 1
Achilles Heel Cleavage with Oct2A/M.NlaIII/R.NlaIII on linearized plasmid pAC1.

lane 1: Molecular weight marker III (BM).
lane 2: Molecular weight marker VI (BM).
lane 3: pAC1, linearized with R.AflIII and digested with R.NlaIII.
lanes 4 to 9: Achilles Heel Cleavage with increasing concentrations of Oct2A.
lane 4: no Oct2A, lane 5: 680 ng Oct2A, lane 6: 1.2 μg Oct2A, lane 7: 1.7 μg Oct2A,
lane 8: 2.2. μg oct2A, lane 9: μg oct2A.
Increasing amounts of Oct2A were bound (15 min.) to linearized pAC1 (500 ng) and
methylated with M.NlaIII. Oct2A and methylase were removed by phenol extraction,
the DNA was isolated by ethanol precipitation and cleaved with R.NlaIII.

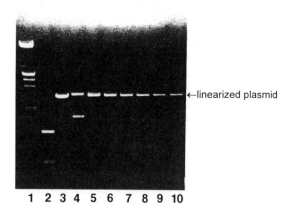

Figure 2
Achilles Heel Cleavage with MerR protein/M.SssI/R.MaeII and the plasmid pMR1.

lane 1: Molecular weight marker III (BM).
lane 2: pMR1 digested with R.MaeII.
lane 3: pMR1 digested with R.AflII, size marker for the linear form of the plasmid.
lane 4 to 10: Achilles Heel Cleavage with increasing concentrations of MerR protein.
lane 4: no MerR, lane 5: 750 ng MerR, lane 6: 1.5 μg MerR, lane 7: 2.25 μg MerR,
lane 8: 3 μg MerR, lane 9: 4.5 μg MerR, lane 10: 6 μg MerR.
After repressor binding (30 min.) the plasmid (500 ng) was methylated with 8 U of
M.SssI. Repressor and methylase were removed by phenol extraction and ethanol
precipitation. Then the plasmid was digested with R.MaeII.

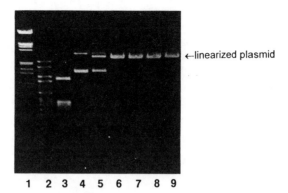

←linearized plasmid

Figure 3
Achilles Heel Cleavage with raf repressor/M.SssI/R.MaeII and the plasmid pRA1.

lane 1: Molecular weight marker III (BM).
lane 2: Molecular weight marker VI (BM).
lane 3: control, pRA1 digested with R.MaeII.
lane 4 to 9: Achilles Heel Cleavage of pRA1 (500 ng) with increasing amounts of raf repressor.
lane 4: no repressor, lane 5: 1 µg, lane 6: 2 µg, lane 7: 3 µg, lane 8: 4 µg, lane 9: 5 µg.
After repressor binding (20 min.) the plasmid was methylated with 8 U of M.SssI. Repressor and methylase were removed by phenol extraction and the DNA was isolated by ethanol precipitation. Subsequently the plasmid was digested with R.MaeII.

Contract number: GENO-CT91-0011 (SSMA)
Contractual period: April 1992 to March 1994

Coordinator
Dr. G. Schmitz-Agheguian
Boehringer Mannheim GmbH
Werk Penzberg
Nonnenwald 2
D - 82372 Penzberg
Germany
Tel: 49 8856 60 2745
Fax: 49 8856 60 3180

Participants
Professor B. Dujon
Institut Pasteur
Unite de Génétique Moleculaire des Levures
25, rue du Docteur Roux
F - 75724 Paris Cedex 15
France
Tel: 33 1 45 68 8482
Fax: 33 1 45 68 8521

Professor N. L. Brown
University of Birmingham
School of Biological Sciences
UK - Edgbaston, Birmingham B15 2TT
United Kingdom
Tel: 44 21 414 6556
Fax: 44 21 414 6557

Dr. V. Bouriotis
IMBB - Institute of Molecularbiology
and Biotechnology
GR - 71110 Heraklion
Greece
Tel: 30 81 210 235
Fax: 30 81 210 234

Human Genome Analysis Programme
M. Hallen and A. Klepsch (Eds.)
IOS Press, 1995

NORMALISED AND CHROMOSOME SPECIFIC cDNA LIBRARIES AS A SOURCE OF TISSUE-SPECIFIC SEQUENCES

F. Gannon
University College Galway, Ireland

1. Background Information

There are many methods which have been described to achieve partial normalisation of cDNA libraries. The most durable of these involves the use of liquid hybridisation followed by hydroxylapatite chromatography. This project aimed to streamline aspects of these procedures by the use of characteristics of the PCR method. If successful this would yield representative or normalised cDNA libraries of a complexity which reflects the genes which are transcribed in a cell but not the level at which they were expressed. The PCR method was evaluated by comparison to the liquid hybridisation approach. The feasibility of using chromosome 21 DNA immobilised on solid matrices as a way of selecting sequences transcribed from it was also evaluated.

Keywords: Normalisation, cDNA, PCR, immobilised DNA, reannealing.

2. Objectives and primary approaches

This project is driven by the search for new methodologies and a comparison of their efficiencies to achieve the goals of normalised cDNA libraries enriched in chromosome specific and as an extension, tissue specific sequences. Variations of two different approaches to obtaining normalised libraries were used; the well established process of liquid hybridisation to different CoT values followed by differentiation between those highly reiterated sequences that had reannealed and those less frequently occuring sequences that had not, by hydroxyapatite chromatography (IMBB). In parallel the frequently observed fact that PCR amplification continues until the concentration of the predominant sequence reaches a plateau was used as the basis for a potentially novel normalisation procedure (UCG). The potential for chromosome specific selection of sequences was performed by enriching for unique sequences from chromosome 21, immobilising these and then hybridising them with a pool of cDNA sequences. The retained cDNA sequences were subsequently used to generate cDNA libraries and the success of the approach assessed by hybridisation with known chromosome 21 probes (IMBB).

3. Results and discussion

3.1 PCR Methodology (UCG):

This project was predicated on two widely held and frequently reported aspects of PCR; (a) the products of multiple cycles of PCR do not accurately reflect the starting amounts and (b) after a finite number of cycles the PCR reaches a plateau. The aim of this project was to convert these disadvantages into an attractive procedure to achieve normalisation in the expectation that once the predominant sequences, in a mixed population of a cDNA library, had reached their plateau, the minor sequences would continue to be amplified thereby ultimately reaching a normalisation of the cDNA population from which libraries could be generated.

The underlying presumptions of the approach were confirmed by showing that following 35 cycles of PCR an equivalent amount of product was obtained from a thousand fold range of unique template DNA. PCR is therefore not quantitative in this case. However, when 2 targets of slightly different size were used as templates, the DNA which was present at the lower initial concentration was not amplified once the plateau was reached by the predominant template. The "window" for equivalent amplification was very narrow (approximately a 10 fold difference of starting concentrations). This in turn puts a cap on the degree to which normalisation can occur by this method. Many experiments were performed to establish the reasons for the plateau and its apparent inhibitory effect on any further amplification. No satisfactory solution either based on the addition of potentially depleted reagents or on a build up of inhibitory substances was found. Similar results were obtained with different polymerases and further biochemical studies will be needed to clarify this matter. (Morrison and Gannon, in press).

3.2 Generation of PCR "normalised" libraries: (UCG)

The end point for the above PCR experiments was the analysis of DNA bands on agarose gels using a variety of combinations of pairs of template DNA fragments. To see if the approach was more fruitful with starting material of greater complexity, cDNA libraries were prepared with or without a PCR "normalisation" step using human uterus, cervix, brain or ovary cell RNA as the start point. In different experiments up to 10 probes selected to represent low (approx. 0.05%), medium (0.175% or high (1.25%) sequences were used to hybridise the standard or "normalised" library. There was a good degree of normalisation between the medium and high level cDNAs but only occasional low sequences were altered in levels relevant to medium or high level sequences. The general thrust of these results are in keeping with the model studies and indicate that the PCR based method is not going to yield normalised libraries as had been hoped. The exceptional "normalisation" of some of the minor sequences could be related to sequence (but did not correlate with size) but the basis for this was not examined. (Pope, Morrison and Gannon, submitted).

3.3 Liquid hybridisation and hydroxyapatite normalisation: (IMBB)

In parallel with the attempts to normalise using PCR, RNA from human erythroleukemia or a glioblastoma-astroblastoma cell line was used in CoT hybridisation experiments to achieve the same goal. Following hybridisation for different time periods of the previously denatured ds cDNA inserts, hydroxylapatite columns were used to remove the reannealed most frequently occuring sequences. The selected sequences which should correspond to a normalised population were sized and libraries generated. A cDNA library of 1.74×10^6 recombinants which resulted from the 24 hour hybridisation was most thoroughly analysed using 10 distinct probes. The results show that the rare cDNAs were increased approximately 3.5 fold relative to medium sequences or 36 fold in relation to high level sequences. This is not an adequate degree of normalisation. Multiple possible reasons can be advanced for the failure of a trend towards normalisation to be completed. These include the use of random priming to generate the cDNA with consequent partial overlapping of all of the mRNA fragments, which could influence reannealing patterns, sequence variation and its effect on hybridisation rates and the initial extreme complexity of the starting RNAs especially from the glioblastoma-astroblastoma cell lines. Nonetheless some normalisation was achieved. The cDNA library is made available and characterisation of some of the clones is ongoing.

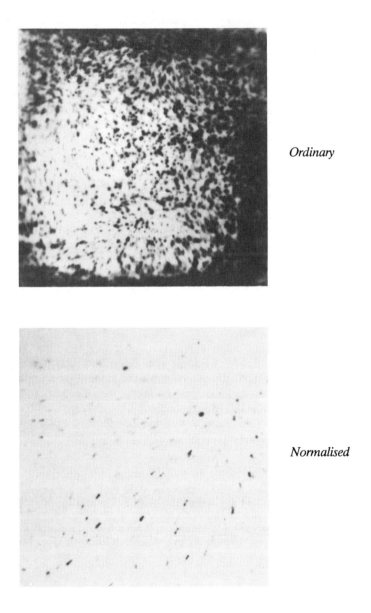

Ordinary

Normalised

Figure 1

Erythroleukemia K562 cDNA Libraries
Probe: *Alu* I repeat sequence (100,000 pfus)

4. Selection of chromosome specific cDNA Libraries (IMBB)

To achieve an enrichment of Chromosome 21 sequences, initial experiments were performed in which the human Glud, b-globlin and actin genes were immobilised on cellulose, sepharose F/F and nylon matrices. A five hundred to one thousand fold enrichment was found on one round of selection. Using the optimal conditions from these experiments, the inserts from a chromosome 21 library were immobilised on the activated sepharose. Prior to immobilisation the DNA was digested by Sau3A, denatured, reannealed for controlled periods and the unique non annealed sequences isolated using hydroxylapatite chromatography. After two cycles of selection, libraries were prepared and screened for enrichment of 3 chromosome 21 sequences. A very minimal enrichment was achieved. Careful examination of the literature would suggest that the complexity of the chromosome DNA may be the problem. At a complexity of 35-45 Mb, the times required for hybridisation may be such that the specific binding to noise ratio was not adequate. The fact that 8×10^6 equivalents of the chromosomal 21 DNA was used suggests difficulties in overcoming this limitation in the future.

5. Major scientific breakthrough and /or industrial applications

The data obtained in this project gave unequivocal results which indicated that the novel approaches proposed were not superior to more standard procedures. Although this was disappointing, some widely useful insights were obtained in terms of the limitations of hybrid selection using very complex target DNA and in the fine detail of PCR amplification of mixed populations of DNA. A specific context in which this will be useful is in the quantitative use of PCR amplification in diagnostic assays.

6. Major cooperative links

Two laboratories from the geographic extremes of the E.U. participated in this project. Experiments were of necessity of a comparative rather than a joint nature. Nonetheless there was very extensive phone and fax interaction in particular as unexpected results were encountered. The IMBB provided cell lines and libraries to UCG. 2 visits of the contractors to each others laboratories for meetings took place.

References

- C. Morrison and F. Gannon. BBA. The impact of the PCR plateau on quantitative PCR. (In press).
- C. Morrison, C. Pope, and F. Gannon. The study of the usefullness of PCR in the normalisation of cDNA libraries. (In preparation).
- A. Puciriov, K.Chroniary and N.K. Moschonas. Construction and preliminary screening of a normalised cDNA expression library of human erythroleukemia K562 cells. (In preparation).

Contract number: GENO-CT91-0016 (SSMA)
Contractual period: 1 February 1992 to 31 January 1994

Coordinator
Professor Frank Gannon
University College Galway
University Road
Galway
Ireland
Tel: 353 91 586 559
Fax: 353 91 586 570

Participant
Dr. Nicholas Moschonas
Institute of Molecular Biology & Biotechnology (IMBB)
Division of Mammalian Molecular Genetics
P.O. Box 1527
71110 Heraklion
Crete
Greece
Tel: 30 81 210 079
Fax: 30 81 230 469

Number of joint/ Individual publications: 2

Author Index